R25.00

Mind–body Medicin

In memory of my sister Karen who taught me so much even when I thought I was teaching her.

For Churchill Livingstone:

Publisher: Inta Ozols
Project manager: Valerie Burgess
Project development editor: Valerie Bain
Project controller: Derek Robertson
Copy editor: Carolyn Holleyman
Design direction: Judith Wright
Promotions manager: Hilary Brown

Mind-body Medicine

A Clinician's Guide to Psychoneuroimmunology

Edited by

Alan Watkins MD

Lecturer in Medicine, School of Medicine, Southampton General Hospital,
Southampton, UK

Foreword by

Wayne B. Jonas MD

Associate Clinical Professor in Family Practice and Preventive Medicine/Biometrics,
Uniformed Services University of Health Sciences,
Bethesda, Maryland, USA

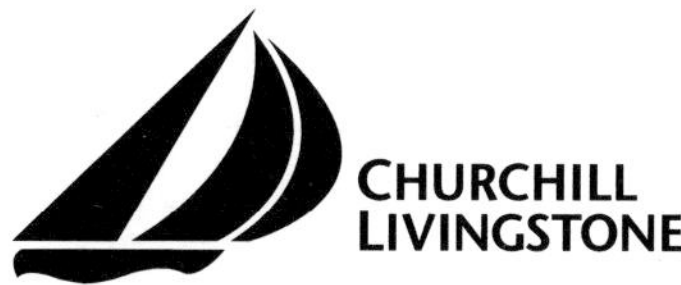

NEW YORK EDINBURGH LONDON MADRID MELBOURNE SAN FRANCISCO AND TOKYO 1997

CHURCHILL LIVINGSTONE
Medical Division of Pearson Professional Limited

Distributed in the United States of America by Churchill Livingstone, 650 Avenue of the Americas, New York, N.Y. 10011, and by associated companies, branches and representatives throughout the world.

First published 1997

ISBN 0 443 05526 2

British Library Cataloguing in Publication Data
A catalogue record for this book is available from the British Library.

Library of Congress Cataloging in Publication Data
A catalog record for this book is available from the Library of Congress.

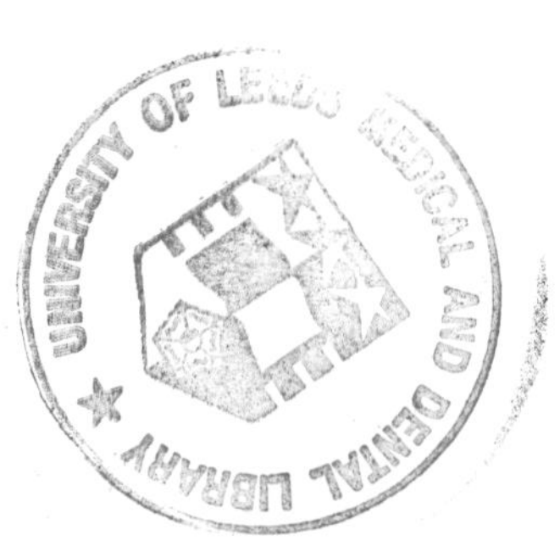

Note
Medical knowledge is constantly changing. As new information becomes available, changes in treatment, procedures, equipment and the use of drugs become necessary. The editor, authors and the publishers have, as far as it is possible, taken care to ensure that the information given in this text is accurate and up to date. However, readers are strongly advised to confirm that the information, especially with regard to drug usage, complies with latest legislation and standards of practice.

Neither the publishers nor the authors will be liable for any loss or damage of any nature occasioned to or suffered by any person acting or refraining from acting as a result of reliance on the material contained in this publication.

The publisher's policy is to use **paper manufactured from sustainable forests**

Printed by Bell and Bain Ltd., Glasgow

Contents

Contributors

Michael H. Antoni PhD
Professor of Psychology and Psychiatry, University of Miami, Florida, USA

Ruth Bolletino PhD
Psychotherapist specializing in working with people with cancer, New York, USA

Tacey Ann Boucher BA
Research Assistant, Center for Addiction and Alternative Medicine Research, Minneapolis, Minnesota, USA

Gregory A Carlson BA
Director, Addiction Medicine Program, Hennepin County Medical Center, Minneapolis, Minnesota, USA

Patricia Culliton MA LicAc
Director of the Alternative Medicine Division, Department of Medicine, Hennepin County Medical Center, and Co-director, Center of Addiction and Alternative Medicine Research, Minneapolis, Minnesota, USA

Simon Easton BSc MA CPsychol
Senior Lecturer, Department of Psychology, University of Portsmouth, Portsmouth UK

Michael J. G. Farthing MD FRCP
Professor of Gastroenterology, St Bartholomew's Hospital and the Royal London School of Medicine and Dentistry, London UK

Jennifer Gomborone BSc MSc PhD
Consultant Clinical Psychologist, Wellington Hospital, and Honorary Research Fellow in Gastroenterology, Digestive Diseases Research Centre, St Bartholemew's Hospital, London, UK

Sandra Goodman BSc PhD
Publisher and Director, Positive Health Publications Ltd, Bristol, UK

Gail Ironson MD PhD
Professor of Psychology and Psychiatry, University of Miami, Florida, USA

Derek Johnston MA PhD
Professor of Psychology, School of Psychology, University of St Andrews, St Andrews, Fife, UK

Jenny King MSc DipCOT
Senior Lecturer, Department of Health Studies, Brunel University College, Isleworth, Middlesex, UK

Lawrence LeShan BS MS PhD
Research Psychologist, New York, USA

Frederic Luskin MS
Research Fellow, Complementary and Alternative Medicine Program, Stanford University, Stanford, California, USA

George Lewith MA DM MRCP MRCGP
Honorary Senior Lecturer, Department of Medicine, University of Southampton, Southampton, UK

Kathryn A Newell MA
Research Assistant, Complementary and Alternative Medicine Program, Stanford University, Stanford, California, USA

Peter G F Nixon FRCP
Honourary Consulting Cardiologist,
Charing Cross Hospital, London, UK

David Peters MB ChB DRCOG MFHom MRO
Principal Lecturer in Complementary Therapy Studies, Centre for Community Care and Primary Health, University of Westminster, London, UK

Michael Sharpe MA MB MRCP MRCPsych
Senior Lecturer in Psychological Medicine, University of Edinburgh, Edinburgh, UK

Alan Watkins MD
Locum Lecturer in Medicine, School of Medicine, Southampton General Hospital, Southampton, UK

Simon Wessely MA BM BCh MSc MD FRCP MRCPsych
Professor of Epidemiology and Liaison Psychiatry, King's College School of Medicine and Dentistry, London, UK

Teresa E. Woods MS PhD
Department of Psychology,
University of Miami, Florida, USA

Foreword

Complementary, alternative, and unconventional medical practices are growing in popularity around the world. As the prevalence of these practices increases, it behooves the practitioner and scientist to sharpen both their critical thinking skills and their compassion to distinguish between what is useful and may become the medicine of the future and what is fanciful and should be discarded with the other ineffective methods of the past. In this volume, Dr Watkins has provided us with descriptions from various perspectives of one aspect of complementary medicine, namely mind–body medicine. This also may serve as a model for how new disciplines and modalities emerge in the future.

Much of what we consider unconventional medicine was relegated to the scientific fringe at one time or another. The incredibly powerful tools off reductionism and materialism and their formalization into scientific and technological methods in the last century have banished many of our more dreaded diseases and this still leaves us in awe. With the proliferation of detailed and specialized knowledge comes an awareness of interconnection and interdependency; what we find in one field of science and medicine may depend upon another field for its interpretation. This growing recognition of the holism of life has led to a resurgence of interest in systems and systems theory as a method of studying biology. A decision by some psychologists, immunologists and neuroscientists to begin a dialogue, ask questions of mutual interest and investigate the answers to those questions across disciplines has led to a remarkable transformation in each of those fields. Not only has the discipline of psychoneuroimmunology, as it is now called, led to a new approach in understanding how the mind and the immune system work, but it is increasingly shedding light on the ancient medical practices and what meaning they have for the modern world. The realization that lymphoid and immune tissues are enervated, that they contain receptors to neuropeptides whose sensitivity can be altered by hormone levels and cycles – cycles often controlled by the brain – and the parallel realization that immune cells produce cytokines, steroids and peptides that influence specific and global regions of the brain has forever changed our perception of the unity of mind and body. We now know, and can demonstrate with the most rigorous modern science, that the perceived separation between mind and body is, in fact, an illusion, and that we as whole persons function like ecosystems, responding to every stimuli in global ways. How this new-found, unconventional scientific knowledge will assist us in better understanding both conventional and complementary medicine is not yet known. This knowledge is a tool being sharpened for use as we examine these complex areas.

Any book that is a compilation by multiple authors will be of varied quality and value, and in this book some chapters are shining stars. Its main strength, however, is in the topic of its title – mind–body medicine. There are chapters that have pulled together new syntheses and helpful common sense and evidence-based understandings. These chapters make the book a 'must read' for all those concerned with healing.

Chapter 1, by Alan Watkins, is a brilliant synthesis of the underlying scientific basis of mind–body medicine. Here he elucidates the pathways whereby mind and body not only communicate with each other but function as an integrated whole. The implications of the classic research which he describes, such as the mental and social modulation of susceptibility to upper respiratory tract viruses, wound healing, environmental toxins and dietary poisons, powerfully illustrate that we must take the mind seriously. The research descriptions showing the immunosuppressive and immunostimulatory effects of classical conditioning also open up new questions about not only the placebo effect, but the mechanism of action of all conventional and complementary medications.

Chapter 2, which explores the use of complementary medicine and some of the underlying reasons for its use, demonstrates how ordinary people and patients, unsophisticated in the scientific method, understand intuitively the value of care, social support, love and stress management on their health. The fact that complementary practitioners are found to be more friendly and that patients are generally more satisfied with complementary medical care serves as an important lesson for us all.

Chapter 9 is, in my opinion, one of the most important chapters on mind–body medicine ever written for the practicing physician. If we learn anything from our increased awareness of the network of psychoneuroimmunological patterns, it is that the diagnostic categories that have arisen from subspecialization in conventional medicine are largely irrelevant when these patients come into general practice. Ian Heath has said, 'in hospitals, diseases stay and patients come and go; in general practice, patients stay and diseases come and go'. And so it is, that in general practice, be it specialized or in primary care, the powerful nonspecific effects that occur on multiple diseases and, indeed, the susceptibility to chronic disease in general makes the use of mind–body approaches an important and compelling element in the integrated medicine of the future. The nonspecific nature of these effects makes the diagnostic category into which the patient falls almost irrelevant, as it appears that all such patients can, at least on some level, improve by being managed in a way that utilizes the intimate integration of mind and body. This does not mean that psychotherapy is required for all patients, as Chapter 10 shows. In this chapter the limitations and strengths of psychotherapy are nicely outlined and the distinction between psychotherapy and mind–body medicine incorporation in general medicine is made.

After discussing the theoretical underpinnings, the book addresses how mind–body medicine influences a number of specific clinical conditions. Especially noteworthy and important are the chapters on heart disease, GI disease, allergies and aging. Whereas the utility of the science and the scientific clinical connection may still be fuzzy in a number of areas for this emerging discipline, the leaders appear to be in these areas and the authors do a commendable job.

Finally, mind–body medicine may not be solely for our patients but may have implications for how we manage our own lives as health care professionals and how we teach, learn and deliver medicine. We know, for example, that doctors who smoke less and engage in more health promoting habits will counsel their patients more in these areas. So it may be that in mind–body medicine, to utilize it to its maximum benefits for the health care system, the health care practitioners, and the education systems for practitioners, will need to incorporate these activities into their daily lives. Holism, after all, means not only that we see the world as a whole but also experience it that way.

1997 W.B.J

REFERENCE

1 Heath I 1995 British Medical Journal 311:372

Preface

The 20th century has been witness to a revolution within science and medicine. The revolution has produced a very considerable increase in our understanding of the basic cellular mechanisms involved in virtually all the major disease states. But, despite wars on cancer and massive amounts of research into every cause of ill health from allergies to arthritis, and heart disease to HIV, modern medicine is frequently reduced to a polypharmacy palliation of suffering. It is clear, as we approach the next millenium, that modern medicine stands at a cross-roads. The current biological approach is limited in its perception and in its ability to explain the human condition. It has had its day and we now need to embrace a new approach.

In the last 20 years there has been a growing awareness amongst scientists and clinicians of how the different systems within the body interact and how the breakdown in cooperation between these different systems can set the stage for the development and progression of disease. The rapid evolution of new areas of scientific research, such as neurocardiology, neuroendocrinology, neuroimmunology, neuropsychology, psychophysiology, immunopsychiatry and psychoneuroimmunology, demonstrates the importance of understanding the human system as an integrated whole. These areas of research also provide evidence to support the view that the health of any individual not only depends on physical health but also on the unique mental, emotional and spiritual aspects of that individual.

This book was born out of a desire to bring these areas of research to the attention of all health care professionals, and to encourage the adoption of a new approach to health and well being. A more human approach, one that embraces new ideas and a variety of therapeutic strategies, is detailed here under the banner of 'mind–body medicine'. It argues that we can integrate the proven benefits of modern medicine with the best mind–body medicine has to offer, and that this integration should be driven by sound scientific principles and research.

The momentum for change is accelerating in all walks of life, and medicine is no exception. Health care is at a cross-roads, and practitioners have a choice. They can follow their current path or they can explore a new path to a broader understanding of health by adopting a systems approach, integrating new ideas, alternative techniques and new research into their practice. Many have already been guided by their intuition down this path. For the more cautious, I am pleased to say that there are sound scientific reasons for following them, and these reasons are chronicled in the pages of this book. I hope it will serve as a useful reference guide for the journey and illustrate some of the joys of life that this path reveals, as we enter the next millenium.

Southampton, May 1997 A. D. W.

Acknowledgements

I would like to acknowledge those key individuals who have personally inspired me over the years and who have supported me professionally in what I have been trying to achieve: Dr Hilton Davis and Professor John Gruzelier, who helped to expand my interest in behavioural medicine as a medical student; Dr Peter Nixon, whose pioneering work at Charing Cross taught me that a biopsychosocial approach could not only work in practice but was also a much more rewarding approach for the doctor and patient – his foresight and wisdom has never received the recognition it richly deserves, and I am delighted he could contribute a chapter to this volume; Mr Mike House, who taught me there was meaning beyond medicine; more recently, Professor Stephen Holgate, who has been a source of considerable encouragement and professional support – his vision and courage are a testimony to his brilliance and an example to us all; Dr George Lewith, for his energy, drive and for being a good sounding board; Doc Lew Childre, for helping to bring coherence to my understanding and perspective to my vision; Rollin McCraty and Mike Atkinson, my research partners and good friends, who are helping make the implicate explicate; and, finally, Mr Chris Sawicki, business partner, joke-swapper and good friend, whose own intuition and wit help make visions a reality.

A special thanks to all those unsung heroes whose writings and teachings have influenced me. A thanks to the numerous pioneers who have conducted the research chronicled in this book, often under trying financial circumstances and scientific discrimination. It takes courage to pursue difficult questions and brilliance to produce results.

Finally, I would like to thank my wife Sarah. Her love and support have been my greatest source of inspiration; I am blessed by her presence. Lastly, my three sons, Jack, Sam and Joe, who keep me in touch with love, compassion and humor, vital tools for survival in today's world.

CHAPTER CONTENTS

1

Mind–body pathways

Alan Watkins

INTRODUCTION

The whole area of mind–body medicine is a complete jungle. It is awash with numerous self-help books, written by lay therapists, and some doctors, who advocate a wide variety of largely untested remedies for every ailment from corns to cancer. The more bizarre therapies, such as rebirthing and high colonic lavage, have distorted the perception of the whole field to such an extent that most physicians and scientists have steered well clear, and rightly so. However, there is now a substantial amount of sound scientific evidence from the fields of neuroendocrinology, neuroimmunology, neurobiology, nutrition and behavioral medicine to suggest that our autonomic, endocrine and immune systems are not autonomous, but engage in an interactive dialog with each other and with higher perceptual centers and limbic emotional centers to maintain health and fight disease. Because of the distorted perception that most physicians and scientists have of mind–body medicine, this research has gone largely unnoticed. This book is designed to guide physicians through the field of mind–body medicine and provide sound scientific advice on what, if anything, mind–body techniques can offer their patients, thus enabling them to make appropriate treatment choices based on science and state of the art research.

There is an enormous variety of opinion as to what constitutes mind–body medicine. This book uses the term in its broadest sense, seeing mind–body medicine as a metaphor for an approach to health that focuses not just on the physical body and the conscious mind, but also incorporates unconscious emotional life and an individual's spiritual dimension. Therefore mind–body interventions cover a wide variety of therapeutic practices, from counseling and cognitive – behavioral therapy to various alternative medical practices such as homeopathy and acupuncture. This liberal definition includes alternative medicine not because of its philosophical emphasis on the mental, emotional and spiritual side of ill health, but because it is widely believed that many alternative therapies may have an effect through an altered perception of disease, as assessed by subjective outcome measures, via an enhanced expectancy effect, or even through direct activation of mind–body pathways[1]. The greater emphasis placed on psychosocial or mind-body factors by alternative medical practitioners, compared with orthodox medical practitioners, is one of the major reasons why patients are drawn to them[2].

HISTORICAL PERSPECTIVE

The early custodians of health in most cultures treated both the mind, with trances and rituals, and the physical symptoms of the body, with herbs and natural remedies. With the advent of civilization, treatments for the mind and spirit became separated from treatments for the body, and this separation gave birth to two schools of thinking, namely the mechanists and the vitalists. The mechanists concentrated on the physical reality, and administered physical treatments and herbal remedies. They became the dominant providers of health. In contrast, priests, magicians and healers took the vitalistic approach and concentrated on the mind, energy and the more spiritual dimension of health. The mechanistic school of thought spawned the subsequent development of reductionism and the biomedical approach to ill health, with its emphasis on physical disease, while vitalism was more aligned to the principles of alternative and complementary medical practice[3].

However, it has been recognized for some time that mechanistic and materialistic ideas are insufficient to explain the human condition and the genesis of disease. The astrophysicist and philosopher Sir Arthur Eddington observed (cited in[4]):

> The materialist, who is convinced that all phenomena arise from electrons and quanta and the like, controlled by mathematical formula, must presumably hold the belief that his wife is a rather elaborate differential equation, but he is probably tactful enough not to obtrude this opinion on domestic life.

Since Eddington's day there have been various attempts to reconcile vitalistic and mechanistic approaches to health. The concept of 'wellness' evolved out of the idea that a healthy mind produced a healthy body and reduced the risk of disease. This concept was embraced by some arms of the medical community under the guise of holistic medicine. Holistic medicine sought to address the social, psychological and spiritual dimensions of life, believing that they were important to 'wellness' and recovery from illness. Mind and body were seen as part of the same whole, connected and related in function. This book similarly attempts to reconcile the reductionist and vitalistic approaches to health and illness. It draws on reductionist research while seeking to demonstrate the importance of the whole. This first chapter will concentrate on the scientific (reductionist) evidence which has accumulated over the last 20 years, which clearly demonstrates that the mind and the body are intimately connected.

PSYCHONEUROIMMUNOLOGY

There is now a substantial amount of evidence from research into the mind (psychology), the brain (neurology) and the body's natural defenses (immunology) to suggest that the mind and body communicate with each other in a bidirectional flow of hormones, neuropeptides and cytokines[5]. The investigation of the pathways connecting mind and body is now a rapidly emerging field of research in its own right, called psychoneuroimmunology (PNI)[6].

The last 20 years have seen a rapid advance in scientific understanding of the immune system. The fact that many immune processes were originally demonstrated in a test tube, in vitro, led to the early assumption that the immune system was autonomous. However, PNI research has successfully challenged this assumption and a wealth of hard scientific data has provided irrefutable evidence that virtually all of the body's defense systems are under the control of the central nervous system (CNS). Thus, every idea, thought and belief has a neurochemical consequence, and neuropeptides flow from the CNS, impinging on specific receptors on virtually all leukocytes, regulating their function. The CNS has the potential to critically inhibit or enhance immunity through two major neuroimmunomodulatory pathways; neuroendocrine and autonomic[7]. PNI research has painstakingly characterized these pathways and demonstrated their importance in a wide variety of disease models in animals. Scientists who work in the field are in no doubt about the fundamental importance of these pathways in immune regulation; however, their role in pathogenesis and progression of major disease states in humans has yet to be elucidated. There is substantial circumstantial evidence suggesting that these pathways are critically important in maintaining health and fighting disease, but until this area of research receives increased recognition and funding of high quality interdisciplinary research teams, 'conclusive scientific proof' will not be forthcoming.

This chapter discusses what is presently known about mind–body pathways, and it argues that mind–body connections are crucial to survival since they enable an organism to mount an integrated response to threats, be they immunological or psychological. Furthermore, this chapter argues that dysfunction in one part of the whole system can promote dysfunction in another.

The other chapters in this book will discuss the evidence for the effectiveness of mind–body therapies, which may be harnessing neuroimmunomodulatory pathways, in the management of commonly encountered clinical problems.

AUTONOMIC NEUROIMMUNOMODULATORY PATHWAYS

Autonomic innervation of lymphoid tissue has been extensively studied[8]. The bone marrow and thymus, where immune cells develop, are richly supplied by sympathetic, parasympathetic, and non-adrenergic non-cholinergic (NANC) nerves[9,10]. These nerves also irrigate fields of lymphocytes in secondary lymphoid organs, and modulate the maturity and activation of immune cells in the tertiary lymphoid tissue of the airway and intestine, where antigens and allergens are first encountered. Although the exact role of autonomic innervation in regulating immunity has not been clearly defined, there is sufficient evidence to suggest that autonomic nerves are capable of regulating almost all the cells involved in inflammation[11–13].

Autonomic innervation of lymphoid tissue is very complex. For example, parasympathetic nerves may release acetylcholine or the inhibitory NANC neuropeptides, nitric oxide and vasoactive intestinal polypeptide (VIP). Similarly, sympathetic nerves can release the excitatory NANC neuropeptide Y. Thus a single population of nerves is capable of storing and co-releasing several neuropeptides, and the same neuropeptide can be released from sympathetic, parasympathetic or NANC nerves. The factors determining whether classical transmitters or neuropeptides are released from autonomic nerves are unknown. It is also clear that the pattern of autonomic innervation is dynamic, and may change during the course of an inflammatory response.

The effects of autonomic innervation on lymphoid tissue primarily depend on the specific neuropeptide released and the type of cell targeted by that neuropeptide. For example, tachykinins released by excitatory NANC nerves may impair inhibitory NANC or adrenergic nerve activity and therefore reduce their specific effects, such as bronchodilation. Similarly, capsaicin may deplete tachykinin stores and promote an increase in adrenergic transmission[14]. Positive and negative feedback loops exist as some neuropeptides augment their own synthesis from their cell of origin or other inflammatory cells[12]. For example, mast cell tryptase degrades VIP, which would normally inhibit tryptase release[15].

The complex array of checks and counterbalances between the autonomic networks and the cells involved in inflammation varies within individual lymphoid compartments. Thus in regional lymph nodes, T cells may be regulated by sympathetic nerves, whereas the antigen presenting ability of Langerhans cells is inhibited by calcitonin gene-related peptide NANC nerves[16]. Similarly, the contractile response of peripheral airway smooth muscle is modulated by neurokinin A, whereas central airway smooth muscle is more affected by cholinergic innervation.

NEUROENDOCRINE NEUROIMMUNOMODULATORY PATHWAYS

Not only are there direct neural connections between brainstem autonomic nuclei and lymphoid tissue, but there is also substantial evidence indicating that a wide range of leukocyte functions can be inhibited or stimulated by hormones released by the CNS and peripheral endocrine tissue. Growth hormone, thyrotropin releasing hormone, thyroid stimulating hormone, human chorionic gonadotrophin, arginine vasopressin, gonadotrophin releasing hormone, androgens and prolactin are all capable of immunoregulation[17,18]. Also, the opiates produced following expression of the pro-opiomelanocortin gene, (α-, β-, and γ-endorphin, enkephalins, and adrenocorticotrophic hormone (ACTH) have wide reaching effects on immune cells[19]. For example, opiates have been shown to inhibit neurogenic microvascular leakage, mucus secretion and cholinergic transmission[13], and corticotrophin releasing factor (CRF) may modulate sensory nerve transmission.

Circulating leukocytes possess high and low affinity receptors for all these neuroendocrine steroids[20]. The level of sophistication seen in the autonomic regulation of immunity is mirrored by neuroendocrine perturbations of immunity. For example, the immune response to ACTH is different from the response to truncated ACTH molecules. Similarly, the response to α-endorphin differs from that to β-endorphin, and the response to met-enkephalin or β-endorphin differs from the response to morphine or α-endorphin[21,22].

Furthermore, it is clear that autonomic and neuroendocrine neuroimmunomodulatory pathways may regulate each other's function (Fig. 1.1). For example, the hypothalamus, which synthesizes many of the releasing hormones acting on the pituitary, receives a rich autonomic innervation from a variety of brainstem nuclei and is capable of synthesizing catecholamines[23]. Similarly, the central and basomedial nuclei of the amygdala can synthesize both catecholamines, serotonin and corticotrophin releasing hormone (CRH)[24]. In addition, electrolytic lesions or electrical stimulation of the hypothalamus can profoundly affect peripheral catecholamine production and subsequent cellular immunity[25]. Similarly, neurohormones can have a profound effect on autonomic function[26].

Thus there is a very wide potential repertoire of responses to stress. Different stressors may not only produce subtle differences in the autonomic outflow to different vascular and lymphoid target tissues, but also subtle differences in neuropeptide and neurohormone production. All these potential autonomic and neuroendocrine responses may interact at a tissue and cellular level to initiate, terminate, dampen or augment an immune response. Such complexity provides great potential for modulating any immune reaction in any organ of the body to a greater degree than any presently available immunosuppressant.

IMMUNONEUROMODULATORY SIGNALS

Cytokine-induced neuroendocrine changes

Not only does the CNS modulate immunity, but immune cells also modulate CNS function

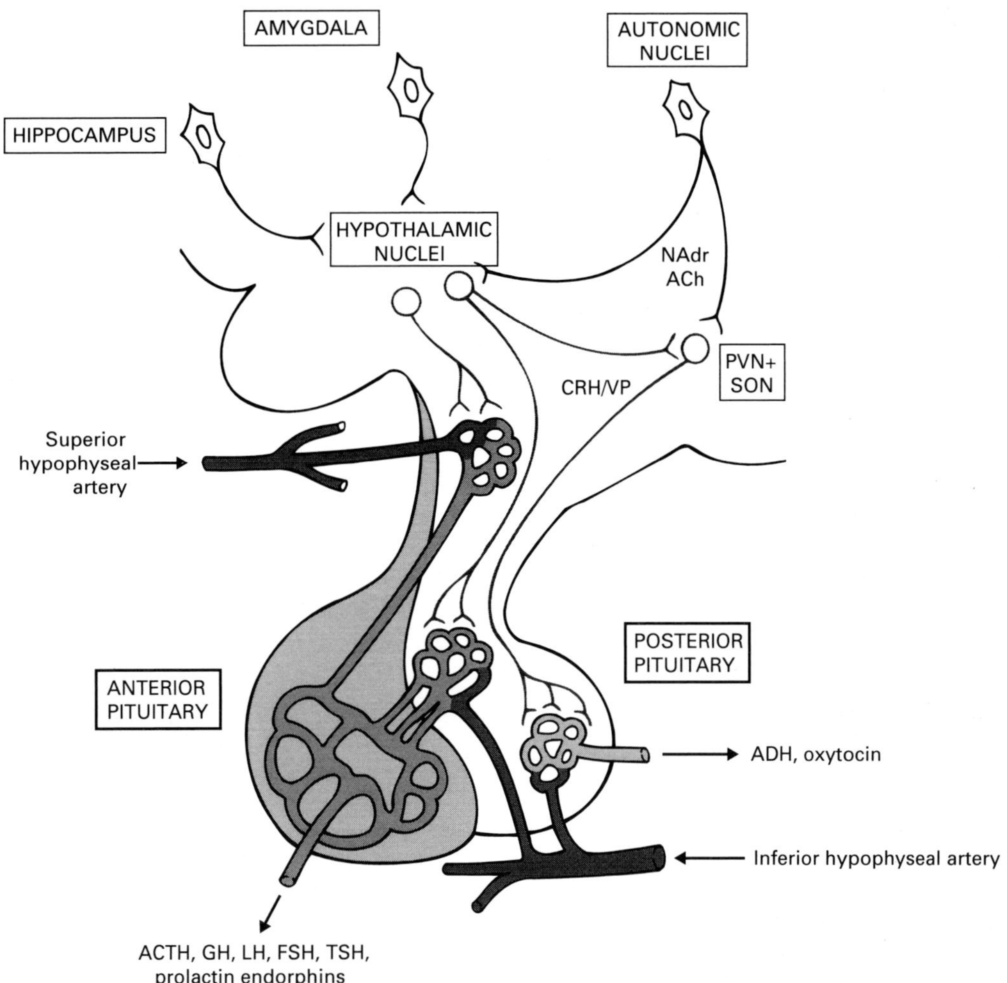

Figure 1.1 The interaction between autonomic and neuroendocrine systems. The emotional nuclei of the limbic system (the hippocampus and the amygdala) are connected to the hypothalamus and the autonomic nuclei in the brainstem demonstrating how emotions may regulate hormonal and autonomic function. CRH = corticotrophin releasing hormone; VP = vasopressin; ACTH = adrenocorticotrophin releasing hormone; GH = growth hormone; LH = leutenising hormone; FSH = follicle stimulating hormone; TSH = thyroid stimulating hormone; ADH = anti-diuretic hormone.

(Fig. 1.2). Peripherally produced immune signals have been shown to affect a wide variety of CNS functions. For example, leukocyte-derived interleukin (IL)-1, IL-6 and tumor necrosis factor (TNF)-α modulate neuropeptide and neurosteroid synthesis and central noradrenergic activity[16,22,25,27,28]. Cytokine-induced activation of the neuroendocrine axis is believed to occur mainly by promoting the release of CRH, or vasopressin (VP) from the paraventricular nucleus of the hypothalamus[29–31]. Two hours after lipopolysaccharide (LPS) administration c-fos immunoreactivity can be detected in the emotional, autonomic and neuroendocrine nuclei of the brainstem[32]. In addition, leukocyte-derived cytokines may act directly on pituitary cells promoting hormone release[33]. There is some evidence to suggest that leukocyte-derived cytokines may be more potent than endogenous CRH in eliciting ACTH release[34].

In addition to their direct action on hypothalamic nuclei, leukocyte-derived cytokines

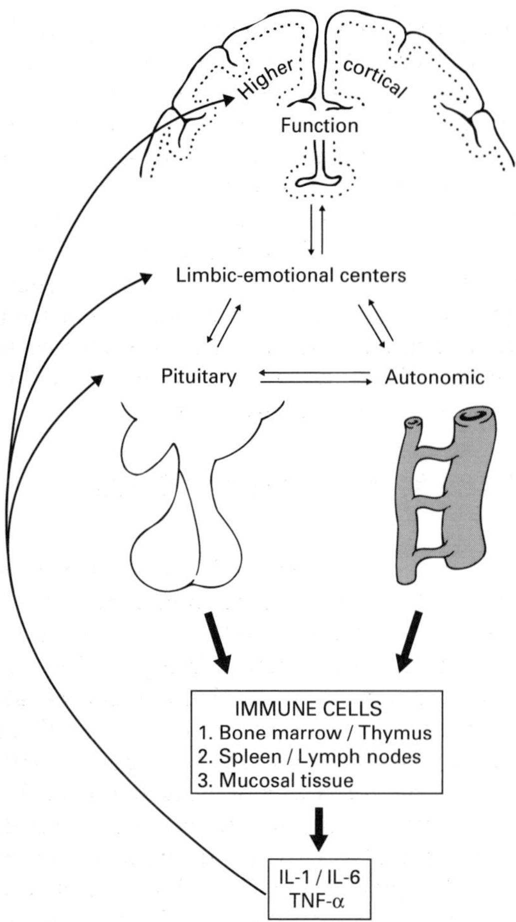

Figure 1.2 Bi-directional communication between the CNS and the immune system. Cytokines from the immune system communicate information to the brain, regulating its function and the brain talks back in a bi-directional flow of cytokines, hormones and peptides. IL-1 = interleukin-1; IL-6 = interleukin-6; TNF-α = tumor-necrosis factor-α.

may also have an indirect effect on hypothalamic CRH production, by modulating the activity of afferent innervation of the paraventricular nucleus. Thus, cytokine-induced CRH synthesis is lost following the destruction of hypothalamic autonomic innervation using 6-hydroxydopamine[35]. Alternatively, leukocyte-derived cytokines may alter CRH synthesis by changing neuronal or endothelial expression of nitric oxide synthetase (NOS) within the hypothalamus. Nitric oxide has been implicated in the regulation of CRH production, although its exact role remains unclear. Recent evidence has demonstrated that the nitric oxide precursor L-arginine and the synthetic nitrate molsidomine inhibit IL-1-induced CRH production[36]. In contrast, NG-monomethyl-L-arginine, a competitive inhibitor of NOS, completely suppressed IL-2-induced CRH release[37]. These immunoneuromodulatory signals can also be blocked by adrenalectomy and T cell depletion[38].

Cytokine-induced behavioral changes

Peripherally derived immune signals not only affect central neuroendocrine axis activation, but they can also affect behavior. For example, peripheral administration of bacterial LPS, IL-1 and TNF-α are known to promote fever, malaise, fatigue, and reduced interest in feeding, drinking and social behavior.

Transduction of immune signals into the CNS

Cytokines cannot cross the blood–brain barrier; therefore exactly how peripherally generated cytokines gain access to the hypothalamus to alter neuroendocrine activation and behavior is unclear. Four theories have been advanced. Firstly, it has been suggested that there may be a cytokine-specific uptake mechanism within the CNS[39]. Secondly, various authors have suggested that cytokines cross the blood–brain barrier at points of increased permeability, induced by endogenous steroid production[40,41]. More recently, prostaglandins have been implicated in the transduction of the peripheral cytokine signal into the CNS, since cytokine-induced modulation of hypothalamic noradrenaline levels is blocked by pretreatment with a cyclooxygenase inhibitor[22], and hypothalamic CRH production is blocked by epoxygenase and phospholipase A_2 inhibitors[42]. There is some evidence to suggest that both of these theories may be correct, with leukocyte-derived cytokines gaining access to microglia at points of increased permeability and modulating microglial cytokine production through a prostaglandin-dependent mechanism. The subsequent production of cytokines by microglia has been shown to alter CRH synthesis[43–45]. Alternatively, some authors have suggested that prostaglandin (PG)$F_{2\alpha}$ or PGE_2 produced by the microglia in response to peripherally-derived cytokines may upregulate CRH production directly[46,47]. A third possible explanation for how leukocyte-derived cytokines modulate CNS function is that the leukocytes themselves gain access to the CNS at points of increased permeability.

Finally, more recent data have suggested that peripherally derived cytokines may not need to cross the blood–brain barrier in order to alter CNS function. A number of groups have demonstrated that peripheral vagotomy or peripheral IL-1 receptor antagonism blocks the behavioral and neuroendocrine effects of peripherally administered IL-1. Support for the existence of this immunoneuromodulatory pathway has been provided by the discovery of IL-1 receptors on paraganglia of the vagus. Thus, when an inflammatory reaction occurs in the periphery this information is communicated to the CNS by cytokines impinging on peripheral cytokine receptors on the vagus. This results in altered afferent input to the tractus solitarius in the brainstem. This altered neural traffic may then stimulate local cytokine release by the microglia[48,49].

It is quite possible that all four of these pathways may be transducing peripheral cytokine signals into the CNS, and different pathways are employed depending on which cytokine is involved and in which immune compartment the immune response is occurring.

Leukocyte-derived steroids

Leukocytes not only modulate neuroendocrine peptide production by the CNS, but they are capable of producing stress-associated peptides and hormones that were previously thought to reside exclusively in the CNS[50,51]. These leukocyte-derived peptides and hormones may be identical to those produced by the brain, or they may be unique structural and functional variants, or cleaved subunits of the total molecule[52]. Leukocyte stress peptides and hormones may be produced in response to powerful stimulants such as 'superantigens' or viruses; alternatively they may be produced in response to the macrophage IL-1 release that occurs following stimulation of these cells by CNS trophic hormones[16]. The exact role of these leukocyte-derived stress peptides has been the subject of much debate. Some authors have suggested that they convey information to the CNS about the nature of the peripheral immune response[53]; others have suggested that their role is to regulate the immune response in a paracrine fashion, since insufficient plasma levels are produced to modulate the function of other endocrine tissues, such as the adrenal gland[16,54,55].

CORTICAL ACTIVATION OF NIM PATHWAYS

It is clear, therefore, that activation of neuroendocrine cells within the hypothalamus or the brainstem autonomic nuclei and subsequent efferent neuroimmunomodulatory (NIM) signals are regulated by incoming afferent signals from the immune system. In addition to these incoming immunoneuromodulatory signals, there are also a number of cortical and limbic afferent inputs to the autonomic and hypothalamic nuclei that are capable of regulating efferent NIM signals[56], and these inputs utilize a wide variety of neuropeptides[57]. But what is the evidence that higher cortical centers are involved in the activation of NIM pathways?

Firstly there is clear evidence to suggest that at least three cortical centers are intimately involved in regulation of autonomic outflow from the brainstem nuclei. Secondly, the enormous literature on the physiological effects of stress suggests that how we cope can have a profound effect on neuroendocrine and autonomic activity and significantly impair the immune system. Similarly, the research investigating the effects of personality on the development and progression of cancer and chronic inflammatory diseases such as asthma and rheumatoid arthritis support the idea that psychosocial variables play a major role in the disease outcome. The numerous studies on patients with depression suggest that depressive thoughts and a depressed mood can have a significant impact on immunity, and this may be mediated by the neuroendocrine and autonomic changes seen in depression. Finally, there is a substantial body of evidence to suggest that perceptions may be profoundly immunosuppressive, or immunoenhancing. The research implicating higher cortical centers in the regulation of immune function cuts across the fields of psychiatry, immunology, and neurobiology, and provides persuasive evidence that perceptions, thoughts, and feelings play a crucial role in disease onset and progression by activating neuroendocrine and autonomic efferent NIM pathways.

Cortical control of autonomic outflow

It has long been known that autonomic responses frequently accompany motor seizures. Thus, individuals who collapse from a seizure may involuntarily void urine and feces, whereas those collapsing from an arrhythmogenic event rarely lose continence. Attempts to resolve the question of whether the autonomic activity seen following epileptic cortical activity is due to cortical innervation of the autonomic nuclei in the brainstem, or the result of reflexes initiated by the muscular contraction during the seizure were fraught with difficulties. Early work relied on electrical stimulation of the cortex. However, such studies were difficult to interpret, because the area of stimulation was not well described in neuroanatomical terms and the voltages used were large, leading to diffuse spread of current to adjacent areas of the cortex. In addition, many of the autonomic responses observed may have been secondary to stimulation of subcortical regions rather than cortical stimulation. Furthermore, these studies could not exclude the possibility that the muscular contractions produced by cortical excitation were responsible for initiating reflex autonomic discharge. Therefore, the results of these stimulation studies were frequently contradictory.

Even when cortical mapping became more precise, the electrical stimulation may have been producing autonomic effects as a result of stimulation of 'fibers of passage' rather than the cell bodies in the area of cortex stimulated. Alternatively, electrical stimulation may have produced collateral excitation of association areas which then promoted autonomic activity, rather than autonomic activation occurring secondary to stimulation of the targeted area. While chemical stimulation overcame many of these objections, the distinction between primary autonomic responses and reflex autonomic responses secondary to somatic activity remained difficult. Other confounding variables such as type and depth of anesthesia, differences in the behavioral state in conscious animals, or opposing autonomic effects in different body compartments, have made interpretation of single studies very difficult. However, with a multidisciplinary approach, and by cross-correlating a variety of different neuroanatomical and neurophysiological methodologies, it has been possible to establish that there are at least three areas of the cortex which are intimately involved in the regulation of autonomic function[58].

Insular cortex

Results of numerous studies in rats, cats, dogs and primates have identified the insular cortex[59], the medial prefrontal cortex[60], and the sensorimotor cortex[61], as important sites of autonomic control. These studies have suggested that the insular cortex is a visceral sensorimotor area akin to the somatic sensorimotor area and involved in regulating changes in blood pressure, heart rate, gastric motility and peristaltic activity in addition to changes in respiration and adrenaline secretion. It must be remembered that the insular cortex also has extensive connections, particularly to the lateral hypothalamus[62,63], and also to the central nucleus of the amygdala[64], the parabrachial nucleus[65,66], the parasympathetic preganglionic nucleus in the medulla[23,24], and the nucleus of the tractus solitarius[67], where autonomic afferents converge. In addition, connections to thalamic nuclei and the reticular activating system have been identified. Thus the insular cortex is perfectly placed to integrate emotional and autonomic responses and mediate stress-induced cardiovascular responses[68]. In fact phasic stimulation of the insular cortex has been shown to provoke severe arrhythmias.

Medial prefrontal/infralimbic cortex

In contrast to the visceral sensorimotor role of the insular cortex, it has been suggested that the medial prefrontal cortex, and more specifically the infralimbic cortex, acts as a visceral motor center, involved in heart rate, blood pressure and gastric tone regulation[18]. This hypothesis is based on its extensive limbic inputs from the hippocampus and amygdala[69], with few visceral sensory inputs. Furthermore, the infralimbic cortex has a number of significant efferent pathways[70]. A dorsal pathway projects to the prelimbic cortex and the anterior cingulate cortex. A lateral pathway projects to the insular cortex and the perirhinal cortex with a few fibers projecting to the corticospinal tract. The ventral pathway is the largest efferent pathway and innervates the thalamus, the hypothalamus, the amygdala, and autonomic cell groups in the brainstem including the periaqueductal gray matter, the parabrachial nucleus, the dorsal motor nucleus of the vagus, the nucleus of the tractus solitarius, the nucleus ambiguus, the ventrolateral medulla and the intermediolateral cell column in the spinal cord (IML)[69,71,72]. The extensive projections of the infralimbic cortex suggest that it may mediate the visceral motor responses to emotional and stressful stimuli.

Sensorimotor cortex

The third cortical area that has been identified as having an important role in autonomic regulation is the somatic sensorimotor cortex. It has been suggested that the motor cortex acts as a cardiovascular command center, capable of initiating the somatic responses to exercise in addition to altering visceral function in line with the somatic demands[16].

Therefore, although there is clear evidence linking the cerebral cortex with autonomic nuclei, it is not yet clear how, or if, these pathways are involved in integrating cortical, autonomic and behavioral activity.

The complexity of these interactions between cortical centers, autonomic nuclei and peripheral responses is illustrated by the central control of blood pressure. One of the most important central nuclei in blood pressure regulation is the rostral ventrolateral medulla (RVLM). This is believed to be the site of the vasomotor center[73]. Interestingly, neurones in the RVLM not only exhibit 'pacemaker-like' activity[74], but also generate respiratory-related rhythms in their discharge[75]. Furthermore there seems to be a topographic organization within the RVLM with different groups of neurones controlling different vascular beds[76]. However, the RVLM is not the only nucleus influencing blood pressure. Evidence suggests that efferent activity from other central nuclei, such as the raphe nucleus[77], is integrated with RVLM efferent activity by the IML, which then send out an integrated signal to the heart. The raphe neurones have also been shown to exhibit cardiovascular and respiratory rhythms in their discharge[78,79]. The RVLM itself receives afferents from chemoreceptor and baroreceptor neurones via the solitary tract (NTS) in addition to the inputs from higher cortical centers, vide infra. This degree of complexity has led some authors to suggest that different central nuclei may mediate the pressor response to different behavioral stimuli or different emotional states[80].

Cortical control of neuroendocrine activation

Specific centers within the cerebral cortex not only regulate autonomic activity, but also have a significant impact on hormonal production by the hypothalamus and the pituitary. Thus the frontal cortex, believed to be the primary center for rational thought, in addition to the limbic emotional nuclei, modulate neuroendocrine output. Much of the research substantiating the role of the frontal cortex in neuroendocrine activation comes from work with negative emotional states such as depression. There is a considerable amount of research characterizing the neuroendocrine abnormalities in depressed patients. Abnormalities of glucocorticoid (GC) metabolism are the most widely studied. A significant number of depressed patients are known to be hypercortisolemic, with a loss of the normal diurnal variation in cortisol levels[81]. Suppression of plasma cortisol levels with the 11-β-hydroxylase inhibitor metyrapone fails to produce the normal upregulation of type 2 GC receptors on lymphocytes in depressed patients[82]. Dexamethasone-induced suppression of cortisol levels is frequently lost[83,84], and these patients have a poorer clinical outcome and increased risk of relapse[85]. The release of ACTH in response to CRH infusion is also blunted in depression, and this blunting is probably due to a decrease in the number of anterior pituitary CRH receptors[86]; consequently CRH levels are often increased in the CSF[87]. Despite persistently elevated GC levels in many depressives they do not normally become Cushingoid, which suggests that there may be a defect in the type 2 GC receptor[88], resulting in steroid insensitivity.

Corticosteroids and depression

Current thinking holds that depression is secondary to reduced monoamine levels in the brain, and there is a large amount of circumstantial evidence to support this theory[89]. In addition, the release of CRH from the paraventricular nucleus in the hypothalamus is known to be regulated by the two major monoamine neurotransmitters, noradrenaline from the locus ceruleus and serotonin from the raphe nucleus[90]. However, it has been argued that the reduced monoamine levels in the brain of depressive patients are secondary to chronic changes in GC metabolism rather than the cause of the GC abnormalities[91]. This hypothesis is supported by studies in adrenalectomized rats, which revealed a significantly reduced turnover of 5-HT in the dorsal hippocampus, and a reduced number of noradrenaline receptors in the paraventricular nucleus of rat brains, both effects being reversed by corticosterone replacement[92,93]. In addition, monoamine reuptake inhibitors not only increase the availability of monoamines[94], but they have also been shown to increase the number of GC receptor neurones in the locus ceruleus and the raphe nucleus[95,96].

Furthermore, it has been argued that increased hypothalamic corticosteroid tone seen in depressed patients is responsible for the abnormalities in growth hormone, prolactin and thyroid stimulating hormone metabolism[97,98], in addition to the abnormalities in autonomic function[99,100,101]. In addition, the blunting of the *d*-fenfluramine-induced prolactin response, classically thought to be due to 5-HT receptor sensitivity, may in fact be due to chronically elevated GC levels[102,103]. The suggestion that GC activity is central to depression is supported by a 50% prevalence of depression in patients with Cushing's syndrome[104], and a reduction in depressive symptoms following treatment of these patients with metyrapone[105].

The activation of the hypothalamic pituitary adreno-cortical (HPAC) axis may explain the increased incidence of immune dysfunction seen in depressed patients[106,107]. For example, intracerebroventricular injection of CRF has been shown to reduce splenic natural killer cell activity[108]. However, there is considerable variation in the large number of studies investigating immune function in depressed patients[109]. Some, but not all studies have demonstrated reduced lymphocyte proliferation[45], and reduced total lymphocyte count in depressed patients compared with controls[110]. The variability of these results may be due to the heterogeneity of the patient population studied, the lack of stringent immunological controls, and failure to control the level of stress during the experiment. When the variability in immunological assays is controlled for, significant age-related differences between normal and depressed patients are apparent, particularly in the older more severely depressed patients[47]. A number of studies have correlated negative emotional states such as depression with the subsequent development of disease. For example, a 17-year prospective study of 2000 healthy males found that higher depression scores during early adulthood predicted the subsequent development of cancer[111].

Cortical control of immunity

It is clear from the data cited above that the cortex regulates the autonomic and neuroendocrine pathways capable of regulating immunity, but what is the evidence that the cortex directly controls immunity? A substantial amount of circumstantial evidence, from a variety of different sources has suggested that cortical function may directly influence immunity. For example, the effects of stress, perception and personality on immunity have all been extensively investigated (vida infra). In addition, there is a strong relationship between cerebral dominance and allergy and autoimmune disease, with left handers having a 11.5-fold increase in the incidence of self-reported allergy[112,113]. Furthermore, electrolytic lesions of the right or left neocortex have been shown to induce opposite effects on immune function[114]. Left cortical ablation suppresses immune function, while right cortical ablation enhances immunity[115,116]. These studies assessed a wide variety of immune parameters including mitogen-induced proliferation, natural killer cell activity, macrophage activation, secretory IgA and interleukin-2 production. Similarly left cortical stimulation has been shown to enhance immune parameters[117,118], and recent human evidence suggests that individuals with higher resting left frontal cortical activity had significantly higher NK cell activity[119].

The effects of stress and immune function

There is an enormous amount of research characterizing the physiological response to stress. Stressful situations are known to activate central autonomic nuclei and the sympathetic-adreno-medullary (SAM) axis, in addition to the HPAC axis. These two pathways underpin different behavioral responses, and are associated with different emotional moods. The SAM axis is involved in the fight and flight response, and is associated with the feelings of anger and anxiety. Fighting involves noradrenaline and the central nucleus of the amygdala, while the flight response involves adrenaline and the basal nuclei of the amygdala[120]. In contrast, activation of the HPAC axis promotes submission and the emotions of defeat and despair[121,122], and is thought to involve the septohippocampal system[123]. Typically chronically stressful environments promote a vacillation between anger and despair, as individuals fight to gain control over their environment or give up, believing that they have no control. These cycles of anger and despair promote the production of a destructive range of catabolic hormones, injurious to a number of bodily systems, not just the immune system (see Ch. 3).

Animal studies

In contrast to the data on depression, the immunosuppressive effect of stress is remarkably consistent across different populations and different kinds of stressors. There is a substantial amount of animal evidence highlighting the importance of cognitive centers on immunity[124,125]. Furthermore, there is extensive research on the immunosuppressive effects of a wide range of environmental manipulations such as isolation, separation, overcrowding, disrupted dominance hierarchy, introduction of an aggressive intruder, restraint, cold, noise, and inescapable foot shock[126,127]. Most of these studies have employed in vitro assessments of lymphocyte function, such as mitogen proliferation, cytokine production and cellular cytotoxicity or non-specific, in vivo assessments of immunity, such as antibody production[128,129]. Far fewer functional studies have evaluated the effects of stress on the development and progression of animal models of disease.

One such study evaluated the effects of restraint stress on the pulmonary response to nasal infection with the influenza virus. The authors reported that restraint stress virtually abolished the viral-induced mononuclear lung infiltration and significantly reduced mediastinal lymph node IL-2 production, and virus-specific cell-mediated immunity, but did not affect antibody production[130]. Subsequent studies demonstrated that the inhibition of the cellular influx was due to increased corticosteroid levels, while the inhibition of virus-specific effector cells was the result of increased catecholamine levels[131]. The increased survival, following restraint, was due to the combined effect of catecholamines and neuroendocrine steroids[74]. These results confirmed earlier work suggesting that corticosteroids and catecholamines were important in mediating the stress-induced inhibition of T cell response[132,133], and may be crucial to the recovery from certain autoimmune diseases such as experimental allergic encephalomyelitis (EAE)[134].

There is evidence to suggest that acute and chronic stress may have differential effects on T cell sub-populations[135,136]. For example, housing mice individually rather than in groups of four significantly increased the amount of IL-4, but not IL-2 produced by Balb/c mice splenocytes in response to keyhole limpet hemocyanin (KLH). In contrast, isolation increased IL-2, but not IL-4 production by C57BL/6 mice[137].

Human studies

The literature on the effects of stress on immunity in humans is also plentiful[138]. Early research in this field ranked major life events according to how 'stressful' they were. This was based on retrospective data looking at the incidence of these events prior to the development of major illness. Death of a spouse was believed to be the most debilitating, and Bartrop, in a seminal study, demonstrated that bereaved individuals showed significant immunosuppression 2–6 weeks after the death of a spouse compared with non-bereaved individuals[139]. These findings were confirmed in a subsequent prospective study on men whose wives were dying of breast cancer[140]. More recently, traumatic marital separation has been shown to be more immunosuppressive than bereavement[141,142].

Such work relating stress to immune impairment and disease continues to be produced in a variety of different clinical settings. For example, a recent highly publicized study demonstrated that highly stressed subjects were more likely to develop an upper respiratory tract infection, on exposure to five commonly encountered viruses, than subjects experiencing less stress[143]. However, the majority of research in this area now focuses on the effects of acute stress. For example, examinations have been shown to depress humoral and cellular immunity[144], while sleep deprivation inhibits neutrophil phagocytosis[145]. Models of chronic stress in humans have been more difficult to develop[146]. One exception to this trend revealed that chronic stress impairs wound healing and reduces leukocyte cytokine mRNA expression[147]. Current opinion now believes that minor chronic stress, termed 'microstress', is more immunosuppressive than single life events such as bereavement.

This stress-induced immunomodulation in humans has been predominantly attributed to altered neuroendocrine function[148,149]. For example, severe stress may reduce the level of the testosterone precursor, dihydroepiandrosterone sulphate (DHEAS), and reduce humoral immunity in favor of cellular immunity[150]. However, individuals who exhibit the largest catecholamine response to stress also produce the most dramatic alterations in cellular immunity to the same stress[151].

It is clear from both the human and animal literature that the immunological consequences of stress depend on a variety of factors including the nature, duration, intensity and controllability of the stressor. For example, in one study, restraint, heat and cold all exerted different effects on the cell-mediated hypersensitivity[152]. However, extrapolation of animal data to humans must be made with caution since some chronic stressors, which produce immunosuppression in humans, may produce adaptation or even immunoenhancement in animals[153,154]. Such differences serve to emphasize the importance of careful experimental design in setting up studies in animals and humans.

The brain bypass: the importance of perception on immunity

Recent research has demonstrated that our response to stressful events may be neurologically determined. Thus incoming sensory information, which may be stressful, is not only communicated to the higher cortical centers for cognitive interpretation, but the information is also sent, via a small bundle of fibers from the sensory nuclei in the thalamus to the emotional centers in the brainstem, particularly the lateral nucleus of the amygdala[155]. The function of the amygdala has been extensively studied, and it has been shown to be critically involved in emotional memory[156].

Emotional memory involves subconscious learning[157], and the storage of information about the emotional significance of events. The emotional significance of a single event is stored along with all the relevant and irrelevant contextual and environmental cues associated with that event. During emotionally charged events, catecholamine release from the adrenal medulla activates vagal receptors resulting in enhanced afferent input to the amygdala. This increased adrenergic input helps to potentiate the memory for that emotionally charged situation[158]. Such emotionally charged memories are indelible, and very resistant to extinction.

Not only is the emotionally charged memory remembered, but all the contextual cues are simultaneously recalled. For example, many people vividly remember all the details and contextual cues of where they were and what they were doing when President Kennedy was shot. The hippocampus seems to play an important role in recognizing and recalling the contextual cues in animals and man[159,160], while the amygdala has a comparative function and determines the significance of these contextual cues. Thus, while the hippocampus recognizes the features of a dangerous situation, it is the amygdala that determines the significance of these cues and makes us feel uneasy and initiates a behavioral response.

Research suggests that the amygdala is crucial to the acquisition of these subconscious conditioned responses in animals and man[147,161]. Numerous cytoarchitectural and electrophysiological studies have revealed that information about incoming auditory, visual and somatosensory stimuli is sent directly to the lateral nucleus of the amygdala[142,162], which then makes an instantaneous decision about the potential threat that these incoming stimuli represent.

A direct neural connection between the thalamus and the brain's alarm bell, the amygdala, may have substantial survival value. It allows potentially lethal stimuli or environments to be detected instantaneously, and the amygdala initiates an appropriate behavioral response, which ensures survival. The lateral nucleus of the amygdala where sensory inputs are integrated[163], indirectly sends fibers to the central nucleus of the amygdala, via the basolateral nucleus[164].

The central nucleus, through its extensive projections to the motor cortex, the lateral hypothalamus, and other brainstem autonomic nuclei, is then able to hijack all other neural pathways during an emotional emergency[143,165]. Thus the central nucleus of the amygdala acts as a command center activating brainstem autonomic nuclei, neuroendocrine pathways and the motor cortex to initiate the appropriate behavioral response, be it avoidance (flight), readiness (fight), or playing dead (submission), and each one of these responses is underpinned by specific changes in heart rate, blood pressure, catecholamine and stress hormone production[166,167]. If the behavioral response was delayed until the incoming information was processed by the neocortex, valuable seconds would be lost, and this could make the difference between life and death. Not only does the amygdala orchestrate behavioral and physiological responses it is crucially involved in coordinating immunological responses[168].

Emotional imprecision

The processing of incoming sensory information by the amygdala is relatively sophisticated. Electrophysiological studies have shown that acoustically responsive cells within the lateral nucleus of the amygdala can respond to different auditory frequencies[169,170]. However, the comparative function of the amygdala relies on associative matching and is therefore very imprecise. Thus, the amygdala evaluates new stimuli and environments and 'matches' them to previously stored memories. Any similarities in contextual cues or emotional content may provoke a 'match'. The system is designed to err on the side of caution for the sake of survival and it cannot determine whether the 'match' is appropriate or relevant. As a result the amygdala may initiate the same behavioral or physiological response to the new stimulus that it generated during the original 'matched' stimulus. Many of the past experiences that we use to match to are wordless emotional memories from childhood when our language was poorly developed and many events were bewildering[171].

Thus our emotions can have a 'mind of their own', and our reactions to stressful stimuli often bypass the cortex and initiate behavioral and physiological responses independent of rational thought. Hence the brain is neurologically designed to create first impressions and feelings, and designed to think much later.

Cortical override

Fortunately the neocortex does have the capacity to override these instantaneous emotional responses to aversive stimuli. The learned association between a neutral stimulus and a noxious event, such as the pairing of a tone with a footshock, can be extinguished by repeated exposure to the neutral tone on its own. The medial prefrontal cortex has been shown to play a pivotal role in extinguishing classically conditioned emotional and physiological responses[172]. Similarly the cortex may play an important role in conditioning immunological responses by activating the two efferent NIM pathways[173–175].

Conditioned immunological responses

Neutral stimuli that have been previously associated with aversive stimuli can not only elicit unconscious behavioral and physiological responses, but they can also elicit powerful immunological responses[176]. This was first demonstrated in a series of conditioned taste aversion experiments in 1975 by Dr Robert Ader. He was trying to teach rats to avoid sugared water by simultaneously administering cyclophosphamide to induce nausea. When the rats were re-exposed to the sugared water in the absence of the cyclophosphamide, they still developed nausea. This conditioning of a physiological response was not unexpected and had been previously described in a number of animal models. However, what was surprising was that the rats re-fed the sugared water started to die from infectious disease. It seemed that the rats had not only learnt that the cyclophosphamide produced nausea, but also that it induced an immunosuppression. The taste of sugared water had been turned into a powerful immunosuppressive signal[177]. This initial report that the immune system could be classically conditioned in the same way that behavior and physiological responses could be conditioned was met with considerable skepticism. However, these findings have now been extensively replicated in a wide variety of animal models and in man. Thus, animals can learn to suppress, or enhance, their T cell, B cell, cytotoxic cell, natural killer cell and mast cell function in vivo and ex vivo[178–184]. The potential biological significance of conditioning the immune response was highlighted by findings demonstrating that such phenomena could impact mortality rates in some models[185]. There is evidence to suggest that the pathways connecting the thalamus, cortex and the amygdala, and which mediate the conditioned behavioral and physiological responses to neutral stimuli, also mediate conditioned immunomodulation. For example, CRH-induced suppression of natural killer (NK) cell cytotoxicity is correlated with CRH receptor expression in the amygdala[159].

The influence of personality on immune function

One of the major criticisms of the data investigating the immunomodulatory effects of stress is the enormous inter-individual variability in the response to stress[186]. This variability may be due to differences in subconscious or conscious processing of stressful stimuli. Thus an emotionally traumatic childhood may enhance the subconscious emotional responses to stressful stimuli, resulting in enhanced physiological responses to stress, increased production of immunosuppressive neuropeptides and hormones, and submissive behavior. There is some evidence that psychosocial disruption in utero, postnatally and during childhood can have long-term consequences on the immune system[187–189]. Early emotionally traumatic years may be manifested as poorer coping responses to stress in adulthood. Strategies and styles of coping have been used to characterize the personality of an individual. Premorbid personality and coping strategies have been shown to be as important as the characteristics of the stress itself, in determining the immunological consequences of stress. Personality factors may not only exacerbate the symptoms and perpetuate the disability in many chronic conditions[190], but may also play a crucial role in determining the progression and outcome of disease. For example, coping strategies and psychological factors have been shown to be significant predictors of who dies from acute asthma[191–192], in addition to predicting the progression of viral infections[193], AIDS[194], cancer and heart disease[195]. Conversely there is some evidence to suggest that certain coping strategies can minimize the detrimental effects of stressful life events[196].

However, personality is not entirely dependent on early emotional life; subconscious processing of stressful stimuli and cognitive factors come into play. Higher cortical centers, involved in cognition, can override subconscious emotional responses. Therefore inter-individual differences in the response to stressful stimuli may be related to differences in the ability to gain conscious control over emotional responses in addition to the ability of the medial prefrontal cortex to inhibit emotional centers. Such regulation of mental and emotional responses can be taught[197], and there is some evidence to suggest that social support, which encourages the cognitive handling of emotionally charged information, can impact mortality[198,199]. In contrast, non-structured social support and inappropriate cognitive strategies can have a detrimental effect.

DISRUPTED MIND–BODY PATHWAYS

It is apparent that the immune system can no longer be considered as autoregulatory. Virtually every aspect of immune function can be modulated by the autonomic nervous system and centrally produced neuropeptides. These efferent neuroimmunomodulatory pathways are themselves modulated by afferent inputs from the immune system, the cortex and the limbic emotional centers. Thus the brain and the immune system communicate in a complex bidirectional flow of cytokines, steroids and neuropeptides, sharing information and regulating each other's function. This enables the two systems to respond in an integrated manner to environmental challenges, be they immunological or behavioral, and thereby maintain homeostatic balance.

The exact pathophysiological significance of these mind–body pathways and networks is not yet clear. However, the complexity of autonomic innervation of lymphoid tissue, and the widespread distribution of neuroendocrine receptors on leukocytes, suggests that neuroimmunomodulatory pathways may exert subtle control over the balance of pro-and anti-inflammatory forces within individual tissues. Leukocyte-derived cytokines seem to play a particularly crucial role in regulating immunity. Thus a vigorous peripheral immune response would be expected to stimulate the IL-1 receptors on the hepatic branch of the vagus and increase afferent neural activity in proportion to the extent of the immune reaction occurring. This cytokine-induced afferent input induces hypothalamic CRH production, which then promotes ACTH synthesis and corticosterone production, thereby preventing excessive expansion of clones with low affinity for the stimulating antigen, and thus dampening the immune response. In addition, lipopolysaccharide-induced IL-1 production may be fatal if adrenalectomy prevents the normal neuroendocrine dampening of the immune response (Fig. 1.3).

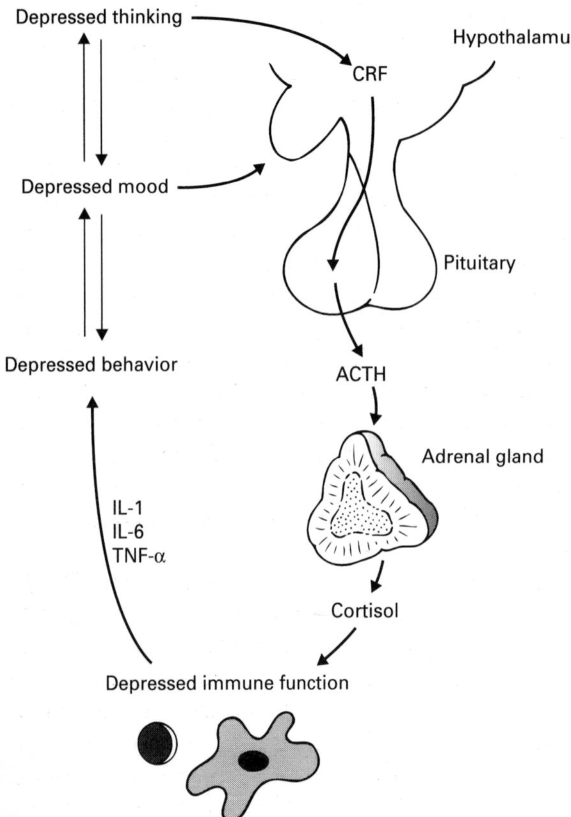

Figure 1.3 The relationship between thought, mood, behavior and immune function. Depressed thinking and mood can alter the autonomic and neuroendocrine output from the brain, potentially modulating immunity. Similarly, immunity and depressed behaviour can alter CNS function thereby altering autonomic and neuroendocrine activity.

Disruption of these afferent or efferent pathways, due to genetic or environmental influences, may upset the homeostatic balance with fatal consequences[200]. For example, some elegant work in rats demonstrated that disruption of afferent input to the hypothalamus produced enhanced immunosuppression. Thus rats stressed by tail shocks suppressed their T cell proliferation and natural killer cell cytotoxicity coincident with an increase in their central IL-1 release and hypothalamic CRH production. The increased CRH then minimized the immunosuppression induced by the tail shock. Interruption of the afferent input to the hypothalamus by intracerebroventricular injection of anti IL-1 antibodies blocked the dampening effects of CRH resulting in enhanced tail shock-induced immunosuppression[201]. Similarly, blocking the transduction of the incoming leukocyte-derived cytokine signals, using prostaglandin inhibitors, has been shown to inhibit hypothalamic noradrenaline and CRH production[202,203]. LPS-induced IL-1 production may be fatal if adrenalectomy prevents the normal neuroendocrine dampening of the immune response. Furthermore, blockade of efferent sympathetic activity with chlorisondamine prevented IL-1-induced immunosuppression[204].

Disruption of mind–body pathways not only impairs immunity in vitro, but there is evidence to suggest that it can also impact animal models of clinical disease in vivo. For example, interruption of autonomic innervation of lymphoid organs has been shown to exacerbate the clinical signs of experimental allergic encephalomyelitis (EAE)[205]. The observed differences in the susceptibility of rats to other autoimmune disease may be related, not to disrupted mind–body pathways, but to genetic differences in their neuroimmunological signaling[206]. Thus Lewis rats possess hyporesponsive hypothalamic CRH neurones compared with F/344 rats, and generate reduced levels of corticosteroid in response to cytokine stimulation, rendering them more susceptible to disease[207]. Such genetic differences may not only determine the susceptibility of rats to EAE, but may also influence their recovery from EAE[208,209]. This genetic alteration in hypothalamic corticosteroid production is analogous to the altered hypothalamic corticosteroid tone seen in depressed patients.

In addition to the above data on genetic differences and pharmacological disruption of neuroimmunological signaling, there is an extensive body of data demonstrating that electrolytic lesions within the limbic nuclei have profound effects on immune effector cell function. Thus surgical ablation of the amygdala in animals enhances immune function, while ablation of the hippocampus suppresses cellular and humoral immunity[210]. Data on the clinical and immunological consequences of limbic lesions in humans are very sparse and somewhat contradictory[211].

Similarly, interruption of cortico-amygdala pathways may have a significant effect on immunity. For example, it has been suggested that structural or functional abnormalities in the communication pathways between the cortex and the emotional centers, as seen in alexithymic individuals, can result in profound immunological[212,213], and behavioral impairment[214,215]. This disruption of the pathways between cognitive and emotional centers can be produced by persistently high levels of ACTH, resulting in damage to hippocampal cells[216]. Furthermore, it has been suggested that the age-related dysfunction that occurs in the autonomic nervous system, including the innervation of lymphoid tissue, may be responsible for the age-related decay in immunological function[217,218].

Therefore interruption or dysfunction in either the incoming immune messages, the efferent neuroimmunomodulatory pathways or the cortical-emotional loops, due to genetic or environmental factors, can not only produce profound immunological dysfunction, but they may perpetuate or attenuate the disease process. Depressive thinking may depress mood, promote depressive behavior, and consequently induce chronic elevation of glucocorticoid levels which then have a significant negative effect on the functional activity of the brain[219]. Conversely, depressive thinking may produce immunosuppression, predisposing to illness which then produces depressed mood (Fig. 1.3).

CARDIONEUROIMMUNOLOGY

Thus, it is becoming increasingly apparent that the breakdown in cooperation between different physiological systems within the body may underlie the pathogenesis of many diseases. In this regard, there is evidence to suggest that the heart plays a hitherto unrecognized key role in balancing the entire human system. For example, the heart is now recognized as an endocrine gland secreting hormones which balance the cardiovascular system[220], and recent evidence suggests that the heart possesses its own intrinsic nervous system which can function independently of the central nervous system[221]. This cardiac nervous system contains catecholamine secreting cells with magnetic properties[222] that operate independently of the sympathetic nervous system[223].

The electrical rhythms generated by this cardiac nervous system and measured by the beat-to-beat variation in heart rate have been shown to affect a number of other organs including the brain and the immune system, and are now widely used to predict the risk of sudden cardiac death[224]. Afferent signals from the heart feed back vital information to the central autonomic nuclei in the medulla oblongata via the baroreceptor network[225]. Different emotional states, positive and negative, have been shown to affect profoundly the electrical rhythms generated by the heart and therefore the nature of the afferent input to the brainstem nuclei[197,226].

In addition to the substantial evidence suggesting that negative emotional states are immunosuppressive, there is now increasing evidence that positive emotional states can enhance immunity[227–229]. Thus it appears that the energy generated by the heart can impact immunity, opening up the possibility of a new field of investigation called cardioneuroimmunology.

Energy

The concept of energy has always been foreign to conventional physicians, and central to complementary therapists. But although conventional medicine claims not to deal in energy, patients frequently visit their doctors complaining of a lack of energy, and doctors investigate such complaints using conventional hematological, biochemical and hormonal tests. In fact physicians have been measuring the electromagnetic energy generated by the heart, brain, nerves and muscles for many years in the form of the electrocardiogram (ECG), the electromyogram (EMG), the electroencephalogram (EEG) and nerve conduction studies. Conventional physicians have also been measuring the energy generated by the cardiovascular and gastrointestinal systems in the form of the blood pressure waves and esophageal and colonic pressure traces.

The heart is the largest producer of rhythmic energy, both electrically and mechanically, in the human system, producing 50 times more electrical energy and 1000 times more electromagnetic energy than the brain. Furthermore the electromagnetic energy emitted by the heart is not confined within the body. This energy can be measured several feet away from the body using sophisticated SQUID-based magnetometers[230].

A greater appreciation of the concept of energy and the fundamental role played by the major energy source in the human body — the human heart — may help not only to establish common ground between conventional and complementary medicine[231], but may also provide significant new insights as we strive to remain healthy and stay balanced during increasingly changing times[232,233].

CONCLUSION

There is now very clear scientific evidence to indicate that the brain regulates immune function through efferent autonomic and neuroendocrine pathways. Furthermore there are a number of afferent pathways by which the immune system modulates brain function. The brain is designed to respond to incoming signals from our senses and it has been suggested that the afferent signals received from the immune system are dealt with in the same way as afferent sensory information. Thus the immune system acts as a sort of sixth sense[16]. The recent finding that the heart also supplies the brain with sensory information raises the possibility that the heart may be our seventh sense.

Just as it is necessary for survival that potentially lethal threats are detected by our five senses, it is also necessary that we detect potentially lethal immunological threats from our sixth sense. The pathways connecting mind and body enable a cohesive integrated response to threats, be they behavioral, physiological or immunological, to be mounted, homeostasis to be established and survival to be maintained. Cognitive, emotional, autonomic or neuroendocrine dysfunction or disruption of the mind–body pathways, whether due to genetic or environmental influences, may upset this homeostatic balance, and therefore increase the likelihood of dysfunction and disease in either system. Thus mind and body can no longer be considered as separate, and we should address both if we are to deliver high quality care into the 21st Century.

REFERENCES

1 Watkins AD 1994 The role of alternative therapy in allergic disease. Clinical and Experimental Allergy 24:813–25

2 Vincent C, Furnham A, Willsmore M 1995 The perceived efficacy of complementary and orthodox medicine in complementary and general practice patients. Health Education and Research: Theory and Practice. 10(4):395–405

3 Watkins AD 1995 Contemporary context of complimentary and alternative medicine. Integrated mind-body medicine. In: Micozzi M (ed) Fundamentals of Complementary and Alternative Medicine. Churchill Livingstone, London, ch 4

4 Dorsey L 1995 What does illness mean. Alternative Therapies 1(3):6–10

5 Felten D L, Cohen N, Ader R et al 1991 Central neural circuits involved in neural-immune interactions. In: Ader R, Felten D L, Cohen N (eds) Psychoneuroimmunology, 2nd edn. Academic Press, San Diego, p 3-19

6 Solomon GF 1987 Psychoneuroimmunology: Interactions between central nervous system and immune system. Journal of Neuroscience Research 18:1–9

7 Brczi I, Nagy E 1991 Effects of hypophysectomy on immune function. In: Ader R, Felten D L, Cohen N (eds) Psychoneuroimmunology, 2nd edn. Academic Press, San Diego, p 3-19

8 Felten SY, Felten DL, Olschowka JA 1992 Noradrenergic and peptidergic innervation of lymphoid organs. Chemical Immunology 52:25–48

9 Calvo W 1968 Innervation of the bone marrow in laboratory animals. American Journal of Anatomy 123:315

10 Williams JW, Peterson RG, Shea PA, Schmedtje JF, Bauer DC, Felten DL 1980 Sympathetic innervation of mouse thymus and spleen: Evidence for a functional link between nervous and immune systems. Brain Research Bulletin. 6:83

11 Barnes PJ 1986 Neural control of human airways in health and disease. American Review of Respiratory

Disease 134:1289–314
12 Joos GF, Kips JC, Pauwels RA 1994 A role for neutral endopeptidases in asthma? Clinical and Experimental Allergy 24:91–3
13 Barnes PJ 1994 Airway neuropeptides. In: Holgate ST, Busse W (eds) Asthma and rhinitis. Blackwell, Oxford, ch 51, pp 667–85
14 Van Ranst L, Lauweryns JM 1990 Effects of long-term sensory vs. sympathetic denervation of the distribution of calcitonin gene-related peptide and tyrosine hydroxylase immunoreactivity in the rat lung. Journal of Neuroimmunology 29:131–8
15 Joos G, Pauwels R 1993 The in vivo effect of tachykinins on airway mast cells of the rat. American Review of Respiratory Disease 148:922–6
16 Hosoi J, Murphy GF, Egan CL, Lerner EA, Grabbe S, Asahina A, Granstein RD 1993 Regulation of Langerhans cell function by nerves containing calcitonin gene-related peptide. Nature 363:159–63
17 Blalock JE 1994 The immune system: Our sixth sense. Immunologist. 2:8–15
18 Reichlin S 1993 Neuroendocrine-immune interactions. New England Journal of Medicine. Oct 21 1246–53
19 Bateman A, Singh A, Kral T, Solomon S 1989 The immune-hypothalamic-pituitary-adrenal axis. Endocrine Review. 10(1):92–112
20 Ader R, Felten D, Cohen N 1990 Interactions between the brain and the immune system. Annual Review of Pharmacology and Toxicology 30:561–602
21 Johnson HM, Smith EM, Torres BA, Blalock JE 1982 Regulation of the in vitro antibody response by neuroendocrine hormones. Proceedings of the National Academy of Sciences of the USA 79:4171–74
22 Mathews PM, Froelich CJ, Sibbitt WL, Bankhurst AD 1983 Enhancement of natural cytotoxicity by beta-endorphin. Journal of Immunology 130:1658–62
23 Terao A, Oikawa M, Saito M 1993 Cytokine induced changes in hypothalamic norepinephrine turnover: involvement of corticotrophin-releasing hormone and prostaglandins. Brain Research 622:257–61
24 Masek K, Petrovicky P, Seifert J 1992 An introduction to the possible role of central nervous system structures in neuroendocrine-immune systems interaction. International Journal of Immunopharmacology 14(3):317–22
25 Janz L, Falk J, Nance DM, Brown R, Li Z, Vriend CY Nirula R, Dyck DG, Greenberg AH 1991 Suppression of splenic macrophage interleukin-1 secretion following intracerebral injection of IL-1: evidence for pituitary adrenal and sympathetic control. Cell Immunology 132:84–93
26 Mason JW, Maher JT, Hartley LH, Mougey EH, Perlow MJ, Jones LG 1976 In: Serban G (ed) Psychopathology of human adaption. Plenum, New York, pp 147–71
27 Rettori V, Jurcovicova J, McCann SM 1987 Central Action of interleukin 1 in altering the release of TSH, GH, and prolactin in the male rat. Journal of Neuroscience Research 18:179–83
28 Kennedy RL, Jones TH 1991 Cytokines in endocrinology: their roles in health and disease. Journal of Endocrinology 129:167–8
29 Grossman A, Costa A, Navarra P, Tsagarakis S 1993 The regulation of hypothalamic corticotrophin-releasing factor release: in vitro studies. Ciba Foundation Symposium 172:129–43
30 Ju G, Zhang X, Jin BQ, Huang CS 1991 Activation of corticotropin-releasing factor containing neurons in the paraventricular nucleus of the hypothalamus by interleukin-1 in the rat. Neuroscience Letters 132:151–4
31 Whitnall MH, Perlstein RS, Mougey EH, Neta R 1992 Effects of interleukin-1 on the stress-responsive and –nonresponsive subtypes of corticotropin-releasing hormone neurosecretory axons. Endocrinology 131:37–44
32 Elmquist JK, Ackermann MR, Register KB, Rimler RB, Ross LR, Jacobson CD 1993 Induction of Fos-like immunoreactivity in the rat brain following *Pasteurella multocida* endotoxin administration. Endocrinology 133(6):3054–7
33 Payne LC, Weigent DA, Blalock JE 1994 Induction of pituitary sensitivity to interleukin-1: a new function for corticotropin-releasing hormone. Biochemical and Biophysical Research Communications 198:480–4
34 Hu SB, Tannahill LA, Lightman SL 1992 Interleukin-1 beta induces corticotropin-releasing factor-41 release from cultured hypothalamic cells through protein kinase C and cAMP-dependent protein kinase pathways. Journal of Neuroimmunology 40:49–55
35 Besedovsky HO 1993 Integrative role of cytokines in immuno-neuro-endocrine interactions. Paper presented to the First Annual Congress of BSI, Brighton, UK, December 6th 1993
36 Costa A, Trainer P, Besser M, Grossman A 1993 Nitric oxide modulates the release of corticotrophin-releasing hormone from the rat hypothalamus in vitro. Brain Research 605:187–92
37 Karanth S, Lyson K, McCann SM 1993 Role of nitric oxide in interleukin 2-induced corticotropin-releasing factor release from incubated hypothalamus. Proceedings of the National Academy of Sciences of the USA 90:3383–7
38 Chover-Gonzalez AJ, Harbuz MS, Lightman SL 1993 Effect of adrenalectomy and stress on interleukin-1 beta-mediated activation of hypothalamic corticotropin-releasing factor mRNA. Journal of Neuroimmunology 42:155–60
39 Banks WA, Ortiz L, Plotkin SR, Kastin AJ 1991 Human interleukin(IL)1α, murine IL-1α and murine IL-1β are transported from blood to brain in the mouse by a shared saturable mechanism. Journal of Pharmacology 259:988–96
40 Katsuura G, Arimura A, Koves K, Gottschall PE 1990 Involvement of organum vasculosum of lamina terminalis and preoptic area in interleukin 1β-induced ACTH release. American Journal of Physiology. 258:E163–71
41 Long JB, Holaday JW 1985 Blood brain barrier: endogenous modulation by adrenal-cortical function. Science 227:580
42 Lyson K, McCann SM 1992 Involvement of arachidonic acid cascade pathways in interleukin-6-stimulated corticotropin-releasing factor release in vitro. Neuroendocrinology 55:708–13
43 Koenig JI, Snow K, Clark BD et al. 1990 Intrinsic pituitary interleukin-1 beta is induced by bacterial lipopolysaccharide. Endocrinology 126:3053–8. [Erratum, Endocrinology 1990 127:657]
44 Romero LI, Lechan RM, Clark BD, Dinarello CA, Reichlin S 1991 IL-1 receptor antagonist inhibits h IL-1

beta but not bacterial lipopolysaccharide (LPS) stimulated IL-6 secretion by rat anterior pituitary cells. In: Program and abstracts of 73rd Annual Meeting of the Endocrine Society, Washington D.C., June 19–22 1991. Endocrine Society, Bethesda, Md., p 150, abstract

45 Vankelecom H, Carmeliet P, Van Damme J, Billiau A, Denef C 1989 Production of interleukin-6 by folliculostellate cells of the anterior pituitary gland in a histiotypic cell aggregate culture system. Neuroendocrinology 49:102–6

46 Cambronero JC, Rivas FJ, Borrell J, Guaza C 1992 Role of arachidonic acid metabolism on corticotropin-releasing factor (CRF)-release induced by interleukin-1 from superfused rat hypothalami. Journal of Neuroimmunology 39:57–66

47 Watanabe T, Morimoto A, Sakata Y, Murakami N 1990 ACTH response induced by interleukin-1 is mediated by CRF secretion stimulated by hypothalamic PGE. Experientia 46:481–4

48 Bluthe RM, Pawlowski M, Suarez S, Pernet P, Pittman Q, Kelley KW, Dantzer R 1994 Synergy between interferon-alpha and interleukin-1 in the induction of sickness behaviour in mice. Psychoneuroendocrinology 19(2):197–207

49 Watkins LR, Wiertelak EP, Goehler LE, Mooney-Heiberger K, Martinez J, Furness L, Smith KP, Maier SF 1994 Neurocircuitry of illness-induced hyperalgesia. Brain Research 639:283–99

50 Blalock JE, Smith EM 1980 Proceedings of the National Academy of Sciences of the USA 77:5972–4

51 Smith EM, Blalock JE 1981 Proceedings of the National Academy of Sciences of the USA 78:7530–4

52 Goetzl EJ 1990 Neuropeptides of the immune system. Paper presented to the American Academy of Allergy and Immunology, 46th Annual Meeting, March 23–28 1990

53 Besedovsky H, del Ray AE, Sorkin E 1985 Immune neuroendocrine interactions. Journal of Immunology 135:750–4

54 Munck A, Guyre PM, Holbrook NJ 1984 Physiological functions of glucocorticoids in stress and their relation to pharmacological actions. Endocrine Reviews 5:25–44

55 Olsen NJ, Nicholson WE, DeBold CR, Orth DN 1992 Lymphocyte-derived adrenocorticotrophin is insufficient to stimulate adrenal steroidogenesis in hypophysectomised rats. Endocrinology 130:2113–9

56 Herman JP, Schafer MK, Young EA, Thompson R, Douglass J, Akil H, Watson SJ 1989 Evidence for hippocampal regulation of neuroendocrine neurons of the hypothalamo-pituitary-adrenocortical axis. Journal of Neuroscience 9:3072–82

57 Tizabi Y, Calogero AE 1992 Effect of various neurotransmitters and neuropeptides on the release of corticotropin-releasing hormone from the rat cortex in vitro. Synapse 10:341–8

58 Cechetto DF, Saper CB 1990 Role of cerebral cortex in autonomic function. In: Loewy AD, Spyer KM (eds) Central regulation of autonomic function. Oxford University Press, NY, pp 208–33

59 Ruggiero DA, Mraovitch S, Granata AR, Anwar M, Reis DJ 1987 Role of the insular cortex in cardiovascular function. Journal of Comparative Neurology 257:189–207

60 Hurley-Guis KM, Cechetto DF, Saper CB 1986 Spinal connections of the infralimbic autonomic cortex. Society of Neuroscience Abstracts 12:538

61 Landau WM 1953 Autonomic responses mediated via the corticospinal tract. Journal of Neurophysiology 16:299–311

62 Saper CB, Loewy AD, Swanson LW, Cowan WM 1976 Direct hypothalamo-autonomic connections. Brain Research 117:305–12

63 Luiten PGM, terHorst GJ, Steffens AB 1987 The hypothalamus, intrinsic connections and outflow pathways to the endocrine system in relation to the control of feeding and metabolism. Progress in Neurobiology 28:1–54

64 Ottersen OP 1982 Connections of the amygdala of the rat. IV. Corticoamygdaloid and intraamygdaloid connections as studied with axonal transport of horseradish peroxidase. Journal of Comparative Neurology 205:30–48

65 Mehler WR 1980 Subcortical afferent connections of the amygdala in the monkey. Journal of Comparative Neurology 190:733–62

66 Price JL, Amaral DG 1981 An autoradiographic study of the central nucleus of the monkey amygdala. Journal of Neuroscience 1:1242–59

67 Schwaber JS, Kapp BS, Higgins G 1980 The origin and extent of direct amygdala projections to the region of the dorsal motor nucleus of the vagus and the nucleus of the solitary tract. Neuroscience Letters 20:15–20

68 Cechetto DF 1994 Identification of a cortical site for stress-induced cardiovascular dysfunction. Integrative Physiological Behavioral Science 29(4):362–73

69 Rosene DL, van Hoesen GW 1977 Hippocampal efferents reach widespread areas of cerebral cortex and amygdala in the rhesus monkey. Science 198:315–17

70 Hurley KM, Herbert H, Moga MM, Saper CB 1991 Efferent projections of the infralimbic cortex of the rat. Journal of Comparative Neurology 308(2):249–76

71 Saper CB 1985 Organization of cerebral cortical afferent systems in the rat. II. Hypothalamic projections. Journal of Comparative Neurology 237:21–46

72 Bacon SJ, Smith AD 1993 A monosynaptic pathway from an identical vasomotor center in the medial prefrontal cortex to an autonomic area in the thoracic spinal cord. Neuroscience 54:719–28

73 Dampney RAL 1994 Functional organization of the cardiovascular system. Physiological Review 74(2):323–364

74 Granata AR, Kitai ST 1992 Intracellular analysis in vivo of different barosensitive bulbospinal neurons in the rat rostral ventrolateral medulla. Journal of Neuroscience 12:1–20

75 Guyenet PG 1990 Role of the ventral medulla oblongata in blood pressure regulation. In: Loewy AD, Spyer KM (eds) Central regulation of autonomic functions. Oxford University Press, New York, pp 145–67

76 McAllen RM, Dampney RAL 1990 Vasomotor neurons in the rostral ventrolateral medulla are organized topographically with respect to type of vascular bed but not body region. Neuroscience Letters 110:91–6

77 Bacon SJ, Zagon A, Smith AD 1990 Electron microscopic evidence of a monosynaptic pathway between

cells in the caudal raphe nuclei and sympathetic preganglionic neurones in the rat spinal cord. Experimental Brain Research 79:589–602

78 Gebber GL 1990 Central determinants of sympathetic nerve discharge. In: Loewy AD, Spyer KM (eds) Central regulation of autonomic function. Oxford University Press, New York, pp 126–44

79 Zhou S-Y, Futuro-Neto HA, Gilbey MP 1992 Do caudal raphe neurones relay central respiratory-related inputs to sympathetic preganglionic neurones in the anaesthetized rat? Journal of Physiology 467:16P

80 Spyer KM 1994 Central nervous mechanisms contributing to cardiovascular control. Journal of Physiology 474:1–19

81 Sachar EJ 1982 Endocrine abnormalities in depression. In: Paykel ES (ed) Handbook of affective disorders. Guildford, New York, pp 191–201

82 Rupprecht R, Kornhuber J, Wodarz N, et al. 1991. Disturbed glucocorticoid receptor autoregulation and corticotrophin response to dexamethasone in depressives pretreated with metyrapone. Biological Psychiatry 29:1099–109

83 Gold PW, Chrousos G, Kellner C, Post R, Roy A, Augerinos P, Schulte H, Oldfield E 1984 Psychiatric implications of basic and clinical studies with corticotrophin releasing factor. American Journal of Psychiatry 141:619–27

84 Gold PW, Goodwin FK, Chrousos GP 1988 Clinical and biochemical manifestations of depression. Relation to the neurobiology of stress. New England Journal of Medicine 319:413–20

85 Carroll BJ, Haskett RF 1985 The DST in newly hospitalised patients. American Journal of Psychiatry 143:999–1000

86 Ur E, Dinan TG, O'Keane V et al. 1992 Effect of metyrapone on the pituitary-adrenal axis in depression: relation to dexamethasone suppressor status. Neuroendocrinology 56:533–8

87 Nemeroff CB, Owens MJ, Bissette G et al. 1988. Reduced corticotrophin releasing factor binding site in frontal cortex of suicide victims. Archives of General Psychiatry 45:577–9

88 Young EA, Haskett RF, Murphy-Weinberg V et al. 1991 Loss of glucocorticoid fast feedback in depression. Archives of General Psychiatry 48:693–9

89 Trimble MR 1985 Biological psychiatry. Wiley, Chichester, pp 241–81

90 McEwen BS 1987 Glucocorticoid-biogenic amine interactions in relation to mood and behavior. Biochemical Pharmacology 11:1755–63

91 De Kloet, Reul JMH 1987 Feedback action and tonic influence of corticosteroids on brain function: a concept arising from the heterogeneity of brain receptor systems. Psychoneuroendocrinology 12:83–105

92 De Kloet ER, Kovacs GL, Szabo G et al. 1982 Decreased serotonin turnover in the dorsal hippocampus of the rat brain shortly after adrenalectomy: Selective normalization after corticosterone substitution. Brain Research 239:659–63

93 Jhanwar-Uniyal M, Leibowitz SF 1986 Impact of circulating corticosterone on alpha-1 and alpha-2 noradrenergic receptors in the discrete brain areas. Brain Research 368:404–408

94 Carlsson A 1977 The influence of antidepressants on central monoamine systems. In: van Praag H, Bruinvels J, (eds) Neurotransmission and disturbed behavior. Bohn Scheltema and Holkena, Utrecht, pp 95–108

95 Kitayama I, Janson AM, Cintra A et al. 1988 Effects of chronic imipramine treatment on glucocorticoid receptor immunoreactivity in various regions of the brain. Journal of Neural Transmission 73:191–203

96 Pepin MC, Beaulieu S, Barden N 1989 Antidepressant regulate glucocorticoid receptor messenger RNA concentrations in primary neuronal cultures. Molecular Brain Research 6:77–83

97 Dinan TG, Barry S 1990 Responses of growth hormone to desipramine in endogenous and non-endogenous depression. British Journal of Psychiatry 156:680–4

98 O'Keane V, Dinan TG 1991 Prolactin and cortisol responses to d-Fenfluramine in major depression: evidence for diminished responsivity to central serotonergic function. American Journal of Psychiatry 148:1009–15

99 Roy A, Pickar D, Linnoila M, Potter WZ 1985 Plasma norepinephrine levels in affective disorders. Archives of General Psychology 42:1181–5

100 Rudorfer MV, Ross RJ, Linnoila M, Sherer MA, Potter WZ 1985 Exaggerated orthostatic responsivity of plasma norepinephrine in depression. Archives of General Psychology 42:1186–92

101 Roy A, Linnoila M, Karoum F, Pickar D 1988 Urinary free cortisol in depressed patients and controls: Relationship to urinary indices of noradrenergic function. Psychological Medicine 18:93–8

102 O'Keane V, O'Laughlin D, Dinan TG 1992 D-Fenfluramine induced prolactin release in major depression: response to treatment. Journal of Affective Disorders 26:43–52

103 Deakin JFW, Pennel I, Upadhyaya AJ, Lofthouse R 1990 A neuroendocrine study of 5HT function in depression: evidence for psychosocial causation. Psychopharmacology 101:85–92

104 Kelley WF, Checkley SA, Bender DA et al. 1983 Cushing's syndrome and depression — a prospective study of 26 patients. British Journal of Psychiatry 142:16–19

105 Kramlinger KG, Peterson GC, Watson PK, Leonard LL 1985 Metyrapone for depression and delirium secondary to Cushing's syndrome. Psychosomatics 26:67–71

106 Kronful A, House JD 1984 Depression, cortisol and immune function. Lancet 1:1026–7

107 Dorian B, Garfinkel P 1987 Stress, immunity, and illness — a review. Psychological Medicine 17:393–407

108 Irwin M, Hauger RL, Brown MR et al. 1988 CRF activates autonomic nervous systems and reduces natural killer cytotoxicity. American Journal of Physiology 255:R744–7

109 Stein M, Miller AH, Trestman RL 1991 Depression and the immune system. Findings in search of meaning. Archives of General Psychiatry 48(2):171–177

110 Denney DR, Stephenson LA, Penick EC, Weller RA 1988 Lymphocyte subclasses and depression. Journal of Abnormal Psychology 97:499–502

111 Shekelle RB, Raynor WJ, Ostfeld AM, Garron DC, Bieliauskas LA, Liu SC, Maliza C, Oglesby P 1981

Psychological depression and 17-year risk of cancer. Psychosomatic Medicine 43:117–25
112 Geshwind N, Behan P 1984 Letrality, hormones and immunity In: Geshwind N, Galaburda AM (eds) Cerebral dominance, the biological foundations. Harvard University Press, Cambridge, MA, pp 211–24
113 Smith J 1987 Left-handedness: its association with allergic disease. Neuropsychologia 25(4):665–74
114 Neveu PJ 1992 Asymmetrical brain modulation of the immune response. Brain Research Reviews 17:101–107
115 Biziere K, Giullaumin JM, Degenne D, Bardos P, Renoux M, Renoux G 1985 Lateralized neocortical modulation of the T-cell lineage. In: Guillemin R (ed) Neural modulation of immunity. Raven Press, New York, pp 81–90
116 Barnoud P, Le Moal M, Neveu PJ 1990 Asymmetric distribution of brain monoamines in left and right handed mice. Brain Research 520:317–21
117 Clow A, Higuchi K, Lambert S, Hucklebridge F, Rothwell JC 1995 Salivary sIgA production can be differentially modulated by left and right transcranial magnetic stimulation (TMS) of the tempero-parieto-occipital (T-P-O) cortex in man. Abstract at Physiological Society, December. Kings College, London
118 Amassian VE, Henry K, Durkin H, Chiee S, Cracco JB, Somasundaram M, Hassan H, Cracco RQ, Maccabee PJ, Eberle L 1994 Magnetic stimulation of left vs right tempero-parieto-occipital cortex acts differently on the human immune system. Journal of Physiology 459:22P
119 Kang D-H, Davidson RJ, Coe C, Wheeler RE, Tomarken AJ, Ershler WB 1991 Frontal brain asymmetry and immune function. Behavioural Neuroscience 105:860–9
120 Henry JP 1985 Neuroendocrine patterns of emotional response. In: Plutchik R, Kellerman H (eds) Emotion, theory research and experience. Academic Press, New York, vol 3, p 36
121 Dunn AJ, Antoon M, Chapman Y 1991 Reduction of exploratory behavior by intraperitoneal injection of interleukin-1 involves brain corticotropin-releasing factor. Brain Research Bulletin 26:539–42
122 del-Cerro S, Borrell J 1990 Interleukin-1 affects the behavioral despair response in rats by an indirect mechanism which requires endogenous CRF. Brain Research 528:162–4
123 Henry JP 1986 Mechanisms by which stress can lead to coronary heart disease. Postgraduate Medical Journal 62:687–93
124 Solomon GF, Amkraut AA, Kasper P 1974 Immunity, emotions, and stress. With special reference to the mechanism of stress effects on the immune system. Annual Clinical Research 6:313–22
125 Coe CL 1993 Psychosocial factors and immunity in nonhuman primates: a review. Psychosomatic Medicine 55:298–308
126 Justice A 1985 Review of the effects of stress on cancer in laboratory animals: Importance of time of stress application and type of tumour. Psychological Bulletin 1:108–38
127 Moynihan JA, Ader R, Grota LJ, Schachtman TR, Cohen N 1990 The effects of stress on the development of immunological memory following low dose antigen priming in mice. Brain Behavior and Immunity 4:1–12
128 Glaser R, Rice J, Speicher CE, Stout JC, Kielcolt-Glaser JK 1986 Stress depresses interferon production by leukocytes concomitant with a decrease in natural killer cell activity. Behavioral Neuroscience 100:675–8
129 Khansari DN, Murgo AJ, Faith RE 1990 Effects of stress on the immune system. Immunology Today 11(5):170–175
130 Sheridan JF, Feng N, Bonneau RH, Allen CM, Huneycutt BS, Glaser R 1991 Restraint stress differentially affects anti-viral cellular and humoral immune responses in mice. Journal of Neuroimmunology 31:245–55
131 Hermann G, Beck FM, Tovar CA, Malarkey WB, Allen C, Sheridan JF 1994 Stress-induced changes attributable to the sympathetic nervous system during experimental influenza viral infection in DBA/2 inbred mouse strain. Journal of Neuroimmunology 53(2):173–80
132 Dobbs CM, Vasquez M, Glaser R, Sheridan JF 1993 Mechanisms of stress-induced modulation of viral pathogenesis and immunity. Journal of Neuroimmunology 48(2):151–60
133 Kusnecov AV, Grota LJ, Schmidt SG, Bonneau RH, Sheridan JF, Glaser R, Moynihan JA 1992 Decreased herpes simplex viral immunity and enhanced pathogenesis following stressor administration in mice. Journal of Neuroimmunology 38:129–38
134 MacPhae IA, Ferenc AA, Mason DW 1989 Spontaneous recovery of rats from Experimental Allergic Encephalomyelitis is dependent on regulation of the immune system by endogenous adrenal corticosteroids. Journal of Experimental Medicine 169:431–55
135 Sei T, McIntyre T, Skolnick P, Arora PK 1991 Stress modulates calcium mobilisation in immune cells. Life Science 49:671–77
136 Rook GAW, Hernandez-Pando R, Lightman SL 1994 Hormones, peripherally activated prohormones and regulation of the Th1/Th2 balance. Immunology Today 15(7):301–303
137 Karp JD, Cohen N, Moynihan JA 1994 Quantitative differences in interleukin-2 and interleukin-4 production by antigen-stimulated splenocytes from individually- and group-housed mice. Life Science 55(10):789–95
138 Herbert TB, Cohen S 1993 Stress and immunity in humans: A metanalytic review. Psychosomatic Medicine 55:364–79
139 Bartrop RW, Luckhurst E, Lazarus L, Kiloh, LG, Penny R 1977 Depressed lymphocyte function after bereavement. Lancet 1:834–6
140 Schleifer SJ, Keller SE, Camerino M, Thornton J, Stein M 1983 Suppression of lymphocyte stimulation following bereavement. JAMA 250:374–7
141 Kiecolt-Glaser JK, Fisher L, Ogrocki P, Stout JC, Speicher CE, Glaser R 1987 Marital quality, marital disruption, and immune function. Psychosomatic Medicine 49:13–34
142 Kiecolt-Glaser JK, Kennedy S, Malkoff S, Fisher L, Speicher CE, Glaser R 1988 Marital discord and immunity in males. Psychosomatic Medicine 50:213–29
143 Cohen S, Tyrrell DA, Smith AP 1991 Psychological stress and susceptibility to the common cold. New England Journal of Medicine 325:606–12

144 Kiecolt-Glaser JK, Glaser R, Strain E, Stout J, Tarr K, Holliday J, Speicher C 1986 Modulation of cellular immunity in medical students. Journal of Behavioural Medicine 9:5–21

145 Palmblad J, Cantell K, Strandler H et al. 1976 Stresor exposure and immunological response in man: Interferon producing capacity and phagocytosis. Journal of Psychosomatic Research 20:193–99

146 Kiecolt-Glaser JK, Glaser R, Dyer C, Shuttleworth E, Ogrocki P, Speicher CE 1987 Chronic stress and immunity in family care givers of Alzheimer's disease victims. Psychosomatic Medicine 49:523–35

147 Kielcolt-Glaser JK, Marucha PT, Malarkey WB, Mercado AM, Glaser R 1995 Slowing of wound healing by psychological stress. Lancet 346:1194–6

148 Calabrese JR, Kling MA, Gold PW 1987 Alterations in immune competence during stress, bereavement, and depression: focus on neuroendocrine regulation. American Journal of Psychiatry 144:1123–34

149 McEwan BS, Stellar E 1993 Stress and the individual: mechanisms leading to disease. Archives of Internal Medicine 153:2:93–101

150 Daynes RA, Araneo BA 1992 Programming of lymphocyte responses to activation: Extrinsic factors, provided microenvironmentally, confer flexibility and compartmentalisation to T-cell function. Chemical Immunology 54:1–20

151 Manuck SB, Cohen S, Rabin BS, Muldoon MF, Bachen EA 1991 Individual differences in cellular immune responses to stress. Psychological Science 2:111–115

152 Blecha F, Barry RA, Kelly KW 1982 Stress-induced alteration in delayed type hypersensitivity to SRBC and contact sensitivity to DNFB in mice. Proceedings of the Society of Experimental Biology 169:239–46

153 Monjan AA, Collector MI 1977 Stress-induced modulation of the immune response. Science 196:307–8

154 Levine S, Strebel R, Wenk EJ, Harman PJ 1962 Suppression of EAE by stress. Proceedings of the Society of Experimental Biology 109:294

155 Bordi F, LeDoux JE 1994 Response properties of single units in areas of rat auditory thalamus that project to the amygdala. II. Cells receiving convergent auditory and somatosensory inputs and cells antidromically activated by amygdala stimulation. Experimental Brain Research 98(2):275–86

156 LeDoux JE 1993 Emotional memory systems in the brain. Behavioral Brain Research 58(1–2):69–79

157 Romanski LM, LeDoux JE 1992 Bilateral destruction of neocortical and perirhinal projection targets of the acoustic thalamus does not disrupt auditory fear conditioning. Neuroscience Letters 142(2):228–32

158 Cahill L et al. 1994 Beta-adrenergic activation and memory for emotional events. Nature, Oct 20, 371:702–704

159 Phillips RG, LeDoux JE 1992 Differential contribution of amygdala and hippocampus to cued and contextual fear conditioning. Behavioural Neuroscience 106(2):274–85

160 Bechara A, Tranel D, Damasio H, Adolphs R, Rockland C, Damasio AR 1995 Double dissociation of conditioning and declarative knowledge relative to the amygdala and hippocampus in humans. Science 269(5227):1115–8

161 Roozendaal B, Koolhaas JM, Bohus B 1993 The central amygdala is involved in conditioning but not in retention of active and passive shock avoidance in male rats. Behavioral and Neural Biology 59(2):143–9

162 Clugnet MC, LeDoux JE 1990 Synaptic plasticity in fear conditioning circuits: induction of LTP in the lateral nucleus of the amygdala by stimulation of the medial geniculate body. Journal of Neuroscience 10(8):2818–24

163 Romanski LM, Clugnet MC, Bordi F, LeDoux JE 1993 Somatosensory and auditory convergence in the lateral nucleus of the amygdala. Behavioral Neuroscience 107(3):444–50

164 Pitkanen A, Stefanacci L, Farb CR, Go GG, LeDoux JE, Amaral DG 1995 Intrinsic connections of the rat amygdaloid complex: projections originating in the lateral nucleus. Journal of Comparative Neurology 356(2):288–310

165 Gray TS 1993 Amygdaloid CRF pathways. Role in autonomic, neuroendocrine, and behavioral responses to stress. Annals of the New York Academy of Sciences 697:53–60

166 Roozendaal B, Schoorlemmer GH, Koolhaas JM, Bohus B 1993 Cardiac, neuroendocrine, and behavioral effects of central amygdaloid vasopressinergic and oxytocinergic mechanisms under stress-free conditions in rats. Brain Research Bulletin 32(6):573–9

167 Falls WA, Davis M 1995 Lesions of the central nucleus of the amygdala block conditioned excitation, but not conditioned inhibition of fear as measured with the fear-potentiated startle effect. Behavioral Neuroscience 109(3):379–87

168 Hauger RL, Irwin MR, Lorang M, Aguilera G, Brown MR 1993 High intracerebral levels of CRH result in CRH receptor downregulation in the amygdala and neuroimmune desensitization. Brain Research 616(1–2):283–92

169 Bordi F, LeDoux J, Clugnet MC, Pavlides C 1993 Single unit activity in the lateral nucleus of the amygdala and overlying areas of the striatum in freely behaving rats: rates, discharge patterns, and responses to acoustic stimuli. Behavioral Neuroscience 107(5):757–69

170 Bordi F, LeDoux J 1992 Sensory tuning beyond the sensory system: an initial analysis of auditory response properties of neurons in the lateral amygdaloid nucleus and overlying areas of the striatum. Journal of Neuroscience 12(7):2493–503

171 Goleman D 1995 Emotional intelligence. Bantam Books, NY

172 Morgan MA, Romanski LM, LeDoux JE 1993 Extinction of emotional learning: contribution of medial prefrontal cortex. Neuroscience Letters 163(1):109–13

173 Rogers MP, Dubey D, Reich P 1979 The influence of the psyche and the brain on immunity and disease susceptibility. A critical review. Psychosomatic Medicine 41:147–64

174 Solomon GF, Amkraut AA, Kasper P 1974 Immunity, emotions, and stress. With special reference to the mechanism of stress effects on the immune system. Annals of Clinical Research 6:313–22

175 Stein M, Keller SE, Schleifer SJ 1985 Stress and immunomodulation: The role of depression and neuroen-

docrine function. Journal of Immunology 135:827s–33s

176 Ader R, Cohen N 1991 Conditioning the immune response. Netherlands Journal of Medicine 39:263–73

177 Ader R, Cohen N 1975 Behaviorally conditioned immunosuppression. Psychomatic Medicine 37:333–40

178 Bovbjerg D, Cohen N, Ader R 1987 Behaviorally conditioned enhancement of delayed-type hypersensitivity in the mouse. Brain Behaviour and Immunity 1:64–71

179 Dark K, Peeke HVS, Ellman G, Salfi M 1987 Behaviorally conditioned histamine release. Annals of the New York Academy of Sciences 496:578–82

180 Husband AJ, King MG, Brown R 1987 Behaviorally conditioned modification of T cell subset ratios in the rat. Immunological Letters 14:91–4

181 Klosterhalfen S, Klosterhalfen W 1990 Conditioned cyclosporine effects but not conditioned taste aversion in immunised rats. Behavioral Neuroscience 104:716–24

182 MacQueen G, Marshall J, Perdue M, Siegel S, Bienenstock J 1989 Pavlovian conditioning of rat mucosal mast cells to secrete rat mast cell protease II. Science 243:83–5

183 Moynihan J, Koota D, Brenner G, Cohen N, Ader R 1989 Repeated intraperitoneal injections of saline attenuate the antibody response to a subsequent intraperitoneal injection of antigen. Brain Behaviour and Immunity 3:90–6

184 Solvason HB, Ghanta VK, Hiramoto RN 1988 Conditioned augmentation of natural killer cell activity. Independence from nociceptive effects and dependence on interferon-β. Journal of Immunology 140:661–5

185 Ader R, Cohen N 1982 Behaviorally conditioned immunosuppression and murine systemic lupus erythematosus. Science 215:1534–6

186 Sklar LS, Anisman H 1979 Stress and coping factors influence tumour growth. Science 205:513–5

187 Coe CL, Rosenberg LT, Fisher M et al. 1987 Psychological factors capable of preventing the inhibition of antibody responses in separated infant monkeys. Child Development 58:1420–30

188 Ackerman SH, Keller SE, Schleiffer SJ et al. 1988 Premature maternal separation and lymphocyte function. Brain, Behavior and Immunity 2:161–5

189 Laum BA, Dukta MA 1987 Early handling enhances mitogen responses of splenic cells in adult C3H mice. Brain, Behavior and Immunity 1:356–60

190 Sensky T 1990 Patients' reactions to illness. British Medical Journal 300:622–3

191 Pinkerton P 1972 Depression v. denial in childhood asthma: equivalent fatal hazards. In: Depressive states in childhood and adolescence. Almquist and Wiskell, Stockholm, pp 187–192

192 Strunk RC, Mrazek DA, Fuhrmann GS, LaBrecque JF 1985 Physiologic and psychological characteristics associated with deaths due to asthma in childhood. A case-controlled study. JAMA 254(9):1193–8

193 Totman R, Kiff J, Reed S, Craig J 1980 Predicting experimental colds in volunteers from different measures of recent life stress. Journal of Psychosomatic Research 24:155–63

194 Solomon GF 1989 Psychoneuroimmunology and human immunodeficiency virus infection. Psychiatric Medicine 7:47–57

195 Grossarth-Maticek R, Bastiaans J, Kanazir DT 1985 Psychosocial factors as strong predictors of mortality from cancer, ischaemic heart disease and stroke: the Yugoslav prospective study. Journal of Psychosomatic Research 29:167–76

196 Kobasa SC, Maddi SR, Kahn S 1982 Hardiness and health: A prospective study. Journal of Personal and Social Psychology 42:168–77

197 McCraty R, Atkinson M, Tiller WA, Rein G, Watkins AD 1995 The effects of emotions on the short term power spectral analysis of heart rate variability. American Journal of Cardiology 76(14):1089–93

198 Spiegel D, Bloom JR, Kraemer HC, Gottheil E 1989 Effect of psychosocial treatment on survival of patients with metastatic breast cancer. Lancet 336:606–10

199 Fawzy FI, Fawzy NW, Hyun CS et al. 1993 Malignant melanoma: effects of early structured psychiatric intervention, coping, and affective state on recurrence and survival 6 years later. Archives of General Psychiatry 50(9):681–689

200 Chover-Gonzalez AJ, Harbuz MS, Lightman SL 1993 Effect of adrenalectomy and stress on interleukin-1 beta-mediated activation of hypothalamic corticotropin-releasing factor mRNA. Journal of Neuroimmunology 42:155–60

201 Saperstein A, Brand H, Audhya T, Nabriski D, Hutchinson B, Rosenzweig S, Hollander CS 1992 Interleukin 1 beta mediates stress-induced immunosuppression via corticotropin-releasing factor. Endocrinology 130:152–8

202 Terao A, Oikawa M, Saito M 1993 Cytokine induced changes in hypothalamic norepinephrine turnover: involvement of corticotrophin-releasing hormone and prostaglandins. Brain Research. 622:257–61

203 Lyson K, McCann SM 1992 Involvement of arachidonic acid cascade pathways in interleukin-6-stimulated corticotropin-releasing factor release in vitro. Neuroendocrinology 55:708–13

204 Sundar SK, Cierpial MA, Kilts C, Ritchie JC, Weiss JM 1990 Brain IL-1-induced immunosuppression occurs through activation of both pituitary-adrenal axis and sympathetic nervous system by corticotropin-releasing factor. Journal of Neuroscience 10:3701–6

205 Smith T, Cuzner ML 1994 Neuroendocrine-immune interactions in homeostasis and autoimmunity. Neuropathology and Applied Neurobiology 20:413–22

206 Mason D, MacPhae I, Antoni F 1990 The role of the neuroendocrine system in determining genetic susceptibility to experimental allergic encephalomyelitis in the rat. Immunology 70:1–5

207 Sternberg EM, Hill JM, Chrousos GP, Kamilaris T, Listwak SJ, Gold PW, Wilder RL 1989 Inflammatory mediator-induced hypothalamic-pituitary-adrenal axis activation is defective in streptococcal cell wall arthritis-susceptible Lewis rats. Proceedings of the National Academy of Sciences of the USA 86:2374–8

208 Chelmicka-Schorr E, Checinski M, Arnason BGW 1988 Chemical sympathectomy augments the severity of experimental allergic encephalomyelitis. Journal of Neuroimmunology 17:347

209 Levine S, Sowinski R, Steinetz B 1980 Effects of experimental allergic encephalomyelitis on thymus and adrenal. Relation to remission and relapse. Proceedings

of the Society of Experimental Biology 165:218
210 Roszman TL, Jackson JC, Cross RJ, Titus MJ, Markesbery WR, Brooks WH 1985 Neuroanatomic and neuroendocrine influences on immune function. Journal of Immunology 135:769s–772s
211 Martin JB, Riskind PN 1992 Neurologic manifestations of hypothalamic disease. Progress in Brain Research 93:31–40; discussion 40–2
212 Krystal H 1988 Integration and self-healing: affect, trauma, alexithymia. Hillsdale Analytic Press,
213 Taylor GJ 1987 Psychosomatic Medicine and Contemporary Psychoanalysis. Madison International Universities Press,
214 Parker JDA, Taylor GJ, Bagby RM 1992 Relationship between conjugate lateral eye movements and alexithymia. Psychotherapy and Psychosomatics 57:97–101
215 Sifneos PE 1991 Affect, emotional conflict, and deficit: an overview. Psychotherapy and Psychosomatics 56:116–22
216 Sapolsky RM, Drey LC, McEwen BS 1984 Stress down-regulates corticosterone receptors in a site-specific manner in the brain. Endocrinology 114:287
217 Ackerman KD, Felten SY, Dijkstra CD, Livnat S, Felten DL 1989 Parallel development of noradrenergic sympathetic innervation and cellular compartmentation in the rat spleen. Experimental Neurology 103:239–55
218 Bellinger DL, Felten SY, Felten DL 1988 Maintenance of noradrenergic sympathetic innervation in the involuted thymus of the aged Fischer 344 rat. Brain Behavior and Immunity 2:133–50
219 Rees LH 1978 Human adrenocorticotropin and lipocortin (MSH) in health and disease. In: Martin L, Besser GM (eds) Clinical neuroendocrinology. Academic Press, New York
220 Cantin M, Genest J 1986 The heart as an endocrine gland. Clinical and Investigative Medicine 9(4):319–27
221 Armour JA 1994 Peripheral autonomic neuronal interactions in cardiac regulation. In: Armour JA, Ardell JL (eds) Neurocardiology. Oxford University Press, Oxford, ch 10, pp 219–44
222 Huang M 1996 May, personal communication
223 Huang M, Friend D, Sunday M, Singh K, Haley K, Austen K 1995 Identification of novel catecholamine-containing cells not associated with sympathetic neurons in cardiac muscle. Circulation 92(8):1–59
224 Task force of the European Society of Cardiology and the North American Society of Pacing and Electrophysiology. 1996. Heart rate variability standards of measurement, physiological interpretation, and clinical use. Circulation 93:1043–65
225 Hopkins DA, Ellenberger HH 1994 Cardiorespiratory neurons in the medulla oblongata: input and output relationships. In: Armour JA, Ardell JL (eds) Neurocardiology. Oxford University Press, Oxford, ch 12, pp 277–307
226 Tiller WA, McCraty R, Atkinson M 1996 Cardiac coherence: a new, non-invasive measure of autonomic nervous system order. Alternative Therapies in Health and Medicine 2(1):52–65
227 Dillon KM, Minchoff B, Baker KH 1986 Positive emotional states and enhancement of the immune system. International Journal of Psychology in Medicine 15(1):13–16
228 Rein G, McCraty RM 1994 Effects of positive and negative emotions on salivary IgA. Advances of Medicine 8(2):87–105
229 McCraty R, Atkinson M, Rein G, Watkins AD 1996 Music enhances the effects of positive emotional states on salivary IgA. Stress Medicine 12:167–175
230 Stroink G 1989 Principles of cardiomagnetism In: Williamson SJ, Hoke M, Stroink G et al. (eds) Advances in Biomagnetism. Plenum Press, New York, pp 47–57
231 Russek L, Schwartz G 1996 Energy cardiology: a dynamical energy systems approach for integrating conventional and alternative medicine. Advances 12(4):4–24
232 Paddison S 1992 The Hidden power of the heart. Planetary Publications, Boulder Creek, CA
233 Childre DL 1996 Cut-Thru. Planetary Publications, Boulder Creek

CHAPTER CONTENTS

2

Mind–body medicine: its popularity and perception

Alan Watkins
George Lewith

INTRODUCTION

At the turn of the century doctors, with virtually no effective drugs at their disposal, were largely powerless observers of illness. They provided care and comfort rather than cure. Effective antibiotics did not become widely available until after the Second World War, but since that time medicine has gone through a technological revolution which is increasing in pace. This revolution has produced dramatic improvements in the management of many illnesses; infants born 3 months prematurely now live; childhood leukemias are now cured; diseased hearts, lungs, livers and kidneys can be replaced; arteries blocked by thrombus and atheroma are reopened; ischemic tissue is revascularized. Modern medicine is able to see more deeply and more clearly into the very fabric of our bodies with nuclear magnetic resonance (NMR) scanning, electron microscopy and immunohistochemistry. It is even able to dissect and genetically engineer the DNA inside the nuclei of our cells. The ability of modern medicine to intervene in illness with some high-tech wizardry is truly staggering.

However, this technological revolution has created new problems. There are ethical problems with genetic engineering; cost-benefit problems of organ transplantation; provision problems, with sophisticated technology often only being readily available to those able to afford it; and scientific problems of proving the benefits of the new technologies. But perhaps the greatest problem of all is confusion.

Faced with a bewildering number of therapeutic options, doctors turn to scientific research to help guide their choices. Unfortunately the volume of scientific information has increased, almost exponentially, resulting in an overwhelming amount of literature relevant to the choices to be made. Swamped by technology and overloaded by information, it is all too easy to lose sight of the patient and their needs, to mistake medical activity for care, to initiate interventions because they are possible rather than determine whether they are necessary, desirable or even effective. All too often there is little real information upon which to base our therapeutic options for the management of chronic disease. If this technological revolution and explosion of information have left doctors confused, what chance have the patients? There is evidence to suggest that the increasing interest in mind–body medicine and complementary medicine in particular is, in part, related to a sense of disillusionment with high-tech medicine and the lack of time or care that over-burdened orthodox physicians can give their patients[1].

It has been shown that the very process of grappling with this overwhelming burden of technology and knowledge during medical training drives the compassion and empathy out of medical students[2]. Undergraduates entering medical school with idealistic notions about 'helping people' are soon lost in a sea of biochemical pathways, physiological mechanisms, anatomical detail and histopathology. Wrestling with a vast array of new words and endless lists of causes of every ailment, it is easy to forget that the original intention of medical education was to care for people. Instead a battle for personal survival begins, with students necessarily focusing their efforts on maintaining their own sanity rather than being primarily concerned with how best to help people. Self-care is not taught to students, rather they are trained to repress their anxiety and insecurities in a show of denial and bravado, a coping style that equips them poorly for the greater pressures they will have to address post-qualification. It is little wonder that those charged with the responsibility of caring for others are lamentably poor at caring for themselves (see Ch. 14).

THE EVOLUTION OF SCIENTIFIC MEDICINE

How did we become obsessed with high-tech, investigation-driven medicine? How did we lose sight of the importance of self-care and care for others? In order to find the answers we must understand a little of the history of western scientific medicine. In earlier times, health care was provided by tribal doctors or shamans. These individuals developed powerful intuitive skills and the ability to enter trance states, often drug induced, in order to consult with the spirit world. Knowing little physiology, illness was attributed to the spirits removing the soul or psyche of the sufferer. The shaman would enter a trance, enter the 'spirit world' in pursuit of the soul and arrange with the spirits for its return. Alternatively evil spirits could manifest within a subject's body and the shaman would exorcize the evil spirit by inducing a trance and a cathartic convulsion in the possessed individual, using herbal drugs and frenzied rituals. The exorcized spirit would often be transferred into an inanimate object, such as a stone, which could then be produced and discarded, leaving the sufferer free from its malign influence.

Thus, the earliest health care practices involved both psychological interventions, in the form of trance, and physical interventions, in the form of herbal drugs. By the time of the early structured civilizations, these two aspects of health care had become separated, with the herbalists becoming the dominant providers of health and the spiritual aspects being left to the priests and magicians. Priests consulted the gods, and magicians had 'psychic powers' that enabled them to divine health problems from the study of entrails or the throwing of bones.

This early separation of spiritual and physical aspects to health spawned two schools of thinking, namely the vitalists and the mechanists.

The vitalists and the mechanists

The vitalists believed in a vital energy, and asserted that illness was the result of a disruption in the vital or spiritual force. In contrast, the mechanists believed in more physical explanations for illness. One of the earliest, and most influential advocates of the mechanistic school was Hippocrates in the 5th Century BC Although Hippocrates and his followers did not deny the importance of spiritual energy and acknowledged that the body had significant recuperative powers, they concentrated on identifying specific physical causes for ill health. They suggested that illness was largely due to an imbalance in one of the four humors, blood, phlegm, black or yellow bile and tested various remedies of the day to 'treat' the imbalance. Gradually mechanistic medicine became synonymous with the administration of herbal remedies. After Hippocrates the next major figure in the development of western medicine was Galen; in the 2nd Century AD Galen was an enthusiastic user of all manner of drugs and herbal remedies, often administered as a bewildering and noxious cocktail. However, Galen also recognized the importance of the psyche in physical disease, and his observation that melancholic women were more likely to develop cancer of the breast is widely quoted as the earliest western record of the effects of the psyche on the immune system.

Because many of the remedies offered by mechanistic physicians were either toxic or ineffectual, the vitalistic approach resurfaced. This re-emergence was partly stimulated by the teachings of Jesus and the early Christians. Jesus was reported to effect instant cures through the power of faith. Christian healers harnessed this 'divine power' and encouraged the spirit to manifest within an individual. Such healers relied on 'inspiration', literally the spirit inside themselves, to guide their healing. For several centuries thereafter the clergy played an active role in healing the sick. However, by the Middle Ages the Vatican, which was the dominant force in society, proclaimed that ecclesiastical intervention in cases of possession, and the induction of convulsions and trance states, was suspect paganism, bordering on witchcraft and possibly satanic. As a result the church retreated from its role in healing, and medicine was left to physicians, who by this stage, were firm followers of the polypharmacy advocated by Galen. Vitalism went into rapid decline in the west although it was still exerting a powerful influence in the east, particularly with respect to traditional Chinese medicine and Ayurvedic medicine.

The birth of reductionism

In the mid-16th Century, polemical changes in thinking were running through society. Copernicus had put forward his view that the sun, not the earth, was the center of the universe and Versalius advocated that the results of medical research, such as the discoveries made from cadaver dissection, should not be twisted to fit the theories of the day, as had previously been the norm. This was really the birth of scientific thinking. At the same time vitalism was somewhat rehabilitated by Paracelsus who suggested that there was a mechanistic explanation for miracles, namely the power of the human imagination. Although there was a shift to more rational thinking, therapeutic intervention lagged behind and was still largely based on Galenic principles of polypharmacy, supported by advocacy and testimonials of prominent and influential individuals, with little recourse to scientific testing. In desperate attempts to alter bodily humors, all manner of tortures were foisted upon those who could afford to pay for them.

During the mid-17th Century, reason began to prevail. Thomas Sydenham made the eminently sensible suggestion that medical training should take place at the bedside, and not in the university classrooms through the study of Greek and Latin texts. Sydenham was also the first to distinguish the symptoms of an illness as separate from the underlying disease. This simple suggestion gave birth to a whole school of 'nosologists' who proceeded to classify diseases in much the same way as Linnaeus was classifying plants.

Descartes' assertion that the mind and body were separate entities encouraged the description of physical diseases that did not involve the mind. By the mid-18th Century, Morgani was suggesting that a patient's symptoms could be traced to physical malfunctions in specific body organs. Bichat demonstrated 40 years later that it was diseased tissues, not organs that were at fault. Virchow completed this reductionist cycle in 1850 by showing that it was, in fact, specific cells within tissue, rather than the tissues themselves that were responsible for disease. Thus, in the late 19th Century, the view that a plethora of symptoms and signs presented by the patient could be reduced to a cellular malfunction became the prevailing attitude of the day. Such an analysis was supported by the current thinking. The pulleys, pistons, pumps, bellows and engines of the industrial revolution became metaphors for the tendons, muscles, heart, lungs and gut of the body.

When the complexity of the body was reduced to simple engineering processes it became possible to measure these processes. Measurement of bodily functions thus became a central part of scientific medical thinking. Reductionist thinking and painstaking measurement started to provide an enormous number of insights into human functioning, and became an extremely effective method for increasing scientific understanding of disease. As a result, the validity of individual experience, which could not be measured, was diminished still further and the intuitive knowledge and wisdom of healers were dismissed as anecdotal, or poor science. The ability to quantify the physical domain and the difficulty in quantifying the psyche or spirit merely reinforced the separation of mind and body. Since changes in the psyche and spirit could not be measured, they were dismissed as irrelevant or non-existent. As a consequence reality, as described by science, was largely based on a physical reality. Illness was explained in terms of measurable physical malfunction and the role of a vital force, the humors and the mind was substantially diminished. Modern scientific treatments relied either on surgical intervention or the still largely untested herbal concoctions of the chemists.

Changing picture

The rise of modern scientific medicine, particularly after the Second World War, marginalized many forms of mind–body and complementary medicine. There were few practitioners of acupuncture and homeopathy, and relatively little public demand. As a result this area of medicine did not attract serious attention, either from the general public or from conventional doctors. Perhaps the one exception to this general trend were the manual medical techniques, such as osteopathy and chiropractic. Although these methods were considered by some as 'quackery' during the 1930s, they have slowly become integrated into conventional medicine over the last 50 years, largely through the efforts of interested rheumatologists such as Cyriax and the physiotherapy profession as a whole[3].

However, since the early 1970s, there has been a growing realization that the reductionist model of illness is inadequate and the public demand for a more vitalistic approach such as offered by mind–body and complementary medicine has grown dramatically. The rise in interest in complementary medicine in Europe was first described by Lewith and Aldridge, and subsequently summarized by Peter Fisher in the *British Medical Journal*[4,5]. Eisenberg raised awareness of the extensive use of complementary medicine in North America[6]. A similar report from Australia confirmed that complementary medicine is now being widely used throughout western medical cultures and emphasized that the economic expenditure on such approaches is enormous[7]. These studies suggested that the USA spends up to $15 billion and Australia $1 billion per year on complementary medicine. This level of interest and economic activity can no longer be ignored and must signify fundamental changes in the public's perception of medicine. Society's perception of the pre-eminent role of scientific medicine has undoubtedly changed and, in spite of the many attacks against acupuncture and related techniques[8], it appears that an increasing number of conventional doctors are interested in learning about these areas of medicine[9].

THE RISE OF COMPLEMENTARY MEDICINE

Before the days of socialized medicine in the UK, many orthodox physicians saw complementary practitioners as potential threats to their income and therefore worked hard to discredit them[10]. What has been interesting about the recent surge of interest in complementary medicine is that it has occurred at a time when the demand for conventional health care, both in terms of patient numbers and total overall budget, has also increased significantly. Rather than depleting orthodox medical services of cash or patients complementary medicine seems to have been financially complementing orthodox medical care. A recent study in the USA suggests that the vast majority of individuals seeking complementary medical care did so without the knowledge of their conventional physicians[6]. It would appear that perhaps 15–20% of individuals in the USA were combining both conventional and complementary medical approaches in the management of a chronic condition, clearly demonstrating that complementary medicine was adding to the overall cost of medical care. Patients presumably backed both horses believing that their quality of life or medical condition was more likely to improve if all treatment options were harnessed, proven or otherwise. Similar information from both Europe[5] and Australia[7] indicates that Eisenberg's observations on the rise of complementary medicine in the USA are not isolated, but part of a larger change within all western societies.

There are varying reasons behind the growth in expenditure on conventional and complementary medicine. Conventional medicine is growing because of the increased number of technical procedures that are now available for a whole variety of illnesses, in addition to the desire of an increasingly aging population to retain an improved quality of life. In contrast, complementary medicine is growing alongside conventional medicine because of the patient's desire to be given time and to be listened to, rather than being rushed by an over-burdened conventional physician. People are increasingly confused by high-tech investigation and intervention, and are reluctant to take powerful tablets with multiple side effects.

Population surveys

The first survey of the use of complementary medicine in the UK was carried out by Fulder and Monro and commissioned by the Threshold Foundation in 1980. Since that time a number of surveys have demonstrated that the interest and number of people consulting complementary therapists have increased significantly. For example, a study carried out for Swanhouse Special Events in 1984 found that as many as 30% of a representative sample of approximately 2000 adults had used one or more of a range of non-orthodox therapies over a period of 1 year[11]. A more recent survey by Market and Opinion Research Information (MORI) in 1989 took a similar sample of approximately 2000 adults in various parts of the UK. They demonstrated that 27% had used non-orthodox medicine at one time or another. Unfortunately, these two surveys are not directly comparable, since the Swanhouse Research Survey looked at herbal medicine whereas the later poll carried out by MORI did not. The MORI survey went on to claim that only 23% of their random sample would not consider using any complementary medical technique.

Another body, the Consumers' Association, published a survey of their members in 1985 and found that one in seven had used some form of complementary medicine[12]. Forty-two per cent of those who had used complementary medicine had used osteopathy and 23% had used acupuncture. A follow-up survey carried out in 1992 suggested that one in four of those now surveyed within the Consumers' Association had used complementary medicine within the previous year[13].

While it is impossible to give an absolutely accurate figure for the number of people using complementary medicine in the UK, it is probable that at least 2 million people are using a range of complementary or unorthodox therapies on a regular basis. It is difficult to determine what the true increase in demand and utilization of complementary medicine has been in the last 20 years since most of the surveys conducted selected different populations and asked very different questions. However, within the biased sub-population of the Consumers' Association, it appears that the use of complementary medicine has almost doubled over a period of 7 years. The surveys published by MORI, *Which?* and Swanhouse all suggest that the three most commonly used therapies are osteopathy, herbal medicine and homeopathy, while acupuncture is used by approximately half the numbers using osteopathy.

Non-medical practitioner surveys

An early survey of non-medical practitioners in seven areas of the UK, located by consulting the *Yellow Pages* telephone directory, registers of professional bodies and notices in local papers, estimated that the number of consultations occurring within the UK in 1980 lay between 11.7 and 15.4 million per year[14]. This represented between 6.5% and 8.6% of the total number of general practitioners' consultations that occurred in that year. The average course of treatment involved 9.7 consultations and therefore they deduced that there were approximately 2 million people using complementary medicine at that time. The main therapists consulted were acupuncturists, osteopaths and chiropractors; about 2 million consultations were occurring within each of these disciplines per annum. A subsequent study carried out by Peter Davies for the Institute of Complementary Medicine in 1984 suggested a more conservative estimate of 4.6 million consultations a year involving about 1 million people[15].

The gap between these two very different estimates may be due in part to the fact that Fulder and Munro considered mind–body practitioners of all kinds, including healers and psychotherapists, whereas Davies drew his sample only from those listed in ten professional registers covering six therapies. Fulder and Munro noted that approximately half the practitioners surveyed in their study were not members of professional bodies and were only in practice on a part-time basis.

Medical practitioner surveys

One of the areas which has probably been grossly underestimated in relation to the published surveys, is the growing use of complementary medicine by medically qualified practitioners as part of their general practice commitment. The UK is not alone in experiencing such growth. Information from throughout Western Europe would suggest that France, Germany, Finland, the Netherlands, Belgium, Switzerland, Denmark and Italy are experiencing similar patterns of growth within complementary medicine[4,5]. There has also been a significant growth of unconventional medicine in the USA. The Eisenberg survey suggested that 34% of the US population used at least one unconventional therapy in the previous year[6]. Eisenberg's study had a significant impact on the orthodox medical establishment in the USA. No-one had realized to what extent Americans were using a whole variety of different healing methods. US physicians were shocked to learn that the vast majority of their patients using complementary medicine felt unable or unwilling to discuss this aspect of their care with their doctor. Eisenberg's findings raised many questions. Did the secret use of complementary medicine have an influence on the outcome and interpretation of some large clinical trials of the day in which complementary medicine users were enrolled? If one-third of their patients are regularly using complementary medicine, why, until very recently has the body of US conventional medicine set its face so firmly against the use of homeopathy, herbal medicine and nutritional supplements?

Over the last 2–3 years, we have seen a huge change in attitude in relation to complementary medicine in the North American continent. An Office of Alternative Medicine (OAM) has been established within the National Institutes of Health (NIH) and has had its budget increased each year, up to the present figure in excess of $14 million per annum. Over 40 US medical schools now run introductory courses to complementary medicine as part of their undergraduate curriculum.

This growth is reflected in the trebling of the proportion of the population using complementary medicine in Holland and France[5]. In 1991 the European 'over the counter' market for homeopathy was £590 million, and that for herbal remedies was £1.45 billion[5]. The rise of the European market for complementary medicine has been documented in a recent book entitled, *Complementary Medicine and the European Community*[16]. It is interesting to note that even within the European countries that officially outlaw the practice of medicine by non-medically qualified complementary practitioners (for instance, France and Belgium) there is an increase in the number of non-medically qualified osteopaths, chiropractors, herbalists, therapists and counselors. Many of these non-medically qualified practitioners are effectively practicing medicine while at the same time breaking national laws. The use of complementary medicine in Germany and the Netherlands is well documented and would appear to far surpass its use in the Anglo-Saxon cultures. Current estimates suggest that over 50% of German patients regularly use some form of complementary medicine[5].

Kate Thomas's recent publication relating to the use of complementary medicine within 1000 general practices in the UK shows that approximately half of UK general practitioners are involved in the provision or practice of complementary medicine at the primary care level. This involves approximately three-quarters of a million consultations per annum and signifies a rapidly growing area of the UK health market[17].

Referral rates by medically qualified practitioners

There is good evidence to suggest that the number of patients being referred to complementary practitioners from primary care physicians has also increased. An early study suggested that trainee general practitioners had a favorable view of complementary medicine; however the views and referral habits of established physicians were unknown[18]. A study performed by Wharton and Lewith in 1986 addressed this issue[9]. This study determined the mode of referral to The Centre for the Study of Complementary Medicine in Southampton in 1986. It revealed that 22% of patients seen were referred by primary care physicians, whereas the same audit conducted in 1990 indicated a 38% referral rate. These figures were borne out by the recent Department of Health survey of 1000 general practices in the UK.

WHY DO PEOPLE SEEK HELP FROM COMPLEMENTARY MEDICINE?

Why are so many people turning to complementary therapy? Do patients really feel lost in the technology and uncared for by orthodox medicine? Or are patients being misinformed by media hype on the effectiveness of complementary therapies? An undergraduate study, conducted in 1983 in Southampton, investigated the reasons behind the growing popularity of complementary medicine[19]. The investigators designed a questionnaire to assess the characteristics of patients seeking treatment, the scope of their presenting problems, the reasons why patients elected to be treated by complementary medicine and finally the patient's knowledge, attitudes and expectations of such treatment. The questionnaire was administered at the patient's first visit to a complementary medical center and then again by post 8 weeks later. Sixty-five new patients attending the center over a 2 week period completed the questionnaire during a 20 minute structured interview. Fifty-six of the original 65 patients completed the follow-up questionnaire. The presenting problems are summarized in Table 2.1.

Table 2.1 Presenting problems of patients

Complaint	No. of patients	Specification of complaint
Pain	30	Arthritis, back pain, abdominal pain, headaches
Allergies	10	Eczema, urticaria, asthma, rhinitis
Non-specific symptoms	9	Malaise, feeling unwell, run down
Psychological	3	Anxiety, smoking
Gynecological	2	Dysmenorrhea, candidiasis
Gastrointestinal	3	Celiac disease, spastic colon, diarrhea, inflammatory bowel disease
Hypertension	2	
Loss of balance	2	
Other disease	6	Loss of voice, catarrhal deafness, Raynaud's, acne, muscle wasting, facial rash

Chronic ill health and failed conventional treatment

The 1983 study found that one of the major reasons for individuals to seek out a complementary practitioner is chronic ill health. The duration of symptoms presented varied from 3 months to 44 years with a mean of 9 years[19]. Of the 65 patients attending the complementary medical center, 8.8% had their problem for less than 6 months, a further 8.8% for less than 1 year, 36.8% between 1 and 5 years and 23.5% between 6 and 15 years. The remaining balance of patients (22%) had had their problem for more than 15 years. A more recent follow-up study developed an Attitudes to Alternative Medicine scale (AAM)[20], and administered it along with a standard Walliston Health Locus of Control (HLC) Scale to 35 patients attending for treatment[21]. The findings confirmed the results of the study conducted 6 years previously indicating that patients sought complementary medicine when conventional medicine failed to bring about a satisfactory improvement in their condition. In addition, the mean duration of symptoms presented was almost identical in both studies, 9 and 9.4 years respectively and the percentage of patients who had suffered symptoms for more than 1 year was 82.3% and 82.4%, respectively.

Seeing a complementary practitioner was therefore not the first port of call for many individuals, but an approach which many wished to try as a method of managing their long-term problem. The vast majority of patients consulted complementary practitioners only after exhausting orthodox medical treatments, or consulted complementary practitioners with conditions where orthodox medicine had achieved only limited success such as back pain, arthritis, multiple sclerosis and headaches. Almost invariably within western cultures, a conventional medical opinion from a family physician is sought prior to a complementary practitioner's opinion.

Talking different languages

A more recent study involving in-depth interviews with 34 patients came to a similar conclusion, that the major reason for seeking complementary medical help was to help a condition in which orthodox medicine had been unable to offer any relief[22]. Sharma identified a number of other common reasons why people seek help from complementary therapists. She noted that many patients perceived that orthodox medicine treated symptoms rather than causes and many patients reported that they were unhappy about the over-liberal dispensation of drugs and that these drugs represented, 'unnatural chemical interventions', and drastic solutions which were therefore rejected[22]. This study seems to suggest that the language in which patients who visit complementary practitioners describe their symptoms, is simply not being addressed by their orthodox physicians, and this language is more coherent with that used by the complementary medical community.

When comparing the HLC and the AAM scales, it became apparent that two types of patient appeared to be seeking complementary medicine. The first group were those who turned to complementary medicine as a last resort and do not appear to embrace the theory or underlying philosophy of this approach. Their HLC scales were very much what one would expect from a normal population, and their AAM scales showed no overt sympathy, understanding or indeed belief in complementary medicine.

The second type of patient showed a much greater commitment to alternative medicine in general. Their AAM scales demonstrated a high degree of fundamental belief in this area of medicine and they appeared to be more likely to choose complementary medicine due to belief in it rather than as a last resort. Their HLC scales were significantly more internal than either the general population or the first group of patients, i.e. they felt a greater than average need to take personal control of their own health rather than leaving it to a doctor to 'fix' their problem[21].

Finnigan's study does not correlate the type of patient attending for complementary medicine with outcome. The study published earlier by Moore and Phipps does. Two-thirds of the patients in the Moore and Phipps study believed that complementary medicine would be an effective approach to their problem, and many had very high expectations of treatment. Expectation of success did appear, in the earlier study, to correlate with outcome, so it is likely that those who understand and believe in complementary medicine, will have a higher internal health locus of control and in turn will be likely to report benefit from a complementary medical approach.

Non-specific ill health

The major presenting problem for patients attending the complementary medical center in 1983 was pain (particularly back pain) with generalized non-specific illness making up only 13% of our sample. The type of problem now presenting to the same center has changed substantially. Patients with musculoskeletal pain were much less common while individuals with symptoms of irritable bowel and other chronic 'internal' illnesses were commonplace. The single largest problem, representing up to 45% of patients attending, was individuals with generalized non-specific ill health such as chronic fatigue, for which no definite diagnosis had been made. Since both these studies were small simple 'snapshots' of the clinical workload over two short periods 6 years apart it is difficult to draw definitive conclusions. However, the evidence suggests that patients, and the physicians referring them, believe that complementary medicine may have a role to play in non-specific illnesses which are not readily understood or diagnosed by conventional methods.

Thus, it seems that the main reason that individuals see complementary practitioners is to try and get help with a chronic or non-specific problem that has thwarted orthodox medicine. In addition, a number of patients express a desire to be managed by a practitioner who shares their philosophy, employs a gentler, less drastic and more 'natural' approach, who has time and is not overburdened and preoccupied with high-tech medicine.

WHO SEEKS HELP FROM COMPLEMENTARY MEDICINE?

Recent research suggests that far from being ignorant and ill-informed, the majority of individuals visiting complementary therapists are, in fact, well educated and affluent individuals[23], perfectly capable of making decisions about the quality and efficacy of orthodox and complementary medicine. Sharma confirmed these findings showing that 50% of those using complementary medicine were from the professional and managerial classes while the rest were equally divided among the other social classes[22]. There were far more women than men and the majority of patients were between 40 and 60 years of age. These findings are in agreement with research conducted in Southampton[19].

PRIMARY CARE PHYSICIANS' VIEW OF COMPLEMENTARY MEDICINE

It seems that primary care physicians, responding to the wishes of their patients, are leading the way in the integration of mind–body and complementary techniques with orthodox medicine. Various studies have been performed to assess the knowledge of primary care physicians and their expertise in mind–body techniques. Wharton and Lewith addressed this problem directly[9]. A 4-page postal questionnaire was sent to every GP in the county of Avon. This was designed to establish: how much general practitioners knew about mind–body medicine; whether they practiced a specific therapy; whether they intended to develop more knowledge and/or skills within this area in the immediate future; whether they had referred patients to a complementary practitioner and whether this had been to a medically trained or a non-medically qualified individual.

Of 193 questionnaires sent out to actively practicing general practitioners, 75% (145) were returned. The non-responders were analyzed for age, sex and location, rural or urban, of practice. There seemed to be no difference in the demography of those who responded and those who did not. Of those who responded, roughly one-third had already gained training in one form or other of mind–body medicine, and a further 15% wished to receive training. Table 2.2 shows those doctors who were trained or intended to train in the six main areas surveyed (acupuncture, homeopathy, herbal medicine, manipulation, hypnosis and healing).

Judging by the number of physicians now attending courses run by the British Medical Acupuncture Society and the Faculty of Homoeopathy, it is safe to assume that a similar survey carried out now would elicit a far larger number of general practitioners who have received training within complementary medicine and a further larger percentage who wish to receive training. The membership of the British Medical Acupuncture Society has grown from 200 in 1985 when the survey was carried out to 800 at the beginning of 1992 and by the beginning of 1995 there were 1500 members. Similarly, in the Faculty of Homoeopathy, the demand for courses has grown substantially during this time. The Faculty have now introduced a primary care homeopathy qualification which has been most successful in Glasgow; over the last 5 years more than 200 doctors have completed the Glasgow course and the numbers of general practitioners seeking information about courses and actually attending introductory courses on homeopathy has tripled over the last 5 years[24].

Table 2.2 Number (%) of respondents with training in, and currently practicing, complementary medicine

	Training received	Practicing	Training intended	No training
Spinal manipulation	38 (26)	34 (24)	14 (10)	93 (64)
Acupuncture	4 (3)	4 (3)	9 (6)	132 (91)
Hypnosis	17 (12)	7 (5)	4 (3)	124 (85)
Herbal medicine	1 (1)	1 (1)	1 (1)	142 (98)
Homeopathy	7 (5)	7 (5)	9 (6)	129 (89)
Spiritual healing	8 (5)	10 (7)	1 (1)	136 (94)

Physicians' knowledge and reasons for referral

Fifty-seven per cent of primary care physicians surveyed considered acupuncture to be useful or very useful, and 89% considered spinal manipulation (osteopathy and chiropractic) to be useful or very useful[25]. Therefore, in spite of the limited clinical trials within these two areas, their perceived value appears to be high. It is quite clear from both this and a wide variety of other data that primary care physicians' views on mind–body medicine are not evidence-based. Their perception of complementary medicine appears to be partly influenced by patient demand as well as their own idiosyncratic and very individualistic experience of this area. For example, if a physician's patient or patient's relative is treated successfully by an acupuncturist this is very likely to have a significant effect on the physician's referral pattern to an acupuncturist. The most significant factor influencing the opinions of general practitioners appeared to be the perceived benefit to patients. A high proportion of general practitioners made the comment that either they or their families had personally benefited from mind–body medicine (38%) and

Table 2.3 Referral patterns for complementary techniques (figures are No. (%) of those responding to questionnaire, *except where indicated)

	Never refer	Refer to doctors	Average No. of patients referred to doctors/year	Refer to non-medical practitioners	Average No. of patients referred to non-medical practitioners of complementary medicine/year
Spinal manipulation	23 (16)	77 (51)	6	62 (43)*	13
Acupuncture	57 (37)	44 (28)	3	45 (30)*	4
Hypnosis	47 (33)	66 (44)	4	40 (28)*	4
Herbal medicine	131 (92)	2 (2)	1	9 (6)	2
Homeopathy	57 (40)	68 (42)	4	18 (13)*	2
Faith healing	115 (80)	2 (2)	2	25 (18)	3

*Not all respondents were able to answer this question with a clear positive or negative response, and some gave more than one answer so the figures do not add up.

this seemed to be an important factor in influencing their referral patterns.

The survey also found that primary care physicians did not know very much about the details of most mind–body therapies. In spite of the fact that 89% of respondents perceived spinal manipulation to be useful, only 44% felt they had a knowledge of this subject that was moderate or better. The figures for acupuncture are even lower, only 22% of respondents felt they had a moderate to very good knowledge of this particular discipline.

This lack of knowledge, however, did not seem to affect referral patterns. Table 2.3 shows rates of referral to medical and non-medically qualified practitioners. In the year prior to the survey, 76% of doctors who responded had referred patients to a medical colleague for mind–body medicine and 72% had referred patients to a non-medical practitioner for some form of mind–body medicine. In terms of the total number of patients referred the vast majority were referred to non-medically qualified practitioners rather than medically qualified osteopaths or homeopaths.

There are a number of factors that influence primary care physicians' referral patterns, not least the availability of trained practitioners. There are far more non-medically qualified complementary practitioners than those with medical qualifications. It is possible that GPs perceive non-medically qualified practitioners, who have usually received much more training than their medical counterparts, to have greater expertise within their individual therapy. In addition, since the majority of doctors who have skills in mind–body medicine are general practitioners, there may be some commercial restraint to cross-referral between local primary care physicians. Such data in relation to non-medically qualified practitioners are particularly surprising and indicate a far greater level of acceptance of mind–body medicine than one would at first suppose. Ninety-three per cent of the GPs who replied believed that mind–body practitioners needed some form of statutory regulation, but only 3% of responding GPs felt that such non-orthodox therapeutic methods should be banned or indeed taken out of the hands of non-medically qualified practitioners.

How widespread is the support?

Thus the evidence from the Avon survey of primary care physicians' attitudes suggests that mind–body medicine is both popular and widely used. A similar survey was conducted at roughly the same time by Anderson and Anderson in the Oxford region[26]. They sent a questionnaire to 274 primary care physicians, and 81% (222) replied. The results were similar to those from the Avon area. Thirty-one per cent said they had a working knowledge of at least one form of alternative medicine and 30% had actively sought and read publications about alternative medical techniques. Forty-one per cent had attended lectures or classes about some form of mind–body medicine, but only 12% (as opposed to 33% in Avon) had a practical working knowledge of one of the major techniques within this area. However, 42% wished to receive some form of training in acupuncture, homeopathy or spinal manipulation.

The majority of doctors (95%) had said that patients had discussed mind–body medicine with them during the past year and 59% had referred patients to some form of complementary or alternative medicine. Forty-one per cent of the Oxford doctors felt that alternative systems of medicine were valid and 54% defined complementary medicine as an additional and useful technique which could aid their patients. Sixteen per cent suggested that alternative medicine was unscientific and improperly validated. The figures from these early studies in Avon and Oxford have been borne out by the more recent Department of Health study[17].

CHANGING PERCEPTIONS

The first report from the British Medical Association's Board of Science (BMA, 1986) analyzed the underlying evidence which sustains complementary medical practice[27]. In effect this report could find very little evidence to support and sustain the scientific use of complementary medicine in the orthodox medical community. The BMA's damning report caused much controversy in orthodox and complementary medical circles, and was in stark contrast to the views of many primary care physicians canvassed at that time[9]. This suggested that the BMA was somewhat out of step both with its membership and society as a whole.

The last decade has seen the BMA's view change dramatically. The most recent BMA report sets out a clear agenda for evaluating, attempting to understand and ultimately integrating a whole variety of complementary medical techniques into conventional medicine. Its title, *Complementary Medicine: New Approaches to Good Practice* (1993) indicates how the BMA's mood has changed since 1986[28]. In fact this BMA publication has become a best seller, and the organization is now taking a leading role in the debate over the integration of complementary medicine into conventional medical practice. It has organized a range of meetings over the last few years in which its Board of Science has looked both critically and very openly at patient demand and the needs and requirements of complementary medical practitioners, as well as the demands imposed on mind–body medicine in relation to ethics and scientific rigor.

Such debates are also occurring in the USA and throughout the world. The rapid evolution of the Office of Alternative Medicine within the NIH with its substantial level of funding, represents a clear political commitment to evaluate and develop mind–body medicine as an increasing part of health care provision within North America. The fact that over the last 3 years one third of US medical schools have developed and integrated courses on mind–body medicine into their undergraduate curriculum seems astonishing when only 5 years ago the very practice of complementary cancer therapy or homeopathy could result in a physician being debarred from practice in some states.

CONCLUSION

It is now clear that mind–body and complementary medicine is in widespread use in Western Europe, Australasia, China and the USA, and its popularity would appear to be increasing. There are certainly millions of consultations per year within mind–body medicine in every western nation for which there is information available. Exact figures vary depending on how each culture defines a mind–body practitioner. They may be medical or non-medically qualified, registered or not registered, and from a wide range of disciplines from psychotherapy to aromatherapy, spiritual healing to osteopathy.

Specific patient groups are seeking mind–body medicine, and it may well be that the type of individual who seeks out this treatment, and believes in it, will have a different response to the therapy than those for whom it is just provided as one of many different therapeutic alternatives. Primary care physicians are clearly leading the way in the integration of mind–body and complementary medicine, despite the lack of clinical trial evidence demonstrating efficacy. This is, in all probability, in response to patients' continual enthusiasm and some anecdotal experience. However, more widespread acceptance will require robust scientific investigation. A recent survey by the National Association of Health Authorities and Trusts in the UK suggested that the lack of information on the effectiveness of mind–body therapies was the single most important factor affecting NHS funding of these therapies[29]. The establishment of eight disease-specific centers of excellence, funded by the OAM at the NIH in the USA and similar developments in the UK, indicate that the repeated calls for more research by the BMA, the Royal College of Physicians, the Royal Society of Medicine, the European Parliament Committee on the Environment, Public Health and Consumer Protection (CEPHCP), the House of Representatives (USA) and the WHO now looks as though it may finally be met[30–35].

In advance of the clinical trial research, we believe that it is incumbent upon all physicians to develop an understanding of what mind–body medical techniques are available, their limitations and in which conditions they may have something to offer. This book is designed to guide physicians in their search for greater understanding of this fascinating area.

REFERENCES

1 Sharma U 1992 Complementary medicine today, practitioners and patients. Tavistock/Routledge, London and New York, 1:70
2 Craig JL 1992 Retention of interviewing skills learned by first year medical students: a longitudinal study. Medical Education 26(4):276–81
3 Schoitz EH, Cyriax J 1975 Manipulation past and present. Heinemann Medical Books, London
4 Lewith GT, Aldridge D (ed) 1992 Complementary medicine and the European Community. CW Daniel, Saffron Walden
5 Fisher P, Ward A 1994 Complementary medicine in Europe. British Medical Journal 309:107–111
6 Eisenberg DM, Kessler RC, Foster C, Norlock FE, Calkins DR, Delbanco TL 1993 Unconventional medicine in the United States. Prevalence, costs, and patterns of use. New England Journal of Medicine Jan 28:246–52
7 MacLennan AH, Wilson DH, Taylor AW 1996 Prevalence and cost of alternative medicine in Australia. The Lancet 347:569–73
8 National Council Against Health Fraud 1991 Acupuncture. The position paper of the National Council Against Health Fraud. Clinical Journal of Pain 7:162–6
9 Wharton R, Lewith G 1986 Complementary medicine and the general practitioner. British Medical Journal 292:1498–500
10 Inglis B 1980 Natural medicine. Fontana/Collins, Glasgow
11 Research Surveys of Great Britain 1984 Omnibus Survey on Alternative Medicine (prepared for Swanhouse Special Events), London
12 Which? 1986 Magic or medicine? Which? October issue; pp 443–7
13 Which? 1992 November issue; pp 445–7
14 Fulder SJ, Munro RE 1985 Complementary medicine in the United Kingdom: patients, practitioners and consultations. The Lancet 2:542–5
15 Davies P 1984 Trends in complementary medicine. The Institute for Complementary Medicine, London
16 Lewith G, Aldridge D 1991 Complementary medicine and the European Community. CW Daniel, Saffron Walden
17 Thomas K, Fall M, Parry G, Nicholl J 1995 National survey of access to complementary health care via general practice. University of Sheffield
18 Taylor-Reilly D 1983 Young doctors' views on alternative medicine. British Medical Journal 287:337–9
19 Moore J, Phipps K, Marcer D, Lewith G 1985 Why do people seek treatment by alternative medicine? British Medical Journal 290:28–9
20 Finnigan MD 1991 Complementary medicine: attitudes and expectations, a scale for evaluation. Complementary Medical Research 5(2):79–82
21 Finnigan MD 1991 The Centre for the Study of Complementary Medicine: an attempt to understand its popularity through psychological demographic and operational criteria. Complementary Medical Research 5:83–8
22 Sharma U 1991 Complementary medical practitioners in a Midlands locality. Complementary Medical Research 5(1):12–16
23 McGuire MB 1988 Ritual healing in suburban America. Rutgers University Press, New Brunswick, NJ
24 Reilly D personal communication, July 1995
25 Doctors Decide 1995 BMA News Review July 1995
26 Anderson E, Anderson P 1987 General practitioners and alternative medicine. Journal of the Royal College of General Practitioners 37:52–5

27 British Medical Association 1986 Alternative therapy. Report of the Board of Science and Education, London
28 British Medical Association Report 1993 Complementary medicine: new approaches to good practice. Oxford University Press for the British Medical Association
29 National Association of Health Authorities and Trusts 1993 Research Paper 10: Complementary Therapies in the NHS. NAHAT Publications, Birmingham
30 Watt J, Wood C (eds) 1988 Talking health: conventional and complementary approaches. Royal Society of Medicine, London
31 British Medical Association 1993 Complementary medicine: new approaches to good practice. Oxford University Press
32 Office of Technology Assessment 1990 Unconventional cancer treatments. Government Printing Office Washington DC (OTA-H-405)
33 The Royal College of Physicians 1992 Allergy: Conventional and Alternative Concepts. London
34 Lannoye P 1994 The state of complementary medicine. European Parliament Committee on the Environment, Public Health and Consumer Protection. Draft Report
35 WHO 1994 Global Strategy for Asthma Management. Draft VI. National Heart, Lung, and Blood Institute, NIH World Health Organization

CHAPTER CONTENTS

3

Ischemic heart disease: homeostasis and the heart

Peter Nixon
Jenny King

INTRODUCTION

Sir James Mackenzie, renowned for his studies of cardiac function, recognized four stages of heart disease. The first was the predisposing stage in which the individual was rendered vulnerable through some intrinsic weakness or external factor. The second was one of symptoms without signs. The third was the advanced stage where the disease revealed its presence by physical changes, and the fourth was death. Mackenzie's professional career was necessarily centered on the third and fourth stages, but from his earliest days as a general practitioner in Burnley he dreamed of the possibility of studying the earlier phases. After retiring from his London practice he moved to Scotland to found an Institute for Medical Research in 1919. His biographer reported that he had the entire staff constantly engaged in an attempt to diagnose the first two stages, to investigate the etiology and significance of minor maladies and study the environmental conditions under which patients lived, with the aim of discovering the relation between the environment, ailments and subsequent disease[1].

The purpose of this chapter is to present Mackenzie's four stages as they appear today in a biopsychosocial system which accommodates the psychological and social as well as the organic aspects of cardiac disease. It is implied that the morbid processes at work in the earlier stages may generate the later, and still require close attention even when physical disease has developed: thus intervention in the earlier stages might prevent the catastrophe of myocardial infarction or sudden coronary death in the later.

Coping and adapting

Health and survival depend upon the individual's ability to defend the order and stability of the internal systems against the onslaught of coping burdens and environmental challenges. These onslaughts are typically severe and prolonged during periods of rapid change, uncertainty and turbulence such as we have today[2].

The defense of the internal systems depends upon the integrity of the individual's homeostatic systems, the coping skills required for contending successfully with activity and change, and the adaptive behavior that provides for healthy adjustment to environmental challenges.

The defensive forces require energy and information for success. Their competence naturally varies from time to time, and differs between individuals. Lack of success at coping and adapting accelerates entropic changes and fosters the loss of order and stability of the homeostatic systems.

The understanding of the relationships between the burdens of coping and adapting and disease is growing. For example, Sir George Pickering supported Wolf and Wolff in the view that a primary pathogenic factor for hypertension and cardiovascular disease was over-use and exhaustion of the normal mechanisms of adaptation[3,4]. In animals, this hypothesis has been confirmed by Henry. From his studies of the induction of acute and chronic cardiovascular disease he concluded:

> It has been established that sustained emotional arousal can accompany the psychosocial stimulation induced by the social interaction of members of a social group as they compete for desiderata, such as food and water ... this arousal of neuroendocrine response patterns can, in turn, lead to disease states and to a fatal outcome. Various experimental observations in pigs, monkeys, baboons, tree shrews and rodents demonstrate both acute and chronic disturbances of cardiovascular function. These conditions can lead to sudden death or to sustained high blood pressure with arteriosclerotic lesions in the heart and blood vessels. It is shown that when social pressure that has been maintained for a sufficiently long period is relieved the organism does not revert to normal[5].

Boyd studied arterial disease in man and focused on the pathological effects of arterial constriction and spasm associated with elevation of the blood pressure[6]. His observations and conclusions supported Henry's work. Sterling and Eyer studied the anabolic–catabolic shifts in states of high and prolonged arousal, and provided an invaluable guide to the mechanisms by which psychosocial influences can induce disease[7].

In cardiological practice, under half of those referred for diagnosis and guidance have detectable organic disease with physical changes[8]. Organic changes are not always the cause of the symptoms, but they are almost bound to become the focus of attention. The remainder of the patients, without detectable organic disease, suffer from disorders of function, and risk being deemed neurotic, or treated with drugs designed to palliate symptoms.

This binary method of classifying heart patients as either suffering from organic disease with physical changes, or from functional-neurotic disorder is unfortunate because the major cause of loss of health in both groups might be the same, namely the entropic homeostatic consequences of failure at coping and adapting.

The reluctance of cardiologists to recognize the cardiovascular consequences of failure at coping and adapting and address their cause is derived from adherence to the biomedical model of practice which is reductionist and focused upon organic disease, the third and fourth stages of MacKenzie's schema. Great achievements have been made through this biomedical model, but it is insufficient because it does not accommodate the mind of the individual, his predicament, and the competence of his defense systems. Gruman and Chesney drew attention to its limitations when they wrote:

Despite an intense focus in disease mechanisms, biological factors fail to account for wide variations in morbidity and mortality. Moreover, biological models are unable to explain complex patterns of medical help-seeking and illness behavior. Therefore, solutions drawn only from the biological model will fall short of meeting the health needs of the public.

Conceptualizations of health and illness have always recognized the contributions of social, psychological, economic and environmental factors to health. What is new is that a critical body of evidence has documented the influences of these factors on morbidity and mortality. The fact is that a group of factors including social isolation, social class and depression predict health outcomes *across* diseases. Yet such evidence finds little favor and no home in mainstream biomedical research, which is organized to explore each disease separately — to identify a single etiology and its underlying mechanisms[9].

For these reasons Engel recommended the adoption of the biopsychosocial model that takes in the psychological and sociocultural needs of the person as well as the biological[10].

The human predicament

Figure 3.1 represents the human predicament. The brain deals with information from the external environment, from the processes of the mind, and from the internal systems of the body. Health and performance are maintained and hardiness fostered through experience that enables successful talents for coping and adapting to develop. Failure of coping and maladaptive behavior can increase arousal beyond physiological tolerance and produce morbid effects.

In this context arousal refers to the general drive state of the brain and mind with its concomitant physiological, emotional and behavioral responses. Arousal is defined variously: by Kahnemann as the general activation of the mind which results from the person's interaction with his environment[11], and by the Russian School as the reflection in the brain of the magnitude and quality of mental, emotional and physical needs, and the possibility of their being satisfied[12]. Lader points out that it can be seen as a continuum ranging from torpor at the lower level to conditions such as rage, terror, revulsion or ecstasy at the higher[13].

The exhaustion and unspecific ill health (Fig. 3.1)[14] that develop when the individual is failing to cope with the activities of life and the demands of adaptation probably account for at least half the general practitioner's workload[15]. Increasingly these days they are accepted as the antecedents of specific conditions such as coronary heart disease[16,17] and disorders of immune competence[18,19]. Some refer to them as stress-related conditions.

It is worthwhile to develop the hypothesis that coronary heart disease can be generated or aggravated by the entropic, homeostatic consequences of failure at coping and adapting, because it enables events such as breakdown of health, myocardial infarction and sudden death to be seen as natural consequences of disorder, i.e. as the sudden discontinuities of catastrophe theory[20]. This perception carries the hope of intervention before the 'last straw', a hope denied by the view that these events are random and arbitrary accidents of atheroma.

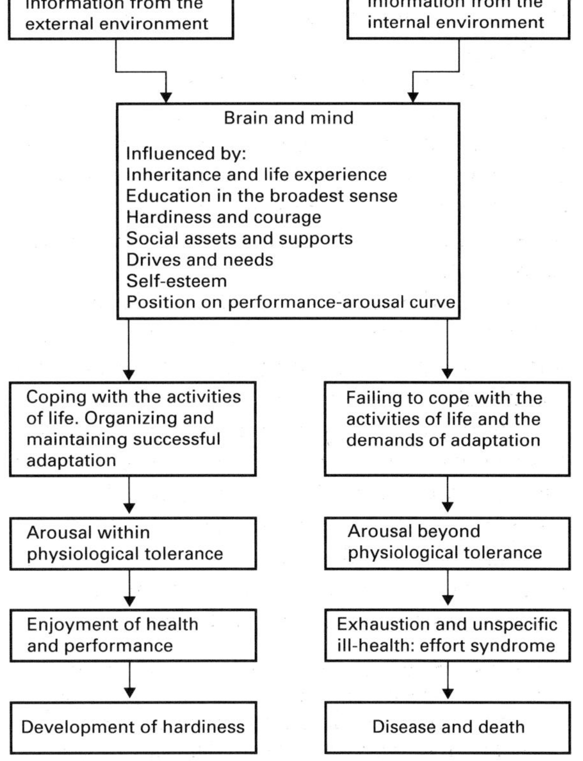

Figure 3.1 A model illustrating a biopsychosocial perspective of health and disease

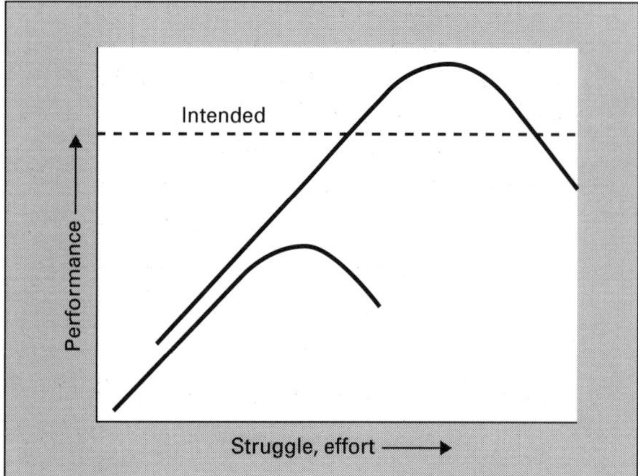

Figure 3.2 Performance increases with effort, to a higher level in some than others, but falls when tolerance is exceeded

The biopsychosocial perspective requires models for clarifying relationships between arousal, performance (the ability to do what has to be done) and health, and the oft-used performance–arousal curves are appealing in their simplicity.

PERFORMANCE–AROUSAL CURVES

In 1908, Yerkes and Dodson experimented with dancing mice and used an inverted U-shaped curve to illustrate the fact that their behavior could be changed with stimuli of optimal strength, whereas weaker or stronger stimuli had a smaller influence[21].

Figure 3.2, the performance–arousal curves, model Lewis's observations of military training: some recruits have a higher potential for performance than others, but all go downhill when effort and distress carry them beyond physiological tolerance[14].

Figure 3.3 illustrates Swank and Marchand's study of battle stress in World War II: the first stage of exhaustion presents with hyper-reactivity and symptoms of anxiety, sleep loss, overbreathing and cardiovascular dysregulation[22]. In civilian practice these changes might be deemed neurotic if the doctor is unaware of the challenges to which the individual has been exposed. Today there is a rapidly growing interest in the prevention of this phase, known in sports medicine as 'overtraining'[23].

Persistence of the arousal beyond the first stage changes the clinical picture. The individual becomes drained of energy, stamina and coping resources and sinks to a lower level of performance. Some may call this chronic fatigue syndrome or ME without realizing that it is not a 'disease' in need of a 'cure,' but a condition of extreme homeostatic depletion amenable to recovery through rehabilitation[24].

The tolerance of arousal varies among individuals. Those with high curves can perform at high levels without generating homeostatic disorders. They are deemed hardy, a quality developed by a successful career of coping and adapting linked with a strong commitment to life's goals, a sense of control over the outcome of life's course, and an abundance of energy that makes it possible to enjoy the challenges of life[25]. Those with lower curves have a lesser capacity for coping and adapting, and a greater propensity to exhaustion and illness.

The onset of exhaustion depends upon the interplay between the initial conditions of the individual's defenses and the magnitude and rate of the challenges to his coping skills and adaptive capacity: for example, post traumatic stress syndrome can begin within minutes, battle exhaustion within days, and the heart attack after 1 or 2 years of the less dramatic but longer drawn-out stressors of everyday life[16,17].

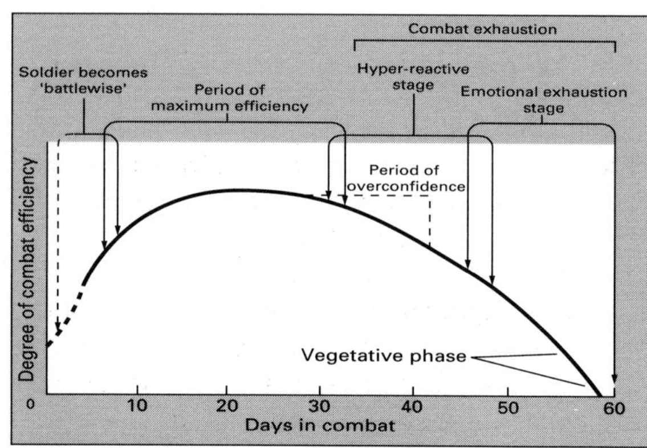

Figure 3.3 The relationship between battle stress and efficiency, and the phases of exhaustion on the downslope. (Reproduced from Swank, Marchand 1946[22])

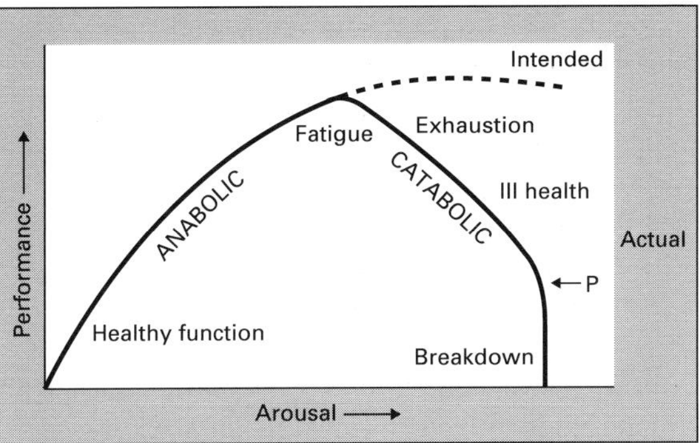

Figure 3.4 The human function curve:[26] a model illustrating the relationships between performance, arousal and health. On the up-slope, performance increases with arousal; the cardiovascular system is in an orderly state and the metabolism anabolic. On the down-slope, every increment of arousal reduces performance. The cardiovascular system is disordered and the metabolism catabolic. Some individuals are hardy and have high curves which permit great performance, whereas others have low curves and are vulnerable to exhaustion, ill health and breakdown (P=breakdown point). The dotted line indicates the intended level of activity and the solid line the actual level of performance. The more the individual struggles to close the gap between what he can do and what he thinks he ought to achieve, the further down he moves and the worse he becomes.

The human function curve (Fig. 3.4)[26]

This is an adaptation of the performance–arousal curves (Figs. 3.2, 3.3) for cardiological practice and rehabilitation. It has heuristic value in the biopsychosocial approach. For example, its peaked top models the conclusions of the British Association for the Advancement of Science's studies of fatigue in World War I[24]: up to a point 'sound physiological recuperation' can be obtained by rest, but beyond that point the individual embarks on an enduring downhill course of loss of performance and health. In other words, the peaked top of the curve represents the watershed between healthy function and reversible fatigue on the upslope, and the enduring degradation of health and performance on the downslope. 'P' represents the point of catastrophe at which the overstrained mechanisms for coping and adapting break down.

The 'intended' line acts as a reminder that maladaptive behavior is often adopted when an individual goes 'over the top': as the gap between his actual ability and his intended performance widens he neglects the need for sleep and rest, arouses himself to greater effort, and drives himself downwards towards breakdown. Sir William Osler used the word nemesis as a metaphor for the coronary catastrophe when it occurred on this downhill course. He regarded its prevention as part of the physician's duty.

High curves and low curves

Psychosocial qualities associated with high curves are thought to include good mothering; and feelings of being competent and in control, secure, well-loved, satisfied with the achievement of needs, successful, appreciated and supported.

The influences which produce low curves in cardiac patients include migration[27]; poor education[28]; failure at school[29]; poor mothering[30]; poverty and struggle in childhood[31]; loneliness[32]; overwhelming coping burdens with lack of support, satisfaction and appreciation[18]; loss of prediction and control of life events[33], and loss of interaction with the 'time and tides of nature in urban industrial life'[34].

Morbid levels of arousal

Movement over the top of the curve (Fig. 3.4) and onto the downslope into exhaustion and ill health can be expressed as a morbid shift to the right. The causative influences can be classified as intrinsic or extrinsic.

Intrinsic causes

These have been described as including high levels of anger, anxiety, exhaustion and tension[16]; sociopsychological exhaustion[35]; lack of assertion skills;[36] restlessness and guilt about relaxation[37]; inability to be satisfied by achievement[38]; and the type A problems of anger, anxiety, aggression, acceleration, haste, hostility, irritation and impatience[39]; loneliness, isolation and widowhood[32].

Extrinsic causes

Environmental factors such as the acceleration

beyond physiological tolerance. In her foreword to the study of the world before 1914, Barbara Tuchman wrote:

> The period of this book was above all the culmination of a century of the most accelerated rate of change in man's record. Since the last explosion of a generalized belligerent will in the Napoleonic Wars, the industrial and scientific revolutions had transformed the world. Man had entered the nineteenth Century using his own and animal power, supplemented by that of wind and water much as he had entered the thirteenth or, for that matter, the first. He entered the twentieth with his capabilities in transportation, communication, production, manufacture and weaponry multiplied a thousandfold by the energy of machines. Industrial society gave men new powers and new scope, while at the same time building up new pressures in prosperity and poverty, in growth of population and crowding in cities, in antagonism of classes and groups, in separation from nature and from satisfaction in individual work. Science gave man new welfare and new horizons while it took away belief in God and certainty in a scheme of things he knew. By the time he left the nineteenth Century he had as much new unease as ease[40].

The pace of change has continued and resulted in a new era of uncertainty for both individuals and organizations, and an unprecedented challenge to their ability to cope with new levels of technological complexity, and social insecurity[41].

Rene Dubos pointed out that profound changes in the way of life, whatever their nature, reduce the resistance of the body and mind to almost any kind of insult. He predicted that the increase in population density and the evolution of even more highly competitive habits would produce an increase in cardiovascular disease[2].

John Cassell in his famous lecture on 'The contribution of the social environment to host resistance' argued that victims of tuberculosis, schizophrenia, heart disease, alcoholism, accident-proneness and suicide have much in common: a marginal place in society caused by social deprivation that made them vulnerable to loss of homeostatic order and stability under the demands of everyday life[18].

Social class may be the most important determinant: men in the lowest grades in the UK have more than treble the coronary mortality of those in the highest[42].

Henry and Stephens recognized that the struggles required to achieve control of one's place in an adverse social environment and to adapt successfully to change may foster unbalanced development of the left cerebral hemisphere[43]: it has been hypothesized that this imbalance may be responsible for the asymmetry and disinhibition of sympathetic input to the heart that can presage the coronary catastrophe[44,45] (see below).

The working environment can also have a major impact on health. Numerous studies have demonstrated that job dissatisfaction can predict myocardial infarction[46,47]. The arousal inherent in a stressful working environment can drain the individual and drive him out of healthy function into exhaustion, ill health or breakdown (Fig. 3.4).

Kagan and Levi studied the reactions of various occupational groups to real-life situations at work and found that these could cause catecholamine production to reach pheochromocytoma-like proportions: the level of adrenaline and noradrenaline excretion roughly paralleled the degree of emotional arousal[48].

Beale and Nethercott examined workers in the 2 year period between their learning that their jobs were insecure and actually losing their posts. They found a 150% increase in consultations with the family doctor, a 70% increase in the number of episodes of illness, a 160% increase in the number of referrals to hospital out-patient departments and a 200% increase in the number of attendances at out-patient departments. The older employees, with poor re-employment prospects, suffered more than younger and more adaptable employees[49].

Karasek's team showed that coronary heart disease and death rates were increased by jobs that combined high demands with little latitude for decision making[47] and Ruberman's group found that the combination of high stress at work with low social support increased mortality after myocardial infarction[50].

Other external factors such as the disruption of biological rhythms have been studied. Shift work increases the risk of ischemic heart disease[51], and irregular hours can induce catabolic bodily changes resembling those found in injury: sea-pilots required to work irregular hours and maintain a high performance while attempting to keep up normal social and domestic commitments are said to suffer from these.

FUNCTIONAL CARDIAC CONDITIONS

Exhaustion and unspecific ill health: effort syndrome

The patients who attend cardiological clinics without detectable organic disease tend to be regarded as neurotic or unwilling to pull their weight. This attitude aggravates the anxiety, anger, frustration and despair that are natural responses to their predicament; and palliative treatment with antidepressant drugs and counseling or cognitive therapy are unlikely to be helpful if the person's metabolic needs and physical requirements for recovery are not taken into account[14].

In the earlier stages the cardinal symptoms are loss of performance; fatigue; overbreathing; chest pain; autonomic instability; cardiac arrhythmia; and sleep disturbance. They result from impairment of homeostatic regulation. In the later stages the clinical picture can be dominated by the effects of depletion of the body's alkaline buffering systems, a consequence of overbreathing (see below). The major symptoms are listed in Box 3.1.

Box 3.1 Disorders characteristic of effort syndrome

- Inability to make and sustain normal levels of effort through fatigue, muscular weakness or aching, and acidotic hyperpnea
- Depletion of alkaline buffering systems and reducation of anaerobic threshold
- Chest pain. Cardiac arrhythmia
- Restlessness foiling attempts to relax
- Anxiety or panic disturbing the first 4 hours of sleep
- Increased neuronal sensitivity and reactivity, e.g. irritability, paresthesiae, photophobia, hyperacusis, tinnitus
- Vasoconstriction or spasm of cerebral, cardiac or peripheral arteries
- Increased contractility of smooth muscle tubes, e.g. esophagus, duodenum, colon and genitourinary tract
- Hypophosphatemia, depletion of potassium and magnesium

This condition was first described by Lewis as a metabolic disorder, to which he gave the name 'effort syndrome'[14,24,52]. An attempt is being made to resuscitate his views because modern equipment enables the buffer depletion to be confirmed by exercise testing with capnography (vide infra), and his principles of rehabilitation to be re-discovered and modified for use today[24]. Thus the majority of cardiological patients without detectable organic disease can hope for restoration of performance and health, and protection from erroneous diagnosis.

CORONARY ARTERY DISEASE

General considerations

Coronary atheroma is a trait of the middle-aged. Moderate and severe stenoses are common in people who seem to be healthy. It is frequently forgotten that the patterns of stenosis in these asymptomatic individuals are no different from those found in patients with angina pectoris. The morbidity and mortality rates associated with angina pectoris are certainly not proportionate to the number of vessels involved. Before the initial onset of symptoms there are long, silent periods when the chronic arterial lesions do not interfere with daily life. Once symptoms have emerged they can disappear for years on end, and the relapses and remissions might not be linked with detectable anatomical changes. It is common to find huge differences of effort tolerance, perhaps 100-fold, between 'good days' and 'bad days' in the earlier phases of angina pectoris, and these cannot be explained by any theory that postulates rigid stenosis as the sole origin of the pain and disability. Even in the case of sudden and unexpected death, pathologists are questioning whether the pathogenesis of the cardiac arrest has much to do with the chronic arterial lesions that might be present[53–56].

Except for the most extreme cases of coronary atheroma, in which rigid stenoses are unarguably and overwhelmingly dominant, it is clear that dynamic factors must play a leading part in the genesis of angina pectoris, and can produce it even when atheroma is negligible or absent.

The dynamic factors include constriction of the venous capacitance vessels, which can dump a

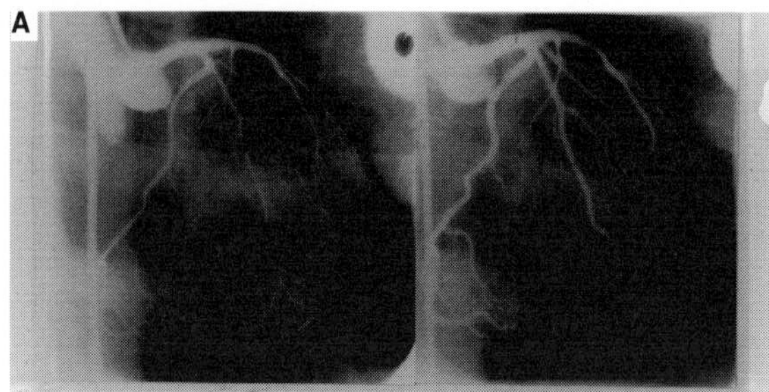

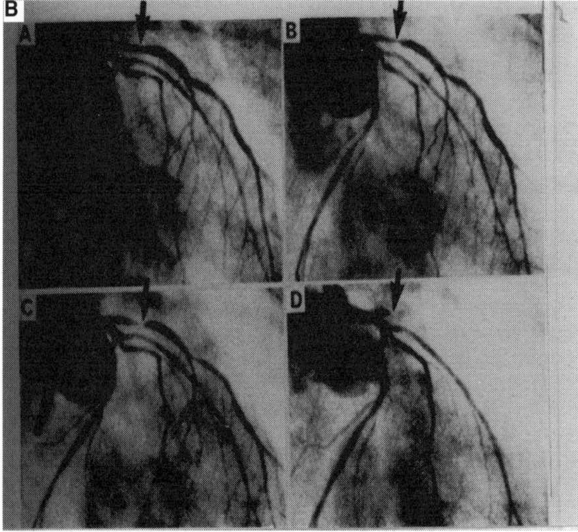

Figure 3.5 Arteriographic appearances in apparently normal vessels. (a) illustrates generalized vasoconstriction. Ischemia can occur if the lumen is compromised by atheroma. (Reproduced from Hackett D et al. 1987 Induction of coronary artery spasm by a direct local action of ergonovine. Circulation 75:577–82, by permission of the American Heart Association, Inc.) (b) shows the development of focal spasm. (Reproduced from Matsuda Y, Moritani K, Ogawa H 1986 Response of the coronary artery to a small dose of ergonovine in variant angina. American Heart Journal 112;947–52)

venous capacitance vessels, which can dump a liter of blood into the thorax; constriction of the systemic arteries increasing resistance to outflow from the left ventricle; constriction or spasm within the coronary system (Fig. 3.5a,b) and reduction of left ventricular compliance. The causes of reduction of left ventricular compliance include overloading; excessive catecholamine and adrenal cortical activity; hypocapnic–sympathetic interactions (see below) and perfusion disorders e.g. ischemic injury (stunning), failure of contractility (hibernation) and subendocardial ischemia such as may occur in blood loss and extreme tachycardia.

These dynamic factors impair the heart's function by altering the left ventricular diastolic-filling pressure relationships. Under normal conditions, the left ventricle fills easily and with little pressure elevation (Fig. 3.6), but in angina the curve is shifted to the left, and the heart's position on it is raised. Effort that was easily accommodated previously now causes greater increases of pressure within the left ventricle. The first indicators are mechanical, as, for example, when the appearance of a palpable and audible atrial gallop rhythm signals the fact that the stiffened left ventricle cannot fill itself easily in early diastole and now must rely upon a powerful left atrial contraction for its filling. ECG changes occur later than the mechanical, and can appear many times a day in individuals who feel no symptoms.

When these changes in the heart are severe enough to bring the person to a standstill during exercise only a minority complain of classical angina pectoris. The majority report the symptoms found in healthy people but at a lower level of effort e.g. breathlessness, exhaustion, and an indefinable compulsion to stop are commonplace.

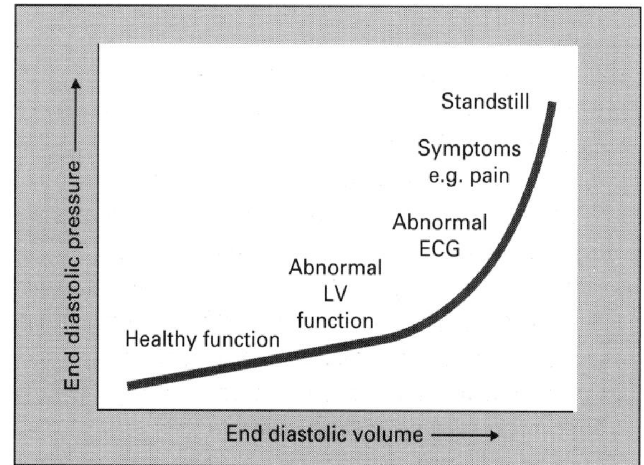

Figure 3.6 A diagram of left ventricular pressure–volume relationships. Normally a large volume is accepted with a minimal rise of pressure. In angina pectoris the distensibility is reduced by reduction of compliance even to a point where small increments of volume cause a steep rise of pressure. The mechanical disturbances are followed by electrical disturbance and then by symptoms.

The differential diagnosis of these symptoms includes debilitating conditions such as anemia and thyrotoxicosis. Hyperventilation can cause both angina pectoris and chest pain that resembles it. Syndrome X is a condition in which normal coronary arteriograms are found in patients with both angina and ischemic ECG changes after exercise: its pathophysiology is not yet determined.

Exercise stress testing cannot distinguish the dynamic causes of angina from the atherosclerotic because the electrocardiographic appearances of ischemia can be the same in both cases.

Genesis

The arousal-related disorders that can contribute to the development or acceleration of coronary heart disease have emotional, pathophysiological, cognitive and behavioral elements. The etiological role of the first two is considered here, before considering the interplay between coronary constriction or spasm and atheroma, and the condition of the culprit coronary artery.

Role of the emotions

The role of emotional arousal in the genesis of heart disease and sudden coronary death is commonly dismissed as anecdotal, but the development of appropriate technology is bringing it into the realm of probability and scientific approbation.

Anger has received the most attention. In animals it can produce delayed myocardial ischemia associated with increased activity of the left stellate ganglion[57]. In man this autonomic disturbance fosters cardiac arrhythmia, coronary vasoconstriction and reduction of the threshold for ventricular fibrillation. It may originate in abnormal function of the left cerebral hemisphere[43,44,45]. In coronary patients anger can induce left ventricular dysfunction with reduction of the ejection fraction[58,59], and it can trigger cardiac arrest[58]. Sinatra described aortic dissection during suppressed rage[60], and we have a patient who suffered the same catastrophe while struggling to lift a heavy weight in a burst of impotent fury.

Unspecified emotional arousal described simply as stress or distress, or upset, has been associated with a variety of cardiological conditions. Deanfield and colleagues linked it with silent myocardial ischemia[61], and Rozanski's group focused upon the role of the personally-relevant stressor[62]. An early editorial on the relationships between the mind and the heart accepted the proposition that about half of the acute admissions to hospital with heart failure were precipitated by gross emotional upset[63].

The first case report of emotional upset causing myocardial infarction with cardiogenic shock was published in 1992. Angiography demonstrated less than than 30% stenosis in the left anterior descending artery without disease elsewhere in the coronary system, and normal left ventricular function[64]. The second case reported had no evidence of atherosclerotic disease at all[65]!

In their examination of the relationship between behavioral stress and cardiac arrhythmia, Verrier and Lown focused on the association of psychological depression (i.e. feelings of abandonment and alienation) with multi-vessel coronary disease, coronary vasoconstriction and sleep loss. They concluded that the treatment of ventricular ectopic activity in some patients is more successful when attention is paid to the brain's neurophysiological trigger rather than its cardiac target: sleep was more effective than antiarrhythmic drugs in reducing the incidence and grade of left ventricular premature beats[66].

With regard to sudden cardiac death, Myers and Dewar examined the circumstances surrounding 100 cases with a coroner's necropsy and concluded that the most significant relationship of the death was psychological distress[67]. A more specific effect of the brain's role in the catastrophe of sudden death was identified by Lown as the 'recall of uniquely individual, emotionally-charged experiences[68].'

The emotional setting which increases the vulnerability to ischemic heart disease was designated as the 'giving-up-given up' complex by Engel[69], and Wolf went so far as to suggest that death might be an adaptive maneuver in intolerable suffering, and not just a matter of the protective systems going awry[70]. Their descriptions would fit a diagnosis of profound exhaustion.

Exhaustion increases cardiovascular vulnerability to the effects of the emotions through failure of habituation. Under the title of 'the emotional eclipse of the heart' Purcell and Mulcahy have drawn fresh attention to its role in the genesis of the cardiac catastrophe[71]. Exhaustion is looked upon as a harbinger of myocardial infarction[16,17], and it appears to play a role in restenosis after coronary angioplasty[72], particularly where hyperventilation adds a vasoconstrictive element[73]. These effects may be dependent upon undamping or disinhibition of the vital regulatory functions discussed below.

This consideration of the relationships between the emotions and the heart opens possibilities for prevention. The first is to increase awareness of hyperarousal and its management. The second is to increase awareness of exhaustion and its management. The third is to employ capnography[74] to identify Rozanski's 'personally-relevant stressors[62]' and Lown's 'emotionally-charged experiences[68]', and thus expose them as targets for counseling or cognitive therapy except in alexithymia (see below).

Pathophysiological mechanisms

A wide variety of potentially pathogenic arousal disorders develop on the downslope of the human function curve (Fig. 3.4), and their interactions can produce cascades of cardiovascular disorder and damage.

Neuroendocrine arousal. Two major pathways can contribute to heart damage, the sympatho-adrenomedullary (S-AM) and the pituitary-adrenal cortical (P-AC) systems[43]. Light effort involves the sympathetic nervous system, but heavier challenges produce adrenal medullary activity and alter cardiovascular regulation, lipid metabolism, glucose production and blood coagulability[75]. When arousal is increased, by heavier and more prolonged effort, unfamiliar problems or loss of control, the P-AC system is activated to secrete cortisol. This is lipogenic and the plasma cholesterol levels can rise up to 60% above baseline[76]. Cortisol also exerts a rapid and 'permissive' effect on catecholamine production[77], and Raab has described the marked potentiation of catecholamine 'toxicity' by adrenal corticoids, particularly where the myocardium has an ischemic handicap[78].

The arousal-induced shift away from a cardioprotective anabolic pattern of metabolism towards a catabolic pattern[7,77,79] fosters the development of diabetes mellitus, obesity, hypertension, hyperlipidemia and atherosclerosis (Box 3.2). Anabolic hormones such as insulin and testosterone decrease during hyperarousal, the latter undermining stamina and the urge to succeed[80]. Clinical observation suggests that the development of a persistent catabolic state can produce a coronary catastrophe in vulnerable individuals within a matter of months. The fact that the progression of atheroma does not follow changes in conventional risk factors[81] may be an indication that they are less powerful than the arousal-induced shifts. It has been noted that the lability or undamping of the serum cholesterol level is an important predictor of coronary morbidity, and this may reflect exhaustion and repeated exposure to high levels of emotional arousal[82].

Sleep disorder. Across a 24 hour period there is normally a balance between catabolism (degradation) and anabolism (renewal): the activities of wakefulness enhance catabolism, while sleep shifts the balance in favor of anabolism. Before they become irreversible[5,83], many of the homeostatic disorders that appear to be resistant to drug therapy, such as elevation of the blood pressure, sugar, uric acid and lipids, revert to base-line normal values when the individual is withdrawn from his usual stressors and enabled to rest well and sleep efficiently at night and in the afternoons for a few days (Fig. 3.7)[84].

Two sorts of sleep disorders are common in effort syndrome and coronary disease. The first is the inability to achieve adequate sleep, probably as a result of going to bed with too high a level of arousal. The second takes the form of wakening during the first 4 hours of sleep — too early for the diagnosis of depression — with symptoms such as anxiety or panic, restlessness, sweating, cerebral vascular disturbances, coronary con-

Box 3.2 Catabolic and anabolic processes

Hormonal pattern during arousal

Catabolic hormones increase	*Anabolic hormones decrease*
Cortisol	Insulin
Epinephrine	Calcitonin
Glucagon	Testosterone
Growth hormone	Estrogen
Antidiuretic hormone	Prolactin
Renin	Luteinizing hormone
Angiotensin	Follicle stimulating hormone
Aldosterone	Gonadotropin releasing hormone (GnRH)
Erythropoietin	Prolactin releasing hormone (PRH)
Thyroxin	
Parathormone	
Melatonin	

Anabolic and catabolic states

Anabolic state

Increased synthesis of protein, fat, carbohydrate (growth, energy storage)
Decreased breakdown of protein, fat, carbohydrate (growth, energy storage)
Increased production of cells for immune system (white blood cells of thymus and bone marrow)
Increased bone repair and growth
Increase in sexual processes (cellular, hormonal, psychological)

Catabolic state (arousal)

Halt in synthesis of protein, fat, carbohydrate
Increased breakdown of protein, fat, carbohydrate (energy mobilization)
Elevated blood levels of glucose, free fatty acids, low density lipoprotein, cholesterol (for energy)
Increased production of red blood cells and liver enzymes (for energy)
Decreased repair and replacement of bone
Decreased repair and replacement of cells with normally high turnover (gut, skin, etc)
Decreased production of cells for immune system (thymus shrinks, circulating white cells decrease)
Decreased sexual processes
Increased blood pressure, cardiac output
Increased salt and water retention

(Reproduced from Sterling and Eyer, 1981)[7]

striction, cardiac arrhythmia, gut disturbance, paresthesiae, pain or cramp in skeletal muscle and other symptoms of hypocapnia and respiratory alkalosis. It is a consequence of hyperventilation compensating for nocturnal acidemia in individuals with buffer depletion[85].

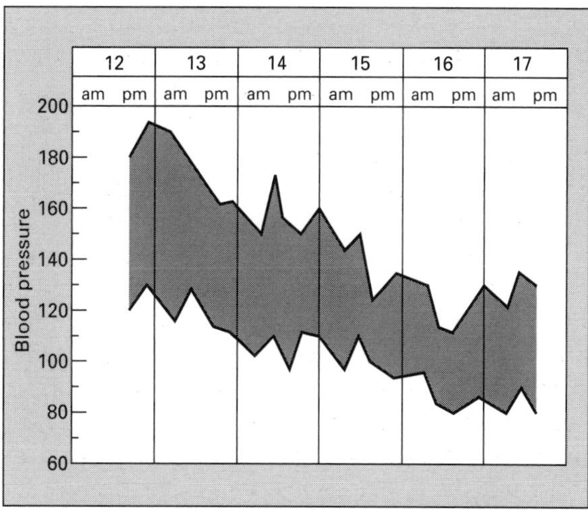

Figure 3.7 The blood pressure response to reassurance, sleep and rest in a male patient with prolonged exhaustion. Elsewhere he had been regarded as a case of hypertension resistant to drug therapy. The recovery represents a shift from catabolic to anabolic dominance. Rehabilitation teaches the skills required for avoiding recurrence

Sleep disturbance is regarded as an important pathophysiological element of angina pectoris[86]. James MacKenzie's view of sleep was simple:

> attacks of angina pectoris may be directly induced by want of refreshing sleep. Whatever form the heart failure may assume, sleep is essential. It may be taken as an axiom that if the patient does not get sufficient sleep he will never get well[87].

Since his day, waking exhausted has been defined as a coronary risk factor[88], and incriminated in restenosis after angioplasty[89].

The autonomic nervous system. This plays an important role in cardiovascular homeostasis[90]. Sympathetic activity is particularly prominent in anterior infarction and afferent impulses can initiate potentially damaging reflexes from the brain[91]. Myocardial ischemia involving the anterior ventricular surface causes greater damage to the right sympathetic nerves than the left and creates a potentially dangerous asymmetry[92] that fosters coronary vasoconstriction during alpha-adrenergic stimulation[93,94]. Beta$_2$ blockade leaves these constrictor influences unopposed and can aggravate angina pectoris[95,96], particularly in the presence of a synergism such as hypocapnia.

The interruption of sympathetic pathways by transmural infarction can establish a 'denervation supersensitivity' to catecholamines[97].

Undamped and asymmetric sympathetic input to the heart from the left stellate ganglion is associated with cardiac arrhythmia, coronary vasoconstriction, shortening of the ventricular refractory period and reduction of the threshold for ventricular fibrillation; and ablation of the left stellate ganglion can provide protection against these disorders[98]. They appear to originate in abnormal function of the left cerebral hemisphere[44,45]. It has long been known that separating the heart from the brain by cervical transection in animals is protective against arrhythmia[99].

Parasympathetic influences can cause bradycardia and hypotension in posterior cardiac infarction[91]. In severe cases the hypotension might not be removed by correction of the bradycardia but yield to fluid infusion[100]. The parasympathetic nerves can be interrupted by subendocardial ischemia, thus reducing the threshold for ventricular fibrillation[97,101], and the effect is long lasting[102]. The inhibition of the parasympathetic system by hyperventilation[103] and pain or emotional distress[104] in acute coronary conditions can also reduce opposition to sympathetic activity. Thus the management of pain and fear in acute myocardial infarction and open-heart surgery, the provision of support, and the elimination of sleep loss may afford greater protection against arrhythmic disorder than antiarrhythmic drugs[100,105].

Bairey's group has shown that the shifts of sympathovagal balance that increase the sympathetic activity and reduce the parasympathetic aggravate the risk of malignant arrhythmia, even to the point where death can be provoked by anger[58]. Conversely the emotions produced by expressions of support and appreciation demonstrably shift the autonomic balance towards cardioprotective parasympathetic activity[106].
Stuart Wolf has written:

> The evidence reviewed supports the thesis that fatal cardiac arrhythmias, with or without associated myocardial infarction, may often be attributable to undamped autonomic discharges in response to either afferent information from below, or to impulses resulting from integrative processes in the brain involved in adaptation to life experience, or both.
>
> In the musculoskeletal system, smooth synergistic responses without excessive irritability are achieved through a well coordinated inhibitory network. Satisfactory visceral control appears similarly to require an autonomic inhibitory network operating at afferent, integrative and efferent levels. The effectiveness of such a regulatory process may be reflected in the degree of variance from day to day and week to week of measured indicators of autonomic function.
>
> Regulatory inhibition appears to be diminished in situations that are interpreted as overwhelming and without hope, such as total social exclusion and other circumstances characterized by hopeless dejection or sudden fear. At times, the loss of regulatory inhibition may provide a mechanism of death.
>
> On the other hand, it would appear that the enhanced lability of autonomic responses associated with weary dissatisfaction, frustration, the feeling of abandonment, and dejection may be damped by emotional support from people and circumstances in the environment. This potentially salubrious effect of a supportive environment may well be further studied and exploited in preventive and curative medicine[107].

Hyperventilation. Many people who are exhausted by failure to cope and adapt hyperventilate. The pathophysiological effects include the aggravation of ischemia (Bohr effect), and an increase in sympatho-adrenal activity[108] (Fig. 3.8). Hyperventilation causes hypophosphatemia, and potassium loss associated with an increase of intracellular potassium ionization and hyper-polarization of the myocardial cell[109]. At the same time the magnesium diuresis induced by the heightened sympatho-adrenal activity reduces intracellular magnesium ionization. This loss of 'nature's own physiological calcium blocker' lessens opposition to the calcium overloading of the myocardial cell[110,111]. The increase of intracellular calcium ionization is aggravated by the respiratory alkalosis[112,113]. The cardiovascular effects of increasing the Ca^{++}/Mg^{++} ratio in the heart include reduction of left ventricular compliance, arrhythmia, platelet agglutination and thrombosis, and increased coronary artery tone (Fig. 3.8). In hyperventilation-induced calcium overloading of the cardiac cell some 70% of the Ca^{++} increase comes from within the cell and only the smaller proportion enters by the slow calcium channels. Calcium-blocking drugs act upon these slow channels and so their protective value is relatively small[112]. The increase of coronary tone rarely occludes normal coronary arteries, but it can rise to a pathological level and contribute to the cracking of an atheromatous plaque and occlusive thrombosis, especially in the presence of neurohumoral vasoconstrictive activity, and damage the endothelium by shear stress: this promotes the formation of atheromatous lesions[114].

Figure 3.5 illustrates the coronary appearances during focal spasm. Ribeiro and Lefer have charted the stimuli that can trigger this dynamic pathophysiologic disorder, and emphasized that calcium mobilization and overloading of the coronary system is the final common pathway (Fig. 3.9)[115]. The calcium-dependent tone of the epicardial coronary arteries and their pH-related cyclical activity is not solely a function of the heart's innervation, and so coronary spasm can occur in the denervated transplanted heart[116]. Hyperventilation's place in cardiology today has been reviewed by Weiner[117], and its specific contribution to failure of angioplasty described by Ardissino and colleagues[73]. Jenkins described it in vivid terms as a distinctive element of 'coronary-prone behavior'[118].

Autonomic–hypocapnic synergy. It is commonly assumed that hyperventilation is a minor consequence of anxiety and increased sympathetic drive, but the evidence suggests that sympathetic activity and hyperventilation are independently triggered[44]. Increased sympathetic drive and hyperventilation can act synergistically,

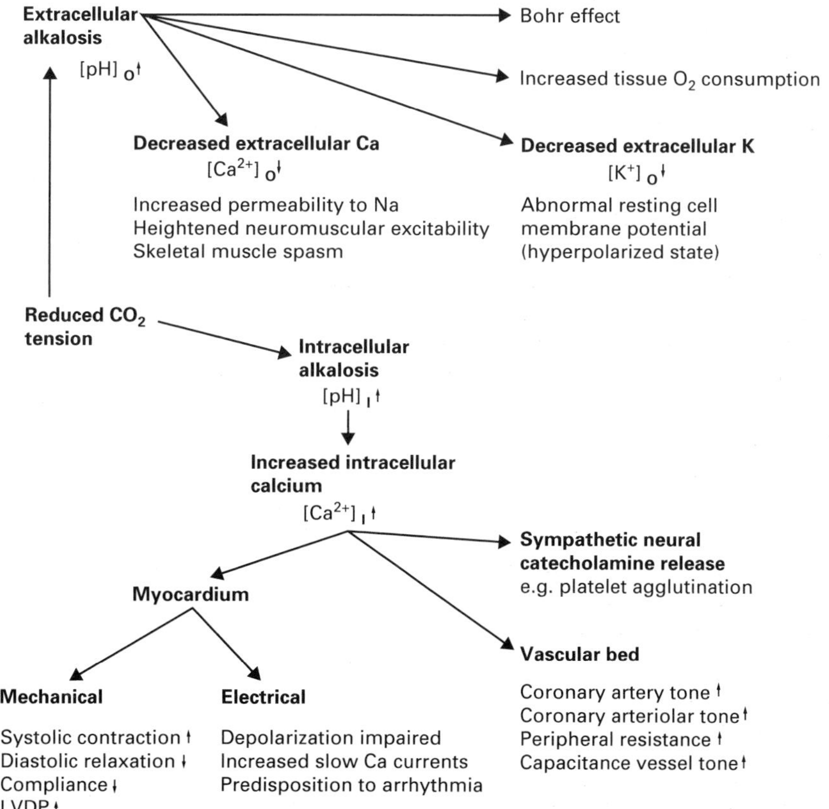

Figure 3.8 Mechanisms by which hyperventilation-induced reduction of CO_2 tension can cause cardiovascular disorder and disease in vulnerable persons. LVDP = left ventricular diastolic pressure. (Courtesy of Hamid Al-Abbasi, 1982)

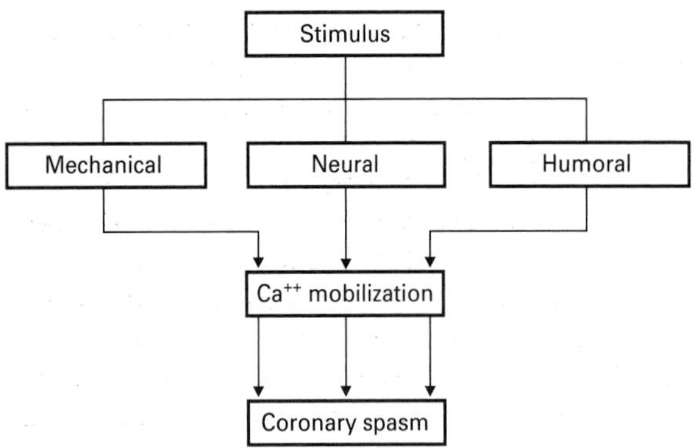

Figure 3.9 Mobilization of Ca^{++} is considered to be the final common pathway by which various stimuli cause coronary spasm. (Reproduced from Ribeiro, Lefer 1983)[115]

and this synergism may have a powerful effect when regulatory inhibition is impaired by exhaustion[107]: sympathetic stimulation amplifies the respiratory response to a given level of blood P_{CO_2}[119] and hypocapnia increases sympathoadrenal activity[108]. The appearance of somatic symptoms aggravates anxiety and increases the activity of the vicious spiral[120]. These symptoms may be misattributed to coronary disease[24].

In one study of sympathetic–hypocapnic synergy it was suggested that hypocapnic reduction of blood flow to the right cerebral hemisphere might contribute to the disinhibition of the left, the consequent overactivity of the left stellate ganglion and the increased risk of cardiac arrhythmia and coronary constriction[44].

Hemostasis and thrombosis. Increased coagulability is now accepted as a major risk factor for coronary heart disease[121]. The increased fibrinogen level might be the consequence of a catabolic metabolism; and the increased adhesiveness of platelets probably reflects calcium overloading due to catecholamine activity and respiratory alkalosis.

Endothelium. The endothelium plays a crucial part in vasomotor regulation. When it is intact dilatation can occur in response to increments of flow, exercise and sympathetic stimulation, and to the intracoronary injection of acetylcholine[114]. When it is denuded or dysfunctional from exposure to the catabolic neuroendocrine factors previously described[7,77], or shear stress[114], vasoconstriction and thrombotic activity can replace the physiological dilatation. Hyperventilation can aggravate these self-injurious mechanisms by increasing intracellular calcium ionization and catecholamine activity (Fig. 3.8).

Coronary constriction and spasm

The idea that the heart can be damaged by coronary vasoconstriction and spasm was accepted by the Victorians because it was as plain as a pikestaff to them that the clinical syndromes could never by explained by the appearances of atheroma at autopsy. Coronary arteriography proved the point: Mason Sones, the pioneer of the technique, filmed vasospasm in his own heart.

The thrombosis causing acute transmural infarction is the result of a dynamic interaction between intimal damage, platelet aggregation and vasoconstriction or spasm[122]. Where the vessel is greatly damaged and stiffened by atheroma, vasospasm might have no role, the catastrophe being caused by thrombosis at the site of a fissured plaque. In such a case the person is likely to have suffered from chronic angina pectoris. In sudden unexpected coronary death, however, the underlying plaque is commonly too small to limit flow or reveal its presence by exercise stress testing[123], and here vasospasm is probably the primary agent of the acute obstruction. An excellent review of vasotonic myocardial ischemia is provided by Bashour[124] and Boyd[6] who present the evidence for its etiological role in atheroma.

Maseri's team studied coronary vasomotion extensively and observed that the constriction or spasm which occurs at the onset of angina at rest is indistinguishable from the appearances at the onset of myocardial infarction[125]. In vasospastic angina the focal spasm is associated with a generalized increase of tone and hypersensitivity to vasoconstrictive stimuli[126] such as can be found in hypocapnia (Fig. 3.8). Increased tone even without spasm can lead to arterial injury: for example the failure to dilate appropriately during increases of cardiac output can cause shear stress which damages the endothelium and thereby fosters thrombosis and atherogenesis[114]. Focal spasm causing serious interruption of blood flow usually appears at sites of atheroma[127], but many descriptions have been published of spasm in radiologically normal arteries[6,65]. Vasoconstriction and spasm can rupture an atherosclerotic plaque, probably by a direct mechanical effect or possibly through occlusion of the vaso vasorum[128], precipitating the thrombotic occlusion of a formerly stable artery[6].

Variable onset and unstable angina, and silent myocardial ischemia can be induced by physiological increases of coronary tone as well as by pathological degrees of constriction and spasm[113], particularly where a critical atheromatous lesion renders the blood flow vulnerable to relatively small dynamic alterations of lumen[6,59,112,124–129].

The culprit artery

In the dynamic interactions between intimal damage, platelet aggregation and arterial constriction or spasm that can precipitate myocardial infarction, the initial conditions of the artery are important determinants of outcome: a plaque ripe for fissuring, constrictivity of the vessel, and homeostatic conditions fostering a shift of the thrombotic–thrombolytic equilibrium towards thrombosis play key roles[122].

In Q wave infarction the culprit artery is totally occluded in over 90% of cases, but subsequently re-opens spontaneously in up to 30% of cases within 12 hours[130]. After thrombolytic therapy the recanalization rate reaches 60–80%[131].

The residual condition of the culprit artery in myocardial infarction has been examined in many centers. Gohlke and his colleagues studied younger patients and found normal coronary arteries at angiography in 31% of those under 30 years of age and in 6% of those between 35 and 39 years[132]. Angiography in these individuals shows focal lesions resembling, and possibly caused by focal spasm (Fig. 3.5). Marzilli described a case where fixed atherosclerotic narrowing developed at the site of recurrent focal spasm and required bypass surgery[133].

Petch reported that 1% of patients following myocardial infarction will have left mainstem stenosis and 26% will have disease of all three coronary vessels. The remainder, nearly three quarters, will not have severe disease[134].

Where myocardial infarction is preceded by chronic angina pectoris the coronary disease is usually severe[135]. In unheralded cases studied 20 days after acute myocardial infarction, 78% showed patency of the infarct-related artery but in chronic angina only 47%. It was concluded that thrombosis can complete the obstruction in severe (≥70%) coronary artery stenosis in long-standing angina, but constriction and spasm are the major agents of obstruction in unheralded cases[136,137].

These studies make it clear that infarction commonly occurs 'unheralded' in patients with the lesser degrees of atheromatous obstruction. Unfortunately the only acknowledged heralds are angina pectoris and evidence of ischemia: exhaustion and failure at coping and adapting were not examined by the authors.

The acceptance of arterial constriction and spasm as major triggers of the coronary catastrophe comes from a series of careful studies in which they were directly observed[125,138–148]. Coronary spasm can also be responsible for cardiac arrest in survivors of infarction who show no evidence of underlying heart disease[148].

The rise in the death rate from ischemic heart disease is now attributed to an increased tendency to myocardial infarction rather than to an increased prevalence of atherosclerosis[149]. This finding can be explained by a rise of the homeostatic disorders that promote coronary spasm, endothelial damage, and increased coagulability.

THE BIOPSYCHOSOCIAL APPROACH IN CLINICAL PRACTICE

The evidence reviewed supports the hypothesis that cardiovascular disorder and disease can result from the emotional consequences of failure to cope and adapt and the concomitant entropic, homeostatic impairment. Accordingly, prevention and rehabilitation require an approach capable of integrating the individual's mind and personal qualities, his behavior, his social circumstances and his predicament with information about the electrophysiological, biochemical and pathological aspects of his 'disease'. The development of such an approach modifies the conventional history taking and clinical examination: it demands information about changes of behavior, and appropriate planning for prevention and rehabilitation.

History taking

In the biopsychosocial approach the clinician is interested not only in the hard information related to the binary medical judgement of 'disease' or 'no disease', but also in the course and shaping of the 'illness' as the patient sees it. In addition, he is interested in the events that might have challenged the patient's adaptive capacity, undermined homeostatic regulation and created the risk of catastrophe. It is a most useful experience to observe a barrister taking a history of the relationships between an external event such as an industrial injury and a heart attack: without leading his client he will take an account of the pivotal event which caused a change of health and performance and the conditions associated with improvement or deterioration.

Some patients are aware of going 'over the top' of the human function curve (Fig. 3.4) and recognize the pivotal influences that cause the shift. Conventionally, doctors decry these insights into the conditions that existed before the appearance of disease, but they are crucial for rehabilitation and the restoration of stability.

A visual analog scale can help the exhausted person to become articulate about his loss of performance: he is asked to express, as a percentage of normal, his present level of 'energy'; the quantum of stamina or endurance that does not depend upon willpower; physical capacity; and efficiency of concentration and memory. After this exercise it will dawn upon many that their ill health may be related to their struggling to keep up a 100% level of achievement with no more than 50–60% of the qualities required. A catastrophe, a breakdown of health, commonly occurs at the 30% level.

The perception of their position on the scale enables many to realise that raising their condition towards the 100% level by rehabilitation should improve performance and health, and thus add a useful strategy to the conventional armamentorium of palliative drugs and surgical intervention

Reading the questionnaire (Box 3.3) without being obliged to provide answers often stimulates an intuitive leap into awareness of the relationships between stressors, feelings, behavior, performance and health; and acknowledgement of social and personal needs.

Awareness can also be achieved by explaining to the person that energy is required for daily

Box 3.3 The human function curve questionnaire

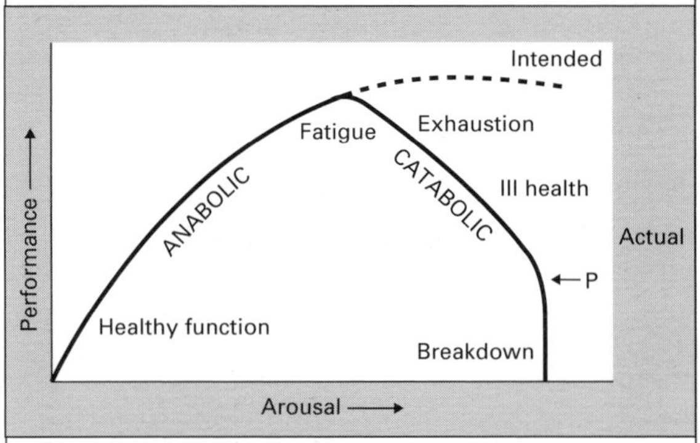

AM I ON THE DOWNSLOPE?

Because too much is demanded of me?
Because I cannot say 'no' when I should?
Because I am not sufficiently in control? Can't cope?
- Too angry, too tense, too upset, too irritable, too indignant?
- Too much people-poisoning?
- Too many time-pressures? Too impatient?

Because I am not sleeping WELL enough to keep well?
Because I am not keeping fit enough to stay well?
Because I am not balancing the periods of hard effort with adequate sleep and relaxation?
Because I am out of real energy and using sheer will-power to keep going?
Because I am infallible, indispensible, indestructible, immortal?

THE PROTESTING HEART

What is it trying to say? Am I listening?
Why is it protesting?
What makes it protest each time? And why so often?
Am I working to make it stronger or am I too upset with myself to succeed?
Am I looking for a drug/operation to keep it quiet?

activities, for the contingencies of life, for self-actualization and achievement, and for the homeostatic needs of the internal systems of the body. If insufficient energy is provided for the maintenance of the internal systems, they must undergo catabolic, entropic degradation, a process serendipitously called 'self cannibalization'[150] or accelerated aging.

The value of providing awareness and insight in the consultation is that it enables many to grasp the idea that they are not essentially 'diseased' but 'over-used', 'over-trained' and inadequately restored, and stand in need of rehabilitation rather than life-long drug therapy or surgical intervention. Those with strong denial or alexithymia may not be able to comprehend this cognitive approach.

Assessment of behavior

The assessment of behavior is an important element of the history taking and observation of the patient. It provides the clinician with a guide to the individual's position on the human function curve (Fig. 3.4). The curve represents a continuum, but there are recognizable stations on the course such as healthy function, acceptable fatigue and exhaustion before illness and breakdown occur. The perception of shifts from one station to another is an important element of diagnoses.

Healthy function

The individual feels well. His manner is relaxed and physical recreation brings pleasure without causing guilty reactions. Burdens and pressures that would cause loss of happiness and health are rejected. Increasing the arousal enhances the performance. Other people look upon him and his relationships as healthy and see him as adaptable and approachable. The qualities required for success, namely rapid and flexible thought, originality, vigor, expansion and capacity for sustained effort, are abundant.

Acceptable fatigue

The individual feels and shows reasonable fatigue, does not deny it, and takes steps to recover as soon as possible. Maladaptive habits that waste time and energy can be modified and inessential drains on the energy can be jettisoned or deferred. Performance can still increase with arousal, but more effort is required. Disciplined effort, youthful conditioning for competition, social pressures and mild stimulants such as coffee and cigarettes play a greater part in sustaining performance. Sleep is adequate. Others see the individual as healthily tired, but they are not made anxious because the qualities required for success are still evident.

Exhaustion

The individual commonly makes strong declarations of health and virility that are at odds with his observed behavior. He rejects the need to maintain a reasonable balance between high endeavor and relaxation, and sees no need to increase his fitness in preparation for periods of unusual effort.

Excessive burdens and pressures, disruptive of health and happiness, are accepted as inevitable because the exhaustion reduces the ability to distinguish the essential from the inessential. Increasing the arousal causes the performance to deteriorate and sets up a vicious circle, because it widens the gap between the actual ability and the intended (Fig. 3.4) and this generates further anxiety and insecurity. Unrealistic views of the gap between actual and intended performance are adopted, errors increase and personal relationships deteriorate. Others can see the growth of unhealthy tension and the symptoms of strain: bad temper, continual grumbling, longer hours worked but less achieved, repeated minor sickness and preoccupation with health, together with insecurity about the future, procrastination, losing sight of long-term goals in preoccupation with minor matters, feelings of frustration and persecution by colleagues, with complaints of lack of cooperation, technical jargon and catch-phrases replacing original thought[26].

Previously acceptable idiosyncracies can reach neurotic proportions and disrupt the peace of mind of others. The qualities required for success disappear. The mind becomes set against change, and adaptability is lost. Leadership comes to depend upon tradition and seniority instead of ability. Eating, drinking, smoking and talking increase, and a compulsive desire for stimulating circumstances may dominate life.

Sleep disorders remove anabolic opportunities and aggravate catabolic deterioration[7,83]. Those exhausted by sleep disorders have to struggle harder for success, and this increases their arousal: they may become incompetent at adapting and habituating. Emotionalism increases, and a rise in hostility undermines social support. Hyperventilation starts, probably as a marker of distress in this predicament, and introduces its own cascades of disorders into the internal system. One of the more important is disruption of sleep by hypocapnia in the first 4 hours. This may be accompanied by cardiac arrhythmia, coronary constriction or panic[24,85].

Biochemical changes associated with exhaustion and a high level of arousal may be seen, such as decreases in serum iron and increases in thyroid and sympatho-adrenal activity[7] and the other catabolic disorders described in Box 3.2. Fluid retention is common.

Attempts to bring about an improvement often make the doctor frustrated and anxious because the more severe the patient's exhaustion, the more he resists attempts to reduce his arousal: righteous indignation and militant enthusiasm are commonly employed to sustain it[26]. Cardiac arrhythmias, heightened awareness of the heart-beat and symptoms such as chest pain are common. Reassurance is usually given, but it cannot provide more than temporary relief if it does not correct the physiological disorders. Reassurance that reduces arousal and thereby improves homeostatic competence should not be dismissed as a placebo, but valued for its physiological effects.

It can be difficult to deal with the exhausted person cognitively because his judgement, concentration and memory are impaired. His perception of his position becomes distorted by such influences as fatigue and sleep disturbance; loss of morale; loss of self-esteem; denial; hostility; and the drive to live 'over the top' in the gap between his actual performance and the level of his intentions.

Some individuals not only deny their predicament and fail to get the rest they need but struggle ever harder, with diminishing reserves, and add displacement activities to their burdens. Some resign themselves to cardiac invalidism because they do not know how to better their condition. In others overwhelming despair promotes fluid retention and heart failure.

Alexithymia

Perhaps a quarter of cardiological patients suffer from alexithymia (PGF Nixon, unpublished observations 1986). This is a consequence of emotional injury in childhood, torture or the psychological battering of a hard life[151]. Such individuals are imperceptive of their emotions and fatigue, and this impairment is associated with susceptibility to disease[43]. Heart patients with alexithymia may be unaware of exhaustion and ill health before they break down. The observer can suspect the condition from the history and behavior. The Toronto Alexithymia Scale[152] is a potentially useful instrument for diagnosis, but its development is not yet complete.

Cognitive therapy is frequently used in attempts to provide awareness in patients who are endangered by their alexithymia, but almost invariably it causes confusion and irritation because they cannot perceive the objectives and so, in rehabilitation, the individual is taught to recognize the boundaries of physiological tolerance of physical and emotional effort through monitoring of the pulse rate responses, respiratory movements and other physical changes.

Clinical examination of the heart

A simple and practical guide to the condition of the left ventricle is the examination of the apex beat with the patient lying on his left side. A normal impulse, the desirable object of therapy, is an unobtrusive outward motion of the apex beat in systole, having a normal area (size of a thumbnail) and no sign of gallop rhythm. Adrenergic overdrive can reveal itself in palpable slapping movements and loud first sounds. In the case of severe left ventricular damage the signs of overdistension may be palpable in an enlarged (4×4 cm) apex beat with paradoxical movement from muscle that has lost its contractility and is expanding passively during systole. Adequate rest and sleep can be employed to prevent this overdistension in the early days of myocardial infarction. The diastolic sounds change with overloading. In mild degrees, atrial systole provides a fourth heart sound, and in more severe cases a palpable shock wave. With further overloading this atrial 'kick' summates with a growing third sound, and in extreme cases the third sound gallop dominates diastole[153].

Investigations

Exercise stress testing

The conventional cardiological examination with exercise stress testing has less value in prevention than is commonly supposed because the majority of persons destined for sudden coronary death will not have enough disease to produce a positive exercise test[123]. On the other hand it has great value in the assessment of physical performance and, if linked with capnography, the respiratory response to the anaerobic threshold.

Capnography

This technique enables the end-expiratory CO_2 level to be measured by drawing expired air through a capnograph. The normal range of end-tidal or end-expiratory carbon dioxide (PET CO_2) is 36–45 mm Hg at rest. It is difficult to draw conclusions from spot readings. One person whose PET CO_2 is 37 mm Hg, but fallen suddenly from 45 mm Hg might suffer symptoms whereas another person accustomed to a level of 30 mm Hg can feel well.

Hyperventilation applies a force — hypocapnia — to the internal milieu. The outcome is influenced by its duration and magnitude, but depends to a major extent upon the initial conditions of the internal milieu. One important factor is the capacity of the alkaline buffering systems, and others include the arousal level; sleep disorder; autonomic imbalance and disinhibition; neuronal sensitivity; the Ca^{++}/Mg^{++} ratio in the myocardium and coronary arteries; and the individual's ability to perceive and correct periods of dysfunctional breathing[24,154,155].

Screening for hyperventilation. The physiological variations produced by these factors have led to disagreement about the way capnography can best be used to determine whether or not hyperventilation contributes to exhaustion and ill health in a given patient. Abnormalities of PET CO_2 can be transient or elusive, and their failure to appear in a consultation does not mean that they are inoperative at other times and places.

Some workers rely upon three tests: the resting PET CO_2 level, the response to a forced hyperventilation provocation test and the level after exercise, but others working in a different clinical field, the cardiological, find that the triad lacks sensitivity and specificity in their patients[156].

In order to overcome these limitations use has been made of the fact that the recall of personally-relevant stressors[62], or emotionally disturbing events from the past[68] causes some individuals to hyperventilate. This respiratory response can be recorded by capnography when it is elicited by imagery[74]: it points to the origin of emotionally-induced myocardial ischemia and arrhythmia, and indicates the target for cognitive and behavioral intervention in cardiac rehabilitation.

Hypnotism is not employed to evoke the response, because early trials showed that it can cause cardiac arrhythmia and myocardial ischemia. Verbal elicitation has not produced these hazards in over 4000 tests except in one individual with enormous anger (Fig. 3.10).

When the breathing behavior remains normal during the recall of powerful stimuli such as anger, loss or bereavement it is reasonable to suspect alexithymia[44].

Perception of hypocapnia. Capnography can be usefully employed to discover how well a subject perceives hypocapnia. Normal controls

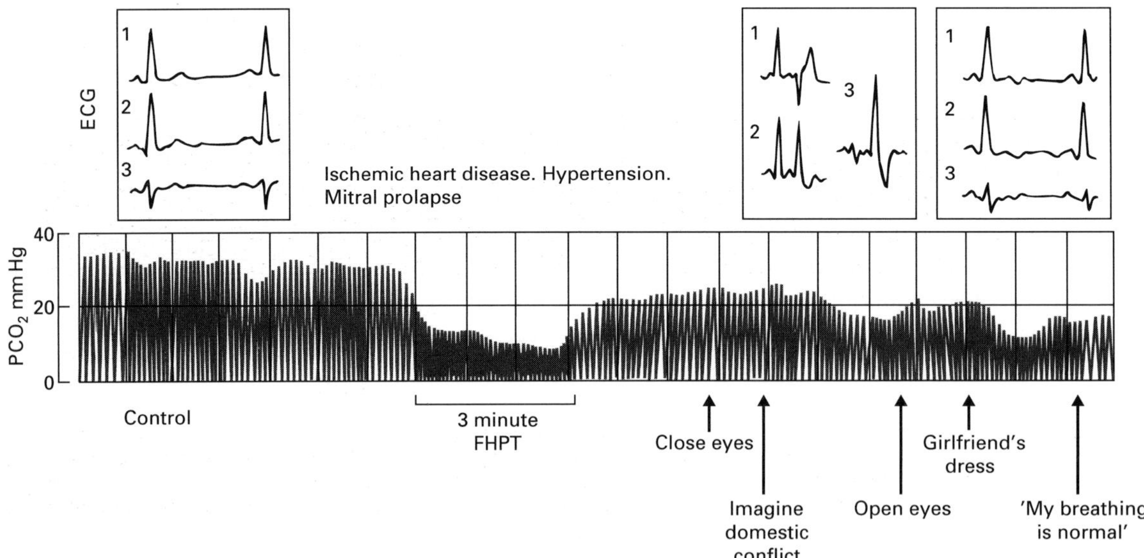

Figure 3.10 A drawing of a capnogram recorded over 21 minutes in a patient (diagnoses shown). (A drawing has been used because the actual respiratory excursions cannot be reproduced exactly.) The upper level (PET CO_2) falls slightly during the control period. It falls to a lower level during the period of imagery (close eyes-open eyes) following the forced hyperventilation provocation test (FHPT). After the period of imagery he is made enormously angry by thoughts of his girlfriend's dress. The PET CO_2 drops to an extremely low level and T wave inversion occurs. Right ventricular ectopy had appeared during the imagery. The patient is certain that his breathing is normal when the PET CO_2 is under 20 mm Hg (normal = 36–45 mm Hg).

are sensitive to small falls of PET CO_2, but those with chronic hyperventilation-related illness may believe themselves to be breathing normally even when they are severely hypocapnic[120,155,156]: they have difficulty in accepting that their symptoms are induced by dysfunctional breathing (Fig. 3.10).

The capnograph can be used as a biofeedback instrument in respiratory training.

Assessment of the anaerobic threshold with exercise. Capnography simplifies the assessment of the respiratory response to the anaerobic threshold during rapidly incremental exercise, and thus provides a useful tool for clinical practice. A bicycle preferably, or a treadmill, is used to increase the work-load every minute in a logarithmic fashion, while the rate of cycling or walking remains constant. At some point the subject experiences discomfort or aching in the legs, presumably from the accumulation of acid metabolites in the exercising muscle, followed soon by acidemic hyperpnea[157,158]. The hyperpnea causes the PET CO_2 level to fall, and the onset of this descent is a respiratory marker of the anaerobic threshold (Fig. 3.11)[159]. The technique makes it possible to assess the capacity of the body's alkaline reserves to buffer the acidic products of exercise. Buffering capacity is high in athletes, and low in the untrained. Extremely low levels characterize effort syndrome where muscular aching and acidemic hyperpnea occur well below the customary levels of everyday activity (Box 3.1).

Assessment of the anaerobic threshold is particularly useful after myocardial infarction, angioplasty and coronary surgery because it is likely to be as low as it is in effort syndrome: without the test the symptoms are usually misattributed to the disease and rehabilitation may not even be considered.

Electrodermal activity

Evidence suggests that arousal asymmetries in the cerebral cortical and sub-cortical structures are transmitted ipsilaterally to the stellate ganglia[160] which distribute efferents to the heart as well as the hands. Thus by employing skin conductance recordings from both hands simultane-

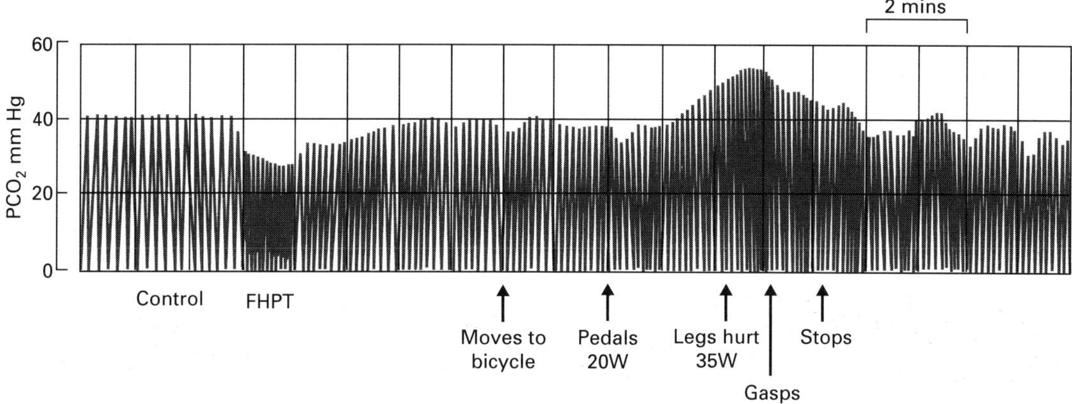

Figure 3.11 Effort syndrome. A drawing of a capnogram before and after exercise testing. (A drawing has been used because the actual respiratory excursions cannot be reproduced exactly.) The PET CO_2 is normal during the control period. Rapid, incremental exercise begins with pedaling at a work-load of 20 watts. At 35 watts the legs hurt. At 3 minutes gasping begins, and the respiratory response to acidemia is indicated by the fall of PET CO_2 (FHPT – 1 minute forced hyperventilation provocation test.)

ously it is possible to obtain information about changes of laterality of function in the cerebral hemispheres. A study employing the imagery of personally-relevant stressors suggests that abnormal processing of arousal in the left cerebral hemisphere is associated with undamped activity of the left stellate ganglion[44]. Cardiovascular consequences include arrhythmias, coronary constriction, shortening of the ventricular refractory period and reduction of the threshold for ventricular fibrillation[45]. It has been suggested that hypocapnic cerebral vasoconstriction may contribute to inhibition of right cerebral hemispheric function and foster greater activity of the left[44].

Combining bilateral skin conductance studies with capnography has revealed that hypocapnia and sympathetic activity go hand in hand in individuals who are facing overwhelming burdens of coping and adapting[44]. They are triggered independently, but act synergistically, and their coupling can be so powerful as to require a few days of resting with judicious use of sedation before the individual can recover from the disorder.

Heart rate variability

The heart rate and blood pressure levels oscillate and the oscillations can be measured in magnitude and frequency with powerful computer resources. In cardiac disease and diabetes mellitus, for example, and under the influence of some drugs, the variability is reduced[161,162]. It can also reflect alterations of parasympathetic–sympathetic balance. It is important to ensure that the observations are not confounded by hyperventilation, a well-recognized suppressor of vagal activity[103], or episodes of subendocardial ischemia that can cause enduring damage to the vagal elements of cardiac control.

McCraty and his colleagues have studied the effects of the emotions and concluded that anger produces a shift towards sympathetic activity, and social support a shift towards parasympathetic activity. Reduction of vagal activity may contribute to the exaggerated blood pressure reactivity to mental stress seen in patients with coronary artery disease[106]. Clinical depression reduces heart rate variability and this appears to increase mortality in coronary artery disease[163].

Metabolic testing

Harmful elevation of blood pressure, lipids and sugar levels and increased coagulability may be biological traits that require long-term treatment of the individual. In cardiological practice there are many in whom they are transient markers of homeostatic impairment that yields to a few days of resting with added sleep (Fig. 3.7).

Traditional cardiac risk factors

There was a period when the traditional risk factors were regarded as causative of coronary disease, but Rose has made it clear that they are not pathophysiological prime-movers[164]. Many of them can be viewed as the behavioral and homeostatic consequences of failure to cope and adapt. Rosenman has provided apt advice:

> It now appears prudent to pay increased attention to the individual who possesses a risk factor, and not merely to the risk factor per se. When full account is taken of the risk factors in prospective studies they account for only about one third of the observed numerical incidence of coronary heart disease (CHD) in subjects undergoing repeated coronary arteriography. The risk factors that are related in epidemiological studies to the incidence of CHD do not appear to be related to the rate of progression of coronary atherosclerosis[165].

In these opinions he supports Petch[81].

Medico-legal implications

A decade ago it was extremely difficult to plead that a work injury might be related to myocardial infarction occurring some months later. The two were regarded as coincidental unless they happened within hours of each other. The view was taken that myocardial infarction is a predestined affair, and expert medical witnesses would demand a scientific level of proof of relationship to injury. Today however when legal rules of admissibility of evidence are adopted, the burden upon the plaintiff is to establish the sufficiency of the work injury and related factors in causation. Absolute proof of such causation is not demanded, and the information about brain–heart relationships is now strong enough to provide plausible explanations for the mechanisms through which stressful events can produce myocardial damage[166].

REHABILITATION

Introduction

The practice of rehabilitation was well-developed in the Victorian era. Effort syndrome and heart disease shared the same principles: sleep and rest were provided for physical and psychological restoration. Relaxation was obtained with massage and baths. Occupation and exercise were employed, and increased at a progressive but tolerable rate until the person had the fitness, stamina and confidence to return to his usual environment. Excess in all things was to be avoided. In heart disease, those who could not afford a restorative regimen had a poor expectation of survival. In this century, the services provided by the military hospitals for effort syndrome in World War I were widely praised. After World War II medicine became oriented towards the discovery of cures for specific diseases, and interest in convalescence and rehabilitation waned. The facilities disappeared.

In the 1960s, a number of cardiologists began to take a fresh interest in rehabilitation, and Hellerstein and Ford published a remarkable paper entitled *Comprehensive care of the coronary patient: a challenge to the physician*[167]. They wrote:

> However skillfully the sociologist, the psychologist and the physiologist dissect him, the patient stubbornly remains an intact human being, struggling back towards homeostasis with all the forces he can muster. The practising physician can help the patient to recognize his needs, ... to measure his resources, and to obtain help. These three functions, consistently performed and flexibly adapted as long as problems ... persist, constitute comprehensive care.

In the 1980s, cardiac rehabilitation received a poor press, viz 'numerous studies failed to identify a direct cardiac mechanism in association with improved functional capacity following exercise training in coronary patients'[168]; 'of little benefit to cardiac function, everyday life or emotional state'[169]; 'no definite evidence that exercise is effective in primary, secondary or tertiary prevention of coronary heart disease'[170]; 'no studies have demonstrated convincing benefit to mortality'[171]; 'it may be that cardiac rehabilitation will join a number of other types of surgical and medical practice whose value has never been definitely proved'[172]. It is possible to attribute these poor results to the general neglect of psychosocial and pathophysiological factors. There were notable exceptions. Frasure-Smith and Prince recognized that life-stress is a precursor of clinical ischemic heart disease, and set up a system to provide monitoring and intervention at the time of need. There were significantly fewer deaths in the monitored than in the control group[173]. Van Dixhoorn and his colleagues allocated patients either to a regimen of exercise plus relaxation and breathing training or to exercise alone; and found the latter to be unsuccessful in some myocardial infarction patients. The relaxation and breathing therapy enhanced the training benefits[174].

Ornish and his colleagues have a unique program of rehabilitation which has been shown to increase blood flow to the heart, to improve cardiac contractility and to permit the regression of atheroma. They employ diet and exercise, and a wide array of psychosocial insights and skills[175]. Their ability to create friendships and to use leadership qualities with devoted patients is possibly unmatched.

Today's problems

Following myocardial infarction, patients can be returned to primary care within a week or less of admission, in a condition of bewilderment, equipped with diet sheet, and pills with functions and side-effects they do not understand. At the out-patient clinics they may meet a succession of junior doctors, none there long enough to get to know them or their family, and none familiar with the problems of managing acute illness at home. The period in the hospital is usually too short and fraught for the cardiac rehabilitation team to assess the patients' psychosocial needs, enable them to deal with the emotional upset and hyperventilation, and guide them in the best possible direction. Furthermore, the early discharge might leave a gap in the care for which the general practitioner is not forewarned and prepared. Rehabilitation may not be available.

Principles

The model of rehabilitation used for 20 years at Charing Cross Hospital was founded upon two principles:

1. There is no close relationship between the anatomy of the coronary arteries and illness such as angina, myocardial infarction and sudden death.
2. The factors which damage the heart's function are derived from the way the individual handles the demands for effort and the physical, psychological and social challenges provided by his external environment.

The belief implicit in these two principles is that individuals can learn to handle effort and emotion without going beyond physiological tolerance and damaging the cardiovascular system. Hence each individual can be assessed and taught what appears to be required for maintaining the heart in the best possible condition.

Furthermore, strategies for anticipation and prevention can be added and integrated with the reactive tactics of conventional cardiovascular medicine and surgery[176,177].

The prescription of a drug to relieve the symptom of angina pectoris leads the patient to believe that it is acceptable to continue to produce chest pain. However, we argue that this course fosters myocardial damage through repeated ischemic battering, and prevents the remission that can so often be obtained by resting and retraining. The essence of the retraining is to keep exercise within 60–70% of the level that would produce pain. This target is just below the anaerobic threshold, beyond which ischemia from coronary constriction or arrhythmia are likely to occur.

Practice

The rehabilitation process starts with an assessment of the biopsychosocial needs of the patients by the doctor working closely with a nurse, occupational- or physiotherapist, hereafter referred to as the therapist. The needs of the individual are defined according to an examination of three factors: the *'disease'*, the distribution and extent of atherosclerosis as gauged by angiography and the degree of left ventricular dysfunction; the clinical *'illness'* which might bear little or no relationship to the disease and the *'predicament'*, an expression of the environmental conditions and social relationships which led to exhaustion, homeostatic impairment and the cardiac catastrophe[178].

The ability of the patient to afford a period of illness, his hardiness, and the quality of his social support are considered to have a strong influence upon the course of the illness and outcome. It has long been understood that morbidity and mortality are lower where the patient can obtain comfort and safety, the best possible conditions for healing, and escape the need to struggle before he is ready for it.

The processes of rehabilitation can be defined as the application of biological, psychological and social (i.e. biopsychosocial) knowledge to patient education. In practice this involves teaching, informing, enabling or training each individual to make the best possible use of himself and his resources, and to reach an optimal level of performance[176,177]. Rehabilitation should begin with a conservation-withdrawal period to permit recovery from exhaustion and energy depletion and promote a return to the healthy function seen on the upslope of the performance–arousal curve (Fig. 3.4).

Conservation-withdrawal

Conservation-withdrawal is the name given by Engel and Schmale to a process of disengagement and inactivity[179]. It is the natural response to hopeless overloading associated with exhaustion and inadequate information, and it provides the appropriate conditions for psychological and physical restoration. This period also provides an opportunity to husband energy, conserve resources and foster anabolic healing processes. Rest and reduction of arousal are essential. Death can occur if sleep is prevented. The necessary introspection that occurs during the conservation-withdrawal period should not be confused with clinical depression. It is inappropriate to jolly the patient out of introspection before his recuperative needs have been met, or to elevate his mood with antidepressant drugs to the point where the ability to rest is lost. The natural reluctance to withdraw from duty is difficult enough to manage without adding iatrogenic obstacles. A widespread difficulty today is the reluctance of the public and the medical profession to accept Moran's aphorism 'if a man is rested in time he will have another summer of high achievement'[180].

From conservation-withdrawal to independence

Adequate rest and sleep during a well-conducted conservation-withdrawal period can achieve a great deal. It provides the opportunity for left ventricular overdistension and dyskinesia to subside, catabolic states such as hypercholesterolemia and hypertension to regress, and homeostatic adaptive capacity to return. It helps the person to move smoothly out of denial without being held up in states of high emotional arousal such as anger, frustration, fear and despair. As the person moves forward he can be encouraged to make the best of his condition and utilize the energy that is beginning to return. The therapist's assessment should include his capacity for assimilating new knowledge and learning how best to take up activities; and the ability of the people around him to accommodate his needs for sleep, rest and peace of mind.

An attitude of patience and optimism should be cultivated. This will enable the individual to outwit the temptations to go 'over the top' (Fig. 3.4) and thereby avoid both the ischemic and arrhythmic consequences of overdistending the left ventricle, and the coronary vasoconstrictive influences of disordered Ca^{++}/Mg^{++} balance. The individual begins to learn that it is usually possible to develop higher levels of performance and hardiness after infarction than could be obtained in the downward spirals of exhaustion and homeostatic disarray before the catastrophe.

The doctor should be available for consultation by the therapist every day, to ensure that action can be taken immediately if the course of rehabilitation is threatened by a physical, psychological or social problem. This freedom of access to the doctor provides the support the therapist needs during the crucial early stages of rehabilitation. In return the doctor gains the advantages of freeing himself from inessential clinic appointments and meeting the patient with the therapist who has already identified the problems and discussed them with the patient and the family. If an intervention such as coronary artery bypass grafting is required, the doctor and therapist can prepare the patient for it and resume rehabilitation afterwards. The outcome of any intervention is likely to be enhanced by the information, support and education provided by the therapist and the doctor. For example, the proper preparation for angioplasty includes the management of exhaustion and hyperventilation[73] in order to reduce the risk of restenosis.

SABRES

The basic educational needs of the patient in biopsychosocial rehabilitation are listed under the acronym SABRES[84,176,177] (Box 3.4). Space does not provide for a full description here, but attention is drawn to points that are often neglected in practice.

Sleep. Each person needs to become aware of the quantity and quality of sleep he requires. Sleep reduces excess catecholamine and cortisol activity[83] and helps the overworked, overdistended left ventricle to return to a proper size[153]. Furthermore, adequate sleep enables emotion and effort to be handled in a much less demanding way. Consequently the general arousal level falls, reducing fatigue and easing the performance of daily activity.

The therapist can take two steps to help. The first is to teach the individual to be aware of the differences in well-being produced by good sleep and bad sleep. The second step is to provide tips and tactics for promoting good sleep, such as unwinding during the evening, setting an 'activity deadline' 90 minutes before bedtime, listening to music, taking a nightcap, avoiding caffeine drinks such as coffee, using a relaxation technique or practicing self-hypnosis. With such tuition most people soon appreciate that the quality of sleep reflects the quality of the day and come to learn that good sleep is a reward for organizing the other elements of SABRES (Box 3.4).

There will be times, particularly in the earlier phases of rehabilitation and in unavoidable periods of effort and distress, when parsimonious but effective doses of sedation are required for success. Small doses of diazepam and or promethazine hydrochloride taken for 2–3 nights can restore the order and stability of cardiovascular regulation when taken before the homeostatic impairment has had the chance to become deeply rooted.

Box 3.4 An acronym listing the essential requirements for restoration and maintenance of health

SABRES

S for Sleep

Awareness of the quality and quantity required for peak performance.

A for Arousal

The ability to manage struggle, hassle and frustration without excessive involvement of the sympathetic nervous system and adrenal medulla.

The ability to accommodate loss, defeat and despair without over-prolonged adreno-cortical activity.

B for Breathing

Awareness of normal patterns and control. Avoidance of the inappropriate and disordered patterns called hyperventilation.

R for Rest

The ability to be still, and at ease.

E for Effort

Awareness of the personal energy cost of physical, mental and emotional effort, and the need for this to be balanced with rest and sleep.

S for Self-esteem

The feeling of worth, confidence and control achieved by the employment of SABRE.

'KNOWLEDGE DISPELS FEAR'

Arousal. In the first stages of recovery the patient's ability to modulate his arousal is low, and so his homeostatic defenses will depend upon external factors such as the well-ordered management of his illness, and a period of conservation-withdrawal that provides for good sleep and protection against overloading. The development of awareness and control of the breathing (vide infra) will help to break the vicious spirals of sympathetic arousal and hypocapnia. As his ability to assimilate information grows he can learn about such things as assertion skills, avoidance of negative 'self-talk', acquisition of flexible attitudes, and the ability to express emotions instead of bottling them up and suffering their somatic consequences. He can learn how to attenuate emotions that interfere with performance, and to avoid over-inflating his emotional responses to contingencies. The lessons are not provided didactically as, for example in a 'stress management' course, but are tailored to his particular needs. The goal is clearly stated to be the improvement of performance and hardiness. Massage may be helpful for teaching arousal reduction, and medical hypnotherapy may be particularly useful in individuals whose hearts continue to be endangered by high levels of anger. A positive emotional focus has been shown to be effective in reducing cardiotoxic sympathetic drive[106].

Breathing. The outcome of a given act of hyperventilation depends upon such factors as arousal level, the quality of sleep, depletion of the body's buffering systems and awareness and control. Most people who suffer from hypocapnia have difficulty in accepting the information that their breathing behavior is abnormal[120,155] (Fig. 3.10), and so they must learn to be aware of what they are doing before they can benefit from breathing lessons. Capnography provides feedback that helps the individual to understand his respiratory dysfunction and recover from it. One simple approach is the use of massage to give the patient the concrete experience of a low arousal state with diaphragmatic breathing. The patient can practice the diaphragmatic breathing to defend himself against the emotional and physical threats of his environment. The somatic symptoms induced by hyperarousal and hyperventilation (anxiety) are a more common cause of post-infarction morbidity than the heart damage itself[181].

Rest. During the recovery from angina pectoris, myocardial infarction and coronary artery bypass grafting the patients cannot afford to be on the go from morning to night. There will be times when being up and about for even an hour will cause obvious fatigue and loss of color. Thus learning to rest is an essential part of restoration. The idea of it is an anathema to most patients: they may have become patients because they were never able to grasp the principle of 'reculer pour mieux sauter.' Rest is important because the goal of optimum performance with order and stability of the internal systems cannot be achieved without a salutary balance of work, play, rest and sleep[182]. The stimulating effects of hyperarousal and hypocapnia can make it impossible for the patient to rest no matter how tired he is[26] and so it is essential to be effective in its management.

Effort. The desire for activity and independence makes it very tempting to return to activity too quickly these days, but it must be borne in mind that both the individual and his heart are susceptible to overloading. Overloading the individual causes exhaustion and homeostatic disorder, and further impairment of the heart through sympathetic overactivity, hypocapnia and disordered Ca^{++}/Mg^{++} ratios.

Overloading the heart causes it to heal with an abnormally large residual volume and a reduced ejection fraction. The benefits of ACE inhibitors in the remodeling processes after ischemic injury should not engender complacency and inattention to the deleterious mechanical effects of overdistending the left ventricle through effort. Angina should be avoided because it inflicts ischemic damage and fosters myocardial fibrosis.

Advice about exercise calls for careful judgement. What sort? how much? how intense? how long? how often? and when to avoid? are the sorts of questions that need to be answered. The guidelines must be flexible because the individual's capacity can vary tenfold according to the quality of sleep and rest, and the presence of hyperarousal and hyperventilation. 'Train not strain' should be the watchwords. In most cases it is reasonable to suggest exercise amounting to about two-thirds of the symptom-limited maximum and to check its safety with an exercise ECG. This check is especially important in the case of those who, through enthusiasm, denial or alexithymia may push themselves into myocardial ischemia without perceiving the usual symptoms of the overtaxed condition. Where assessment of the anaerobic threshold by capnography is available the patient is taught to remain within its limits, thus removing the risks of detraining and cardiac deterioration[158,159].

These exercise guidelines were developed in the early 1960s and the experience at the gymnasium did much to reduce anxiety about the risks of rehabilitation[183]. Today, the activities of daily living such as walking or cycling are popularly used instead of a closely supervised gymnasium for the development of fitness, stamina and confidence and the same guidelines apply. Without guidance confidence is low and every new activity may seem to be a risky adventure. This naturally raises vigilance and arousal and promotes hyperventilation.

Self-esteem. The value one attaches to oneself is badly shaken by the news that the heart is unsound. It may take a year from myocardial infarction before the individual gets up in the morning without wondering momentarily if this day is to be his last. Self-esteem, confidence and security come neither from reassurance nor palliative drugs and operations. They come from the recovery of performance and health that is achieved through guidance out of exhaustion and homeostatic impairment; mastering the self-injurious dynamic factors; and enjoying higher levels of achievement; fulfilling more needs; and adopting a healthier set of compromises. Re-achieving control of life and enjoying increasing ability reduce arousal and its consequences, and restore feelings of worth. A well-guided and successful person who outwits the traps and pitfalls that might cause a relapse may observe 10 years later that the heart attack was the best thing that ever happened to them. Norman Cousins writes well about this aspect of rehabilitation[184].

Impediments to rehabilitation

Doctors and therapists entering rehabilitation encounter a bewildering number of 'heart sink' impediments to success that are rarely included in their training. Outwitting them calls for initiative and leadership, and a great deal of energy. An overtired therapist who depends heavily upon patients' compliance for success courts defeat.

In the exhaustion and uncertainty that attend the coronary catastrophe, the patient may be unable to comprehend or accept the importance of his contribution to recovery. He may be too angry to take part in a cognitive assessment of his needs, and incapable of working out ways of reducing or modifying the burden of his roles in family and social life, and at work. He may 'shop around' for alternatives to the recommended course of rehabilitation in the quest for an easier 'cure' of the disease. He may have little common sense or feeling for the natural order of things, or a chronically low performance–arousal curve (Fig. 3.4) might have minimized his aptitude for coping with novel and complex problems. Some adopt the stance of a detached and distant observer, and use this to avoid involvement with the real problems of the predicament. Others adopt an 'intellectual attitude' and demand 'proof' of the value of every step recommended by the team: they may disdain the attention of juniors who can provide a great deal of time and care, and listen only to the head of the team.

Learning to outwit the impediments develops skills that are extremely useful in the clinical field, and provide great protection for the therapist against the undeniable stresses of the work.

Assessment of outcome

In 1975 the WHO Regional Office for Europe calculated that 68 000 man years of observation in coronary heart disease would be required to demonstrate a 25% improvement of hard end-points (re-infarction and death) by rehabilitation, and no-one could allow for the influence of life events and other variables such as bereavement or loss of work. Funding for rehabilitation has suffered through this apparently impossible system of assessment.

Assessment in small groups such as hospital rehabilitation clinics may depend upon estimates of physical performance, anxiety, hedonic tone, withdrawal from the cardiac surgical waiting list and so forth, but end-points hard enough to justify funding and the choice of rehabilitation vis a vis revascularization procedures are conspicuous by their absence[185]. The problem may be overcome by measuring the respiratory response to the anaerobic threshold[158,159]. In those with effort syndrome it is an appropriate yardstick for the changes brought about by restoration of the body's alkaline buffering systems. In those with coronary heart disease there is a general belief that the benefits of rehabilitation are not derived from alteration of the heart itself but from 'peripheral adaptation'[167]. Pilot studies with small numbers suggest that the crucial peripheral adaptation is the restoration of depleted buffering systems through the biopsychosocial SABRES strategy, the outcome of which can be assessed by measurement of the respiratory response to the anaerobic threshold. After myocardial infarction, bypass surgery and coronary angioplasty it is usual for patients to present for rehabilitation with levels as low as those obtained in effort syndrome and other conditions of chronic fatigue (PGF Nixon, unpublished observations, 1994).

CONCLUSION

It is an age-old belief that the heart 'overtaxed by constant emotional influences or excessive physical effort and thus deprived of its appropriate rest' suffers disorder of function and becomes vulnerable to disease[186].

It is suggested here that the functional disorders are largely derived from the consequences of carrying effort beyond physiological tolerance into a condition of depletion characterized by overbreathing, buffer depletion and dysregulation of the autonomic nervous system. Thomas Lewis gave it the name 'effort syndrome'[24].

It is also suggested that the entropic, catabolic conditions which exist where effort and distress overwhelm homeostatic competence can cause or accelerate coronary heart disease. If this proves to be the case, the heart attack will no longer be regarded simply as a random, arbitrary and unpredictable accident of atheroma, but accepted as a discontinuity in a flawed system, a catastrophe: as such it will become predictable and preventable when there is sufficient information about the interactions between the individual and his social environment, his personal responses and his homeostatic integrity.

A few years ago the information was derived almost entirely from folklore, pattern recognition and intuition, but today the resources for measuring arousal pathology and the consequences of maladaptive behavior are increasing rapidly, and enabling much of the anecdotage to be brought into the mainstream of evidence-based medicine.

The biopsychosocial approach can integrate the newer information about psychological and social influences with the traditional, and open opportunities for exploration such as the 'SABRES' approach to prevention, restoration and rehabilitation.

Doctors may require to deepen their interest in behavior in order to recognize the downhill run to catastrophe; and health education authorities might well consider what syllabus is required for teaching the individual how best to defend his homeostatic integrity when he is overtaxed by the everyday burdens of coping and adapting.

REFERENCES

1 Mair A 1986 Sir James Mackenzie MD. Royal College of General Practitioners, London

2 Dubos R 1980 Man adapting. Yale University Press, New Haven

3 Pickering GW 1955 High blood pressure. Churchill, London
4 Wolf S, Wolff HG 1951 A summary of experimental evidence relating life stress to the pathogenesis of essential hypertension in man. In: Bell ET (ed) Hypertension. University of Minnesota Press, Minneapolis
5 Henry JP 1975 The induction of acute and chronic cardiovascular disease in animals by psychosocial stimulation. International Journal of Psychiatry in Medicine 6:147–58
6 Boyd GW 1989 On stress, disease and evolution. University of Tasmania, Hobart
7 Sterling P, Eyer J 1981 Biological basis of stress-related mortality. Social Science and Medicine 15E:3–42
8 Mayou R, Bryant B, Forfar C, Clark D 1994 Non-cardiac chest pain and benign palpitations in the cardiac clinic. British Heart Journal 72:548–53
9 Gruman J, Chesney M 1995 Introduction for superhighways for disease. Psychosomatic Medicine 57:207
10 Engel GL 1977 The need for a new medical model: a challenge for biomedicine. Science 196:129–36
11 Kahnemann D 1973 Attention and effort. Prentice-Hall, New Jersey
12 Vainshtein II, Siminov PV 1987 Emotiogenic structures of the brain and cardiac activity. Amerind, New Delhi
13 Lader M 1975 Psychophysiological parameters and methods. In: Levi L (ed) Emotions, their parameters and measurement. Raven Press, New York
14 Nixon PGF 1993 The grey area of effort syndrome and hyperventilation: from Thomas Lewis to today. Journal of the Royal College of Physicians of London 27:377–83
15 Lewith GT 1988 Undifferentiated illness: some suggestions for approaching the polysymptomatic patient. Journal of the Royal Society of Medicine 81:563–5
16 Nixon PGF, Bethell HJN 1974 Preinfarction ill health. American Journal of Cardiology 33:446–9
17 Kop WJ, Appels APWM, Mendes de Leon CF, Bar FW 1996 The relationship between severity of coronary artery disease and vital exhaustion. Psychosomatic Medicine 40:397–405
18 Cassell J 1976 The contribution of the social environment to host resistance. American Journal of Epidemiology 104:107–23
19 Henry JP 1983 Coronary heart disease and arousal of the adrenal cortical axis. In: Dembroski TM, Schmidt TH, Blumchen G (eds) Biobehavioural bases of coronary heart disease. Karger, Basel
20 Postle D 1980 Catastrophe theory. Fontana, London
21 Yerkes RM, Dodson JD 1908 The relation of strength of stimulus to rapidity of habit-formation. Journal of Comparative Neurology and Psychiatry 18:459–82
22 Swank RL, Marchand WE 1946 Combat neuroses. Archives of Neurology and Psychiatry 55:236–47
23 Fry RW, Morton AR, Keast D 1991 Overtraining syndrome and the chronic fatigue syndrome Part 1 & 2 New Zealand Journal of Sports Medicine 19:48–52, 76–7
24 Nixon PGF 1995 An appraisal of Thomas Lewis's effort syndrome. Quarterly Journal of Medicine 88:741–7
25 Kobasa SC, Maddi SR, Kahn S 1982 Hardiness and health: a prospective study. Journal of Personality and Social Psychology 42:168–77
26 Nixon PGF 1976 The human function curve. Practitioner 217:765–9, 935–44
27 Editorial 1976 Migrants and cardiovascular disease. British Medical Journal 1:1423–4
28 Weinblatt E, Ruberman W, Goldberg JD, Frank CW, Shapiro S, Chaudhary BS 1978 Relation of education to sudden death after myocardial infarction. New England Journal of Medicine 299:60–5
29 Jenkins DC 1978 Low education: a risk factor for death. New England Journal of Medicine 299:95–7
30 Montagu A 1971 Touching: the human significance of the skin. Columbia University Press, New York
31 Forsdahl A 1977 Are poor living conditions in childhood and adolescence an important risk factor for arteriosclerotic heart disease? British Journal of Preventive and Social Medicine 31:91–5
32 Lynch JJ 1977 The broken heart. Basic Books, New York
33 Weiss JM 1972 Influence of psychological variables on stress-induced pathology. In: Physiology, emotion and psychosomatic illness. Ciba Foundation, Symposium 8. Elsevier, Amsterdam
34 Halliday JL 1949 Psychosocial medicine: a study of the sick society. Heinemann, London
35 Paffenbarger RS, Wolf PA, Notkin J, Thorn MC 1966 Chronic disease in former college students 1: early precursors of fatal coronary heart disease. American Journal of Epidemiology 83:314–28
36 Harburg E, Julius S, McGinn NF, McLeod J, Hoobler SW 1964 Personality traits and behavioural patterns associated with systolic blood pressure levels in college males. Journal of Chronic Diseases 17:405–14
37 Russek HI 1967 Role of emotional stress in the etiology of clinical coronary heart disease. Diseases of the Chest 52:1–9
38 Arlow JA 1945 Identification mechanisms in coronary occlusion. Psychosomatic Medicine 7:195–209
39 Friedman M, Rosenman RH 1974 Type A behavior and your heart. Knopf, New York
40 Tuchman B 1980 The proud tower. Macmillan, London
41 Trist EL 1967 The relation of welfare and development in the transition to post-industrialism. Unpublished monograph. University of Pennsylvania, Pennsylvania
42 Marmot MG, Rose G, Shipley M, Hamilton PJS 1978 Employment grade and coronary heart disease in British civil servants. Journal of Epidemiology and Community Health 32:244–9
43 Henry JP, Stephens PM 1977 Stress, health, and the social environment. Springer-Verlag, New York
44 King JC 1991 Sympathetic and hypocapnic pathways between the brain and the heart: implications for health care. MSc thesis. Roehampton Institute, University of Surrey
45 King JC, Nixon PGF 1995 Effects of non-right-handedness on risk for sudden death associated with coronary artery disease. The American Journal of Cardiology 75:1187
46 Theorell T 1992 The psychosocial environment, stress, and coronary heart disease. In: Marmot M, Elliott P (eds) Coronary heart disease: from aetiology to public health. Oxford University Press, Oxford
47 Karasek RA, Theorell TG, Schwartz J, Pieper C, Alfedsson L 1982 Psychosocial factors and coronary disease. Advances in Cardiology 29:62–7
48 Kagan A, Levi L 1974 Health and environment — psychosocial stimuli: a review. Social Science and

Medicine 8:225–41
49 Beale N, Nethercott S 1986 Job loss and health — the influence of age and previous morbidity. Journal of the Royal College of General Practitioners 36:261–4
50 Ruberman W, Weinblatt E, Goldberg JD, Chaudhary BS 1984 Psychosocial influences on mortality after myocardial infarction. New England Journal of Medicine 311:552–9
51 Knutsson A, Akerstedt T, Jonsson BG, Orth-Gomer K 1986 Increased risk of ischaemic heart disease in shift workers. Lancet 2:89–92
52 Lewis T 1918 The soldier's heart and the effort syndrome. Shaw, London
53 Baroldi G, Mariani G, Falzi G 1978 Degree of coronary obstruction at autopsy in patients with coronary heart disease compared with control population. In: Maseri A, Klassen GA, Lesch M (eds) Primary and secondary angina pectoris. Grune and Stratton, New York
54 James TN 1983 Chance and sudden death. Journal of the American College of Cardiology 1:164–83
55 Sowton E 1979 The treatment of angina pectoris. Practitioner 223:471–6
56 King JC, Nixon PGF 1988 Cardiac rehabilitation: psychophysiological basis and practice. British Journal of Occupational Therapy 51:378–84
57 Verrier RL, Hagestad EL, Lown B 1987 Delayed myocardial ischemia induced by anger. Circulation 75:249–54
58 Bairey CN, Krantz DS, Rozanski A 1990 Mental stress as an acute trigger of ischemic left ventricular dysfunction in coronary artery disease. American Journal of Cardiology 66:28G–31G
59 Ironson G, Taylor CB, Boltwood M et al. 1992 Effects of anger on left ventricular ejection fraction in coronary artery disease. American Journal of Cardiology 70:281–5
60 Sinatra ST, Chawla S 1986 Aortic dissection associated with anger, suppressed rage, and acute emotional stress. Journal of Cardiopulmonary Rehabilitation 6:197–9
61 Deanfield JE, Shea M, Kensett M et al. 1984 Silent myocardial ischaemia due to mental stress. Lancet 2:1001–4
62 Rozanski A, Bairey CN, Krantz DS et al. 1988 Mental stress and the induction of silent myocardial ischemia in patients with coronary artery disease. New England Journal of Medicine 318:1005–12
63 Editorial 1971 The murmuring heart. British Medical Journal 4:125–6
64 Gelernt MD, Hochman JS 1992 Acute myocardial infarction triggered by emotional stress. American Journal of Cardiology 69:1512–3
65 Hachamovitch R, Chang JD, Kuntz RE, Papageorgiou P, Levin MS, Goldberger AL 1995 Recurrent reversible cardiogenic shock triggered by emotional distress with no obstructive coronary disease. American Heart Journal 129:1026–8
66 Verrier RL, Lown B 1984 Behavioral stress and cardiac arrhythmias. Annual Review of Physiology 46:155–76
67 Myers A, Dewar HA 1975 Circumstances attending 100 sudden deaths from coronary artery disease with coroner's necropsies. British Heart Journal 37:1133–43
68 Lown B 1987 Sudden cardiac death: biobehavioural perspective. Circulation 76 (suppl. 1):186–96
69 Engel GL 1968 A life setting conducive to illness: the giving-up — given-up complex. Annals of Internal Medicine 69:293–300
70 Wolf S 1967 The end of the rope: the role of the brain in cardiac death. Journal of the Canadian Medical Association 97:1022–5
71 Purcell H, Mulcahy D 1994 Emotional eclipse of the heart. British Journal of Clinical Practice 48:228–9
72 Kop WJ, Appels APWM, Mendes de Leon CF, De Swart HB, Bar FW 1994 Vital exhaustion predicts new cardiac events after successful coronary angioplasty. Pychosomatic Medicine 56:281–7
73 Ardissino D, Barberis P, De Servi S et al. 1991 Abnormal coronary vasoconstriction as a predictor of restenosis after successful coronary angioplasty in patients with unstable angina pectoris. New England Journal of Medicine 325:1053–7
74 Nixon PGF, Freeman LJ 1988 The 'think test': a further technique to elicit hyperventilation. Journal of the Royal Society of Medicine 81:277–9
75 van Doornen L 1991 Stress and the dynamics behind hypertension, cholesterol and atherosclerosis. In: Appels A (ed) Behavioral observations in cardiovascular research. Swets and Zeitlinger, Amsterdam
76 Dimsdale JE, Herd JA 1982 Variability of plasma lipids in response to emotional arousal. Psychosomatic Medicine 44:413–30
77 Brindley DN, Rolland Y 1989 Possible connections between stress, diabetes, obesity, hypertension and altered lipoprotein metabolism that may result in atherosclerosis. Clinical Science 77:453–61
78 Raab W 1969 Myocardial electrolyte derangement: crucial feature of pluricausal, so-called coronary heart disease. Annals of the New York Academy of Sciences 147:627–86
79 Karasek RA, Russell RS, Theorell T 1982 Physiology of stress and regeneration in job related cardiovascular illness. Journal of Human Stress 8:29–42
80 Henry JP 1982 The relation of social to biological processes in disease. Social Science and Medicine 16:369–80
81 Petch MC 1981 The progression of coronary artery disease. British Medical Journal 283:1073–4
82 Groover ME Jr, Jernigan JA, Martin CD 1960 Variations in serum lipid concentration and clinical coronary disease. American Journal of Medical Science 239:133–8
83 Adam K, Oswald I 1984 Sleep helps healing. British Medical Journal 289:1400–1
84 Nixon PGF 1989 Human functions and the heart. In: Seedhouse D, Cribb A (eds) Changing ideas in health care. Wiley, Chichester
85 Ley R 1988 Panic attacks during sleep: a hyperventilation-probability model. Journal of Behavior Therapy and Experimental Psychiatry 19:181–92
86 Jenkins CD, Stanton B-A, Klein MD, Savageau JA, Harken DE 1983 Correlates of angina pectoris among men awaiting coronary by-pass surgery. Psychosomatic Medicine 45:141–53
87 MacKenzie J 1908 Diseases of the heart. Hodder and Stoughton, London
88 Appels A, Schouten E 1991 Waking up exhausted as a risk indicator of myocardial infarction. American Journal of Cardiology 68:395–8
89 Appels A, Kop W, Bar F, De Swart H, Mendes De Leon C 1995 Vital exhaustion, extent of atherosclerosis, and the clinical course after successful percutaneous

transluminal coronary angioplasty. European Heart Journal 16:1880–5

90 Kleiger RE, Miller JP 1978 Decreased heart rate variability and its association with increased mortality after acute myocardial infarction. American Journal of Cardiology 59:256–62

91 Malliani A, Lombardi F 1978 Neural reflexes associated with myocardial ischemia. In: Schwartz PJ, Brown AM, Malliani A, Zanchetti A (eds) Neural mechanisms in cardiac arrhythmias. Raven Press, New York

92 Schwartz PJ 1984 Sympathetic imbalance and cardiac arrhythmias. In: Randall WC (ed) Nervous control of cardiovascular function. Oxford University Press, Oxford

93 Ricci DR, Orlick AE, Cipriano PR, Guthaner DF, Harrison DC 1979 Altered adrenergic activity in coronary arterial spasm: insight into mechanism based on study of coronary hemodynamics and the electrocardiogram. American Journal of Cardiology 43:1073–9

94 Jones CE, Thomas JX Jr 1984 Neural influences in myocardial ischaemia: effects of neural ablation. In: Randall WC (ed) Nervous control of cardiovascular function. Oxford University Press, Oxford

95 Braunwald E 1981 Coronary artery spasm as a cause of myocardial ischaemia. Journal of Laboratory and Clinical Medicine 97:299–312

96 Robertson RM, Wood AJJ, Vaughn WK, Robertson D 1982 Exacerbation of vasotonic angina pectoris by propranolol. Circulation 65:281–5

97 Zipes DP 1991 Ischemic modulation of cardiac autonomic innervation. Journal of the American College of Cardiology 17:1424–5

98 Malliani A, Schwartz PJ, Zanchetti A 1980 Neural mechanisms in life-threatening arrhythmias. American Heart Journal 100:705–15

99 Levitt B, Cagin N, Kleid J, Somberg J, Gillis R 1976 Role of the nervous system in the genesis of cardiac rhythm disorders. American Journal of Cardiology 37:1111–3

100 Nixon PGF 1968 Cardiac infarction and cardiac resuscitation. In: Baron DN, Compston N, Dawson AM (eds) Recent advances in medicine. Churchill, London

101 Net B, Kolman S, Verrier RL, Lown B 1976 Effect of vagus nerve stimulation upon excitability of the canine ventricle. American Journal of Cardiology 37:1041–5

102 Ryan C, Hollenberg M, Harvey DB, Gwynn R 1976 Impaired parasympathetic responses in patients after myocardial infarction. American Journal of Cardiology 37:1013–8

103 Lum LC 1976 The syndrome of chronic habitual hyperventilation. In: Hill OW (ed) Modern trends in psychosomatic medicine, 3. Butterworth, London

104 Jiang W, Hayano J, Coleman ER et al. 1993 Relation of cardiovascular responses to mental stress and cardiac vagal activity in coronary artery disease. American Journal of Cardiology 72:551–4

105 Lown B, Tykocinski M, Garfein A, Brooks P 1973 Sleep and ventricular premature beats. Circulation 58:691–701

106 McCraty R, Atkinson M, Tiller WA, Rein G, Watkins AD 1995 The effects of emotions on short term heart rate variability using power spectrum analysis. American Journal of Cardiology 76:1089–93

107 Wolf S 1969 Psychosocial forces in myocardial infarction and sudden death. Circulation 39 (suppl. 4):74–81

108 Groen JJ 1975 The measurement of emotion and arousal in the clinical physiological laboratory and in medical practice. In: Levi L (ed) Emotions, their parameters and measurement. Raven Press, New York

109 Knochel JP 1984 Diuretic-induced hypokalemia. In: Stollerman CH (ed) Advances in internal medicine, 30. Year Book, Chicago

110 Seelig M 1989 Cardiovascular consequences of magnesium deficiency and loss: pathogenesis, prevalence and manifestations — magnesium and chloride loss in refractory potassium repletion. American Journal of Cardiology 63:4–21

111 Iseri LT, French JH 1984 Magnesium: nature's physiologic calcium blocker. American Heart Journal 108:188–93

112 Ginsburg R, Bristow MR, Schroeder JS, Harrison DC, Stinson EB 1980 Potential pharmacologic mechanisms involved in coronary artery spasm. In: Bristow MR (ed) Drug-induced heart disease. Elsevier, Amsterdam

113 Yasue H, Omote S, Takizawa A, Nagao M, Nosaka K, Nakajima H 1981 Alkalosis induced coronary vasoconstriction. Effects of calcium, diltiazem, nitroglycerin and propranolol. American Heart Journal 102:206–10

114 Vita JA, Treasure CB, Ganz P, Cox DA, Fish RD, Selwyn AP 1989 Control of shear stress in the epicardial coronary arteries of humans: impairment by atherosclerosis. Journal of the American College of Cardiologists 14:1193–9

115 Ribeiro LGT, Lefer AM 1983 Etiology and pathophysiology. In: Chahine R (ed) Coronary artery spasm. Futura, New York

116 Kushwaha S, Mitchell AG, Yacoub MH 1990 Coronary artery spasm after cardiac transplantation. American Journal of Cardiology 65:1515–8

117 Weiner H 1991 Stressful experience and cardiorespiratory disorders. Circulation 83 (suppl. 2):2–8

118 Jenkins CD 1975 The coronary prone personality. In: Gentry WD, Williams RB (eds) Psychological aspects of myocardial infarction and coronary care. CV Mosby, Saint Louis

119 Schaefer KE 1958 Respiratory pattern and respiratory response to CO_2. Journal of Applied Physiology 13:1–14

120 Lewis B 1954 Chronic hyperventilation syndrome. Journal of the American Medical Association 155:1204–8

121 Meade TW, Brozovic M, Chakrabati RR et al. 1986 Haemostatic function and ischaemic heart disease: principal results of the Northwick Park heart study. Lancet 2:533–7

122 Oliva PB 1981 Pathophysiology of acute myocardial infarction. Annals of Internal Medicine 94:236–50

123 Epstein SE, Quyumi AA, Bonow RO 1989 Sudden cardiac death without warning. New England Journal of Medicine 321:320–4

124 Bashour TT 1991 Vasotonic myocardial ischemia. American Heart Journal 122:1701–22

125 Maseri A, L'Abbate A, Baroldi G et al. 1978 Coronary vasospasm as a possible cause of myocardial infarction. New England Journal of Medicine 299:1271–7

126 Hoshio A, Kotake H, Mashiba H 1989 Significance of coronary artery tone in patients with vasospastic angina. Journal of the American College of Cardiology 14:604–9

127 Maseri A, Newman C, Davies G 1989 Coronary vasomotor tone: a heterogenous entity. European Heart Journal 10:2–5

128 Barger AC, Beeuwkes R 1990 Rupture of coronary vasa vasorum as a trigger of acute myocardial infarc-

tion. American Journal of Cardiology 66:41–3
129 Yasue H, Takizawa A, Nagao M et al. 1986 Pathogenesis of angina pectoris in patients with one vessel disease: possible role of dynamic coronary obstruction. American Heart Journal 112:263–72
130 Davies MD 1989 The pathophysiology of ischaemic heart disease. In: Julian DG, Camm AJ, Fox KM, Hall RJC, Poole-Wilson PA (eds) Diseases of the heart. Balliere Tindall, London
131 Maseri A, Chierchia S, Davies G 1986 Pathophysiology of coronary occlusion in acute infarction. Circulation 73:233–9
132 Gohlke H, Sturzenhofecker P, Thilo A, Droste C, Gornandt L, Roskamm H 1981 Coronary angiographic findings and risk factors in postinfarction patients under the age of 40. In: Roskamm H (ed) Myocardial infarction at young age. Springer-Verlag, Berlin
133 Marzilli M, Goldstein S, Trivella MG, Palumbo C, Maseri A 1980 Some clinical considerations regarding the relation of coronary vasospasm to coronary atherosclerosis: a hypothetical pathogenesis. American Journal of Cardiology 45:882–6
134 Petch MC 1986 Investigation of coronary artery disease. Journal of the Royal College of Physicians of London 20:21–4
135 Ogasawara K, Aizawa T, Nakamura F, Kato K 1989 Angina preceding myocardial infarction and residual coronary narrowing after intracoronary thrombolysis. American Heart Journal 117:804–8
136 Sarmiento RA, Bluguermann JJ, Mora RCAG, Riccitelli MA, Bertolasi CA 1989 Acute myocardial infarction-related coronary artery residual narrowing after intravenous streptokinase: relationship with previous coronary symptoms. American Heart Journal 118:888–92
137 Matsuda Y, Fujii B, Takashiba K et al. 1989 Presence of angina pectoris before acute myocardial infarction and degree of residual stenosis after coronary thrombolysis. American Heart Journal 117:1014–7
138 Kawai C 1994 Pathogenesis of acute myocardial infarction. Circulation 90:1033–43
139 Engel HJ, Page HL Jr, Campbell WB 1976 Coronary artery spasm as the cause of myocardial infarction during coronary arteriography. American Heart Journal 91:501–6
140 Maseri A, L'Abbate A, Baroldi G et al. 1978 Coronary vasospasm as a possible cause of myocardial infarction. New England Journal of Medicine 299:1271–7
141 Dalen JE, Ockene IS, Alpert JS 1982 Coronary spasm, coronary thrombosis, and myocardial infarction: a hypothesis concerning the pathophysiology of acute myocardial infarction. American Heart Journal 104:1119–24
142 Benacerraf A, Scholl JM, Archard F, Tonnelier M, Lavergne G 1983 Coronary spasm and thrombosis associated with myocardial infarction in a patient with nearly normal coronary arteries. Circulation 67:1147–50
143 Hackett D, Davies G, Chierchia S, Maseri A 1987 Intermittent coronary occlusion in acute myocardial infarction. New England Journal of Medicine 317:1055–9
144 Little W 1990 Angiographic assessment of the culprit coronary artery lesion before acute myocardial infarction. American Journal of Cardiology 66:44G–47G
145 Kahn JK, Hartzler GO 1991 Evidence for dynamic coronary vasoconstriction in the early minutes of acute myocardial infarction. American Heart Journal 121:188–90
146 Kuga T, Tagawa H, Tomoike H et al. 1993 Role of coronary artery spasm in progression of organic coronary stenosis and acute myocardial infarction in a swine model. Circulation 87:573–82
147 Fukai T, Koyanagi S, Takeshita A 1993 Role of coronary vasospasm in the pathogenesis of myocardial infarction: study in patients with no significant coronary stenosis. American Heart Journal 126:1305–11
148 Igarashi Y, Tamura Y, Suzuki K et al. 1993 Coronary artery spasm is a major cause of sudden cardiac arrest in survivors without underlying heart disease. Coronary Artery Disease 4:177–85
149 Anderson TW 1970 Role of myocardium in the modern epidemic of ischaemic heart-disease. Lancet 2:753–5
150 Ross RJM, Miell JP, Buchanan CR 1991 Avoiding autocannabilism. British Medical Journal 303:1147–8
151 Lesser IM 1985 Alexithymia. New England Journal of Medicine 313:690–2
152 Bagby RM, Parker JDA, Taylor GJ 1994 The twenty-item alexithymia scale –1. Item selection and cross validation of the factor structure. Journal of Psychosomatic Research 38:23–32
153 Nixon PGF 1974 Non-invasive techniques in angina pectoris. In: Paul O (ed) Angina Pectoris. Medcom Press, New York
154 Nixon PGF 1995 Pathophysiology of hyperventilation. Quarterly Journal of Medicine 88:295–9
155 King JC, Rosen SD, Nixon PGF 1990 Failure of perception of hypocapnia: physiological and clinical implications. Journal of the Royal Society of Medicine 83:765–7
156 Rosen SD 1994 Hyperventilation and the chronic fatigue syndrome. Quarterly Journal of Medicine 87:373–4
157 Lewis T 1915 Lectures on the heart. Shaw, London
158 Nixon PGF 1994 Effort syndrome: hyperventilation and reduction of anaerobic threshold. Biofeedback and Self Regulation 19:155–69
159 Whipp BJ, Davis JA, Wasserman K 1989 Ventilatory control of the isocapnic buffering region in rapidly incremental exercise. Respiratory Physiology 76:357–68
160 Lane RD, Caruso AC, Brown VL et al. 1994 Effects of non-right-handedness on risk for sudden death associated with coronary heart disease. American Journal of Cardiology 74:743–7
161 Stein PK, Bosner MS, Kleiger RE, Conger BM 1994 Heart rate variability: a measure of cardiac autonomic tone. American Heart Journal 127:1376–81
162 Malliani A, Pagani M, Lombardi F 1994 Physiology and clinical implications of variability of cardiovascular parameters with focus on heart rate and blood pressure. American Journal of Cardiology 73:3C–9C
163 Carney RM, Saunders RD, Freedland KE, Stein P, Rich MW, Jaffe AS 1995 Association of depression with reduced heart rate variability in coronary artery disease. American Journal of Cardiology 76:562–4
164 Rose GA 1990 Reflections on the changing times. British Medical Journal 301:683–7
165 Rosenman RH 1986 Current and past history of Type A behavior pattern. In: Schmidt TH, Dembroski TM, Blumchen G (eds) Biological and psychological factors in cardiovascular disease. Springer-Verlag, Berlin
166 Rosen SD, King JC, Nixon PGF 1994 Hyperventilation in patients who have sustained myocardial infarction

after a work injury. Journal of the Royal Society of Medicine 87:268–71

167 Hellerstein HK, Ford AB 1960 Comprehensive care of the coronary patient. Circulation 22:1166–78

168 Amsterdam EA, Laslett LJ, Dressendorfer RH, Mason DT 1981 Exercise training in coronary heart disease: is there a cardiac effect. American Heart Journal 101:870–3

169 Mayou R, MacMahon D, Sleight P, Florencio MJ 1981 Early rehabilitation after myocardial infarction. Lancet 2:1399–1401

170 Froelicher V 1981 Exercise and health. American Journal of Medicine 70:987–8

171 Clarke RS, Ballantyne D 1981 Physical activity and coronary heart disease. Scottish Medical Journal 26:15–20

172 Burridge P, Logan R 1981 A multi-disciplinary coronary rehabilitation programme three years initial experience. New Zealand Medical Journal 93:411–3

173 Frasure-Smith N, Prince R 1985 The ischemic heart disease life stress monitoring program: impact on mortality. Psychosomatic Medicine 47:431–45

174 van Dixhoorn J, Duivenvoorden HJ, Staal HA, Pool J 1989 Physical training and relaxation therapy in cardiac rehabilitation assessed through a composite criterion for training outcome. American Heart Journal 118:545–52

175 Dienstfrey H 1992 What makes the heart healthy? a talk with Dean Ornish. Advances 8:25–45

176 King JC 1996 Acute cardiovascular disorder and disease. In: Turner A, Foster M, Johnson SE (eds) Occupational therapy and physical dysfunction, 4th edn. Churchill Livingstone, Edinburgh

177 Nixon PGF 1992 Behavioral management and rehabilitation after acute myocardial infarction. In: Byrne DG, Caddy GR (eds) Behavioral medicine — international perspectives. Ablex, New Jersey

178 Taylor DC 1979 The components of sickness: diseases, illnesses and predicaments. Lancet 2:1008–10

179 Engel GL, Schmale AH 1972 Conservation-withdrawal: a primary regulatory process for organismic homeostasis. In: Physiology, emotion and psychosomatic disease. Ciba Foundation Symposium 8. Elsevier, Amsterdam

180 Lord Moran 1984 The anatomy of courage. Keynes, London

181 Cay E, Philip A, Aitken C 1976 Psychosocial aspects of cardiac rehabilitation. In: Hill O (ed) Modern trends in psychosomatic medicine, 3. Butterworth, London

182 Meyer A 1922 Philosophy of occupational therapy. Archives of Occupational Therapy 1:1–10

183 Nixon PGF, Carruthers ME, Taylor DJE, Bethell HJN, Grabau W 1976 British pilot study of exercise therapy II: patients with cardiovascular disease. British Journal of Sports Medicine 10:54–61

184 Cousins N 1983 The healing heart. International Journal of Cardiology 3:57–65

185 Julian D 1995 The angina management programme. British Journal of Cardiology 2:219

186 Hilton J 1863 On the influence of mechanical and physiological rest. Bell and Daldy, London

CHAPTER CONTENTS

4

Hypertension

Derek W. Johnston

INTRODUCTION

Primary hypertension, i.e. raised blood pressure of no clearly identified origin, is found in up to 20% of the adult population in the industrialized world and is associated with an increased risk of cardiovascular disease, including myocardial infarction and stroke[1]. For example, if the conventional figure of a persistent diastolic blood pressure of 90 mm Hg and above is taken as indicating hypertension, then the risk of myocardial infarction is doubled compared with that of normotensives, and the risk of stroke is increased by an even greater amount. With higher pressures these risks increase further[1]. Meta-analysis of pharmacological trials[2] have shown that a reduction in blood pressure has a major effect on the incidence of stroke and a lesser effect on myocardial infarction. However the value of pharmacological therapy for mild hypertension remains controversial.

There is increasing evidence that behavioral and psychological processes play an important part in the etiology and maintenance of high blood pressure. Since these processes are potentially reversible (unlike, for example, a family history of hypertension) they have excited considerable interest. The psychological and behavioral factors can be conveniently separated into health behaviors and more directly psychological factors such as stress or personality patterns. Health behaviors, such as overeating, increased salt intake or lack of exercise lead to elevations in blood pressure via a relatively straightforward physical mechanism. In contrast, psychological factors may promote hypertension through a more complex interaction of cortical, brainstem vasomotor and limbic centers with neurohumoural and adrenomedullary mechanisms. Although health behaviors are of great importance in the etiology and treatment of hypertension, this chapter will focus on psychological factors.

PSYCHOLOGICAL FACTORS: DEFINITION OF STRESS

The central question in this area is whether stress causes hypertension. The first hurdle in tackling this question is defining stress. It is generally accepted that there is no entirely satisfactory definition of stress. Kasl (1984)[3], like many others, has pointed out the term 'stress' is used in a number of different ways in psychological studies. Stress has been considered:

1. An environmental condition;
2. An appraisal of an environmental situation;
3. A response to the environment condition or its appraisal;
4. A description of the interaction between environmental demands and an individual's capacity to meet these demands.

The most widely accepted definitions focus on an individual's inability to meet environmental demands and most textbooks in the field emphasize the psychological and physiological responses that ensue when a situation threatens to exceed the person's capacity to deal with it. However, precise definitions do not capture all the phenomena one wishes to describe under the term 'stress', and it is best to use a more wide-ranging definition that encompasses all the processes and practices that are commonly regarded as stress-related. This includes environments that are either universally accepted as taxing (say a war zone), as well as environments that may only tax some individuals; the processes of appraising these environments which includes the characteristics of an individual that may enhance the perception of the environment as stressful or indeed act to alter the environment in a stress enhancing manner (such as the competitive, hostile behavior characteristic of the Type A Behavior Pattern), and the behavioral and physiological responses to the stressful stimuli. Such a generous definition of stress has to be handled with care and in particular it is important to avoid the error of assuming the presence of stress from a subject's physiological response alone.

ETIOLOGY OF HYPERTENSION

Animal studies

The cardiovascular effects of stress have been studied in animal models of hypertension, in laboratory and field studies of the effects of stress on normotensives, hypertensives and individuals at heightened risk of hypertension, and in epidemiological studies of personality factors and environmental stress in the development of hypertension.

It is likely that only studies of lower animals can show a convincing causal relationship between stress and persistent raised blood pressure. Even the results of these studies are rather mixed and it is likely that the effects are heavily dependent on the exact species or strain of animal studied, the particular stressor used and perhaps even procedure variations such as how blood pressure is measured[4]. In the laboratory rat or mouse a variety of experimental manipulations that common sense and the animal's behavior suggest are stressful; such as handling, electric shock, and social encounters in animals reared in isolation, can lead to elevations in pressure. The central question is whether such elevations persist in the absence of the stressor, as presumably they must if this is to model the persistent hypertension of humans. This has proved difficult to demonstrate. Starting from the pioneering work of Folkow[5], it has been claimed that repeated elevations of pressure can lead to sustained hypertension, perhaps through structural alterations of the blood vessels. Forsyth (1971)[6] showed that, in monkeys, prolonged shock avoidance stress led to an initial increase in blood pressure due primarily to increased cardiac output which was eventually replaced by a sustained increase in pressure due to increased peripheral resistance. This has obvious similarities with one model of the progression of hypertension over time in humans[7].

Henry, Stephens and Santisteban (1975)[8] claimed that mice show persistent elevations in pressure and signs of heart damage after prolonged exposure to social stress. Lawler and colleagues (1980 and 1981)[9,10] demonstrated that rats under a shock avoidance regime showed elevations in pressure if they had a modest genetic propensity to high blood pressure, so-called borderline hypertensive rats. These animals also show reduced baroreflex sensitivity under chronic stress[11]. Such rats do not show equivalent elevations in pressure in benign environments and non-hypertension prone rats survived the avoidance regime with normal pressure. Similar findings come from the work of Anderson, Kearns and Better (1983)[12] showing that dogs that were fed a high salt diet had persistent elevations of pressure in shock avoidant situations, but neither salt alone nor stress alone raised pressure, although others have not found such an interaction of stress and salt in the rat[13,14].

These studies demonstrate a finding of fundamental importance; stress alone rarely produces hypertension rather it does so only in combination with some predisposing, or sensitizing, factor. This defines the 'stress diathesis model' which dominates research on this topic, and in psychosomatics in general. Following Henry[15], Lawler argues that the stressors which produce elevations in pressure in the borderline hypertensive rat involve some form of active coping (see discussion of Obrist's work below) and are associated with increased activity in the sympathetic adrenal medulla axis. They have shown increased levels of noradrenaline in the hypothalamus after chronic stress[13].

Neurophysiology

There has been a considerable amount of experimental work investigating the central regulation of blood pressure. Although there is some debate current opinion holds that blood pressure is regulated centrally by the vasomotor center situated in the rostral ventrolateral medulla (RVLM)[16]. However, central regulation is a complex process with different cell groups within the RVLM controlling different vascular beds[17], and a number of afferent inputs from chemoreceptor and baroreceptor neurones plus higher cortical centers all influencing blood pressure regulation. In fact it has been suggested that different nuclei within the brainstem regulate the blood pressure response to different behavioral stimuli or emotional states[18].

This work provides clear scientific evidence of how thoughts and emotions can regulate blood pressure directly through specific neurophysiological pathways. For example, there is a wealth of neuroanatomical and neurophysiological evidence indicating that the central nucleus of the amygdala, through its extensive projections to the motor cortex, the lateral hypothalamus, and other brainstem vasomotor and autonomic nuclei, acts as a command center coordinating the pressor response, the neuroendocrine response and the behavioral and immunological responses to stressful stimuli[19,20,21]. Thus pathways have been identified which link the emotional and thinking centers to the blood pressure center and therefore provide a mechanism for how chronic stress can lead to hypertension. However, in order to determine whether chronic stress plays an important etiological role, by activating such pathways, in human hypertension we must evaluate the human studies.

Human studies

Cardiovascular hyper-reactivity

Humans, like non-human animals, respond to stress with large elevations in blood pressure. Clearly it is difficult to examine the effects of chronic stress experimentally in humans. Studies of acute stress have, however, been informative. Brod et al. (1959)[22], in a classic study, showed that tasks such as mental arithmetic raised blood pressure in healthy young volunteers and hypertensives. Brod et al. concluded that acute laboratory stress primarily affected blood pressure by altering cardiac output. For almost the next 30 years this remained the dominant view. Obrist and colleagues and successors have demonstrated (see Obrist, 1981)[23] that many subjects showed a large increase in cardiac output, particularly on tasks such as difficult paced choice reaction time, which involved what Obrist termed active coping, i.e. a continuous demanding but possible series of behavioral adjustments. Impossible tasks had little effect on blood pressure once the subject had established that the tasks were impossible, nor did tasks that did not demand an active behavioral adjustment, such as the cold pressor test or viewing a stressful film (so-called passive coping tasks). Beta-blockade studies led Obrist[24] to conclude that these effects were primarily due to the effects of the sympathetic nervous system on the heart.

This distinction between active and passive coping has been critical to research and theorizing on the psychological precursors of hypertension in people and, to a lesser extent, in animal studies. Obrist argued that active coping tasks lead to a metabolically excessive increase in cardiac output and the resulting over perfusion of tissues with oxygenated blood lead to a local increase in peripheral resistance (previously demonstrated by Forsyth (1971))[6]. While subsequent studies involving oxygen consumption, have shown that heart rate, and presumably cardiac output, is increased to beyond the metabolic demands of the task during active coping[25], the actual mechanism linking this to hypertension has not been convincingly established.

As indicated above, studies of the natural history of hypertension, particularly the long-term studies of Lund-Johansen (1977)[7] suggest that young, borderline hypertensives have raised blood pressure that is primarily determined by a raised cardiac output without a compensating lowering in peripheral resistance, while with passage of time cardiac output drops back to normal and hypertension is determined by raised peripheral resistance. The processes that lead to this change in the mechanism underlying the raised pressure are not well understood, but may relate to mechanical changes in the blood vessels as a result of persistent raised pressure. Studies of the effects of stress on people with either borderline hypertension or established hypertension are consistent with the view that active coping is critical in the development of hypertension. A meta-analysis by Fredrikson and Matthews (1990)[26] showed that while both borderline and established hypertensives showed enhanced blood pressure responses to laboratory challenges, the response to active coping tasks was particularly large in the borderline subjects, who are likely to go on to have sustained hypertension.

The returns from studies of the cardiovascular effect of acute laboratory stress have been considerable. However, it is not clear how well such findings relate to cardiovascular responses in real life. Much current research utilizes the great advances in ambulatory physiological measurement to determine if the effects seen in the laboratory relate to elevations in blood pressure in field studies. The results have been very mixed[27]. Most studies have used devices that measure pressure quite infrequently, perhaps every 30 minutes, and might therefore be very insensitive to the transitory effects of stress. Field studies using continuous, intra-arterial measures of blood pressure[28,29], have shown positive relationships between the effects of laboratory stressors on blood pressure and blood pressure variability. Similarly studies of continuously measured heart rate, particularly after controlling for the effects of physical activity on the cardiovascular system[30], have also shown that heart rate responses to laboratory challenge and heart rate variability in the field are sympathetically mediated[31]. Continuous non-invasive ambulatory measures of blood pressure have recently been developed[32]. Using such a device Jain has shown that subjects who produce large elevations in blood pressure and heart rate during an active coping task also have higher blood pressure and heart rate when they claim to be under stress in real life[33,34].

One cannot establish cause and effect relationships in studies of subjects with established hypertension. Rather stronger evidence comes from studies of the offspring of hypertensives, who are known to be predisposed to hypertension. Fredrickson and Matthews (1990)[26] showed in their meta-analysis that the blood pressure at rest of the teenage offspring of hypertensives is little different from subjects with no family history of hypertension, but when stressed they show an greater increase in pressure. They often show a greater increase in heart rate also, suggesting that cardiac output is an important determinant of the raised pressure. Again the combined effects of stress and vulnerability are evident. Vogele and Steptoe (1992)[35] have extended these findings in a recent series of papers, and have shown that a family history (and presumably a genetic predisposition to hypertension) also interacts with personality to produce large pressure increase in response to active coping tasks. Vogele and Steptoe (1993)[36] found that schoolboys who inhibit anger and have parents with raised blood pressure are more likely to show large pressor responses to various mental stress tests. More general issues of personality and hypertension are discussed below.

An obvious implication of the claim that a large cardiovascular response to active coping tasks plays a role in the development of hypertension is that such responses should predict hypertension prospectively in an initially normotensive population. There have been a number of studies that have used the cold pressor test (a task involving passive coping). The results of such studies have been mixed although positive predictions have been reported[37]. Light et al. (1992)[38] have described a 10–15-year follow-up of the predictive power of an active coping task in a small cohort of young men. They found that an enhanced cardiac response did predict raised blood pressure 15 years later. In a recent substantial study of civil servants in Whitehall Carroll et al. (1995)[39] found only the slightest of relationships between the pressor response to a mental stressor and increases in blood pressure over 5 years. However, blood pressure did not rise on average over this period in the middle-aged subjects and it may require a longer follow-up to establish the relationship. Such studies are essential to provide evidence for the view that cardiovascular hyper-reactivity is central to the development of hypertension. However, epidemiological evidence of this kind cannot be conclusive in establishing causality since both the initial response to the active coping task and the later raised blood pressure could reflect the effects of some other process.

Personality and hypertension

It was once thought probable that personality might be an important correlate or even a cause of hypertension. There is now a much greater appreciation of the role of symptoms, diagnosis and treatment in the production of the various personality types thought to be characteristic of particular diseases[40]. However, there has been a persistent interest in the study of anger in hypertension and in heart disease in general. We have argued that the data suggest that hypertension is associated with the inhibition of anger[41]. However the data are not as strong as one might wish. Perhaps the most compelling study is that of Kahn et al. (1972)[42] who examined the precursors of hypertension in a 5-year prospective study of 10 000 people. Suppression of anger at work or home and a tendency to brood were all associated with an increased incidence of hypertension. Other supportive evidence has been provided. Harburg et al. (1973)[43], working in inner city Detroit, showed that males (both black and white) who responded to various anger provoking scenarios with anger suppression or guilt were more likely to be hypertensive. This was not confirmed in a later study using the same anger scenarios in a predominantly white rural community[44]. The latter study did, however, show that anger suppression, combined with pre-existent raised blood pressure, was associated with increased all-cause mortality in a 12-year prospective study of almost 700 middle-aged men and women.

Social and environmental factors

If stress is important in the development of hypertension then one would expect that individuals and communities under most stress would display the greatest prevalence of hypertension. Classic studies have shown that blood pressure rises with unemployment and drops when work is found[45], and that subjects in stressful occupations, such as air traffic controllers, have higher blood pressure than other workers in the same airports[46]. The complexity of such relationships was illustrated by DeFrank, Jenkins and Rose (1987)[47] in a study of the rise of blood pressure in air traffic controllers over a 5-year period. They showed there was a subset of subjects whose pressure rose, but that this related to increased consumption of alcohol. While the latter might well have been stress-related, this study shows that one cannot assume that the direct relationships between stress and blood pressure one sees in the laboratory are translated into similar relationships in other less controlled situations. This is particularly likely when studying the effects of all-embracing processes such as social deprivation which affect diet, housing, employment and education. Nevertheless in the British Regional Heart Study the areas with the greatest social disadvantage had the highest prevalence of hypertension in middle-aged men[48], and children[49].

The complexity of establishing relationships in field studies is neatly illustrated by mounting evidence of the importance of distinguishing subjective and objective stress. Most studies relying on objective measures of stress, such as measures of deprivation or job strain, suggest that stress is associated with an increased prevalence of hypertension. However *lower* subjective levels of stress are also associated with hypertension. Winkleby, Ragland and Syme (1988)[50] found that hypertensive San Francisco bus drivers reported lower levels of stress than their normotensive colleagues. It is possible that elevated pressure is associated with a tendency to minimize the stressful nature of events. This may relate to the persistent finding in animals[51] and people[52] that raised blood pressure is associated with lower sensitivity to pain, possibly mediated by the central effects of baroreceptor activity. It has been suggested that such reduced sensitivity may contribute to a persistent elevation in pressure by attenuating the warning signs of impending or current threat[53].

Despite the complexities of the relationships that have been established and the inevitable need for more information, it appears probable that stress, in combination with a genetic or environmentally induced vulnerability, is likely to be the main determinant of hypertension in a small number of patients and contribute to the raised pressure of many of the remainder.

STRESS MANAGEMENT

If stress is involved in the etiology or maintenance of hypertension then it is clearly attractive to attempt to prevent or treat high blood pressure using different forms of stress management. Not surprisingly stress management is nearly as difficult to define as stress. I have suggested that it can be considered as any behavioral or psychological procedure offered or undertaken that deliberately attempts to alter beneficially any aspect of the stress process, including altering the environment, subjective appraisal of that environment and the subjective, behavioral and physiological responses to the stressful experience[54].

There is now a substantial number of randomized controlled trials assessing the efficacy of various forms of stress management for hypertension. A variety of summary and meta-analyses of these studies have been conducted. Until recently they have been generally positive[55,56]. However, some of the most recent studies appear to contradict these positive views (see below). What then is the current position on the use of stress management with hypertensives?

Firstly it is necessary to consider the procedures used in the more successful studies. The successful therapies are based on relaxation and have a number of key characteristics.

1. They are based on live (rather than tape-recorded) relaxation training;
2. They include regular home practice;
3. Patients apply relaxation in stressful situations;
4. Most successful therapies involve some form of counseling, often simple and informal.

Therapy appears equally effective given individually or in groups. This type of therapy was developed and studied by Patel in a series of pioneering papers in the 1970s and 1980s[57–60]. In these papers Patel showed that relaxation-based stress management was associated with sizeable reductions in blood pressure which persisted for up to 4 years and appeared to lead to a reduced risk of myocardial infarction or related heart conditions.[58] Similar reductions in pressure were reported by researchers in various countries[61,62], in studies that used elaborate control or comparison conditions[63,64], and in studies that measured blood pressure in a variety of ways, including ambulatory measurement of blood pressure at the work place.[65]

In addition to these positive studies, there were a few studies[66] which failed to find any effect of stress management. However, the most important negative evidence has come from more recent studies. Agras and Chesney, in twin studies, examined the effects of various forms of relaxation and biofeedback-based stress management in hypertensive men identified through a factory blood pressure screening programme. Agras et al. (1987)[67] examined men who were poorly controlled on their existing medication while Chesney et al. (1987)[68] examined unmedicated hypertensives. Agras et al. found that relaxation led to an initial drop in pressure that was greater than in the control group (who simply received blood pressure monitoring). However, over the next 2 years pressure continued to drop in the control group so that the relaxation group lost their advantage. Chesney et al. could not find any advantage of relaxation training over a variety of procedures at any time over the 2 years of the study. Pressure dropped equally in trained groups or in subjects who simply received blood pressure monitoring, presumably due to habituation to blood pressure measurement.

Three important subsequent studies also failed to find any advantage of relaxation training over control procedures. Van Montfrans et al. (1990)[69] examined the effects of relaxation training on blood pressure measured continuously over a 24-hour period using the intra-arterial method of determining pressure, the gold standard in blood pressure measurement. All other studies have either relied on blood pressure measured using the usual, very limited, clinic measures or have used the discontinuous ambulatory methods that, while probably better than clinic measures, are far from perfect. Using continuous measures Van Montfrans et al. could find no reduction in pressure over a 24-hour period as a result of relaxation.

Irvine and Logan (1991)[70] compared relaxation-based stress management with supportive psychotherapy, in a substantial study of both men and women recruited from a worksite screening programme. Pressure dropped equally in both groups. In addition there was no difference between the conditions in the pressor response to various psychological challenges. Johnston et al. (1993)[71], following up an earlier study by the same group in which relaxation was more effective than a control treatment[64], compared relaxation and an exercise-based control condition in almost 100 unmedicated hypertensives. Outcome was assessed by clinic blood pressure, discontinuous ambulatory blood pressure, the pressor response to a challenging interview and a measure of left ventricular mass. This is often enlarged in patients with raised blood pressure and reduces when pressure drops over a prolonged period. It might therefore serve as a indicator of a sustained drop in pressure. Johnston et al. could find no difference on clinic or ambulatory blood pressure or left ventricular mass between relaxation and the control condition either over the 6 months of treatment or a 6-month follow-up period. Additionally, and most unusually, there was no reduction in pressure in either group.

There was a slight reduction in the pressor response to the challenging interview in the relaxation trained subjects. While this the effect was small it might indicate that the subjects receiving stress management were able to apply it successfully in a stressful situation. Studies with positive results continue to be reported[72,73], however they are often rather small or on unusual populations. An apparent exception is a recent study by Schneider et al. (1995)[74]. They compared progressive muscle relaxation with Transcendental Meditation (TM) and a lifestyle education program in a substantial sample of elderly black Americans with mild to moderate hypertension. They found that both TM and relaxation lowered both systolic and diastolic blood pressure in the clinic. In addition, TM produced reliably greater reductions. TM also had a greater effect on systolic (but not diastolic) blood pressure at home. This study is discussed further below.

Most, but not all (see Eisenberg et al. (1993))[75], of the various summary analyses have suggested that there may be a modest effect of stress management on blood pressure[55,56]. However, it is clear that there is a temporal trend in the findings which have become less positive in the last 8 to 10 years and it difficult to know how to balance the early positive reports with the more recent negative ones. Jacob et al. (1991)[55], in a helpful analysis of the factors affecting the reduction of pressure in controlled trials of stress management, pinpointed two factors. These are the starting level of blood pressure and the related issue of the length of the baseline period over which pressure was measured before treatment started. They claim that pressure dropped more with relaxation in studies in which initial pressure was highest and in which the baseline period was shortest. In recent years studies have been conducted on patients with only mild elevations in pressure, in part because of the belief that drug treatment could not be withheld from patients with the higher pressures, but also to ensure adequate sample size. In addition, baseline assessment periods have lengthened in an attempt to deal with the increasingly recognized instability of blood pressure. Both factors are well illustrated in our last study[71] in which blood pressure was measured daily for at least 3 months before the patient received treatment. After such a prolonged baseline no further drop in pressure occurred in the patients who entered the study, many of whom had by that time, only mild elevations in pressure.

The results of controlled trials of stress management of hypertension therefore suggest that stress management is most effective in patients with high mild or even low moderate hypertension and in whom blood pressure has not stabilized. It has been pointed out that these are of course the conditions most likely to lead to various forms of experimental error through factors such as regression to the mean, and this has led to some concern that relaxation may be doing virtually nothing.[76] This conclusion may be premature. Random errors in measurement should reduce the power to find differences between interventions and there should be a drop in pressure irrespective of treatment. This is not the finding in the positive studies nor in most of the meta-analyses and suggests there is some form of interaction between relaxation and the natural processes that lead to reductions in pressure over time. Relaxation may lead to faster, or even greater, reductions in pressure in those subjects whose pressure might well have dropped during an extensive baseline. It may be that such subjects are more anxious, either generally or about blood pressure measurement, and relaxation helps to reduce this anxiety and/or its cardiovascular effects.

This hypothesis does not appear to apply to the aberrant findings of Schneider et al. (1995)[74] with elderly black Americans since the baseline period (approximately four measurement visits over 4 to 8 weeks) was reasonably extensive and the final pre-treatment blood pressure levels were as low as 144/89 in the relaxation group. The critical issue, however, may relate to the anxiety or stress levels of their patients. As Schneider et al. point out, his patients come from a disadvantaged, highly stressed group in whom hypertension may be more likely to be stress-related compared with the white samples studied in most of the previous trials. Indeed that was one of the reasons for conducting this study. It would not appear surprising if relaxation and related procedures are beneficial in subjects or populations in whom stress is involved in the observed elevations in pressure. These may be the rather specific processes involved in white coat hypertension or perhaps the more general processes that lead to individuals or a population having an increased risk of hypertension. One might hope that interventions to lower pressure in the latter situation would have significant health benefits.

IMPLICATIONS FOR TREATMENT

It is difficult to determine the practical implications of both the research on the role of stress in the etiology of primary hypertension and the recent randomized trials of relaxation-based stress management. It is very likely that objectively determined stress leads to, or has led to, elevations in pressure in a proportion of patients with high blood pressure. This suggests that stress management should be helpful, however the evidence that stress management can lower raised blood pressure is now markedly less strong than it appeared a decade ago and it would be foolhardy to recommend the widespread use of such procedures. However there are undoubtedly well conducted studies that do show beneficial effects of stress management and I am sure that I am not alone in being impressed with its effectiveness in some patients who were not responding well to other forms of treatment. The obvious solution is to select the appropriate patients, but the literature offers few clues as to who they might be. While patients with high levels of perceived stress or anxiety might seem appropriate the evidence suggests that one should make a particular effort to select patients in objectively stressful situations, even if they do not report heightened stress or distress.

Selection of such patients would, at present, be based on theory rather than firm evidence. This is hardly a satisfactory outcome of at least four decades of research on the psychological etiology of hypertension and two decades of systematic treatment research. However, the picture can be viewed more positively. Research has shown that blood pressure is susceptible to a wide range of psychological, social and environmental influences. It is unlikely that a few measurements of blood pressure in the doctor's surgery can determine if a patient has hypertension requiring treatment and the available research literature suggests that a comparatively simple package of home blood pressure measurement, simple training in relaxation and commonsense advice on health behaviors (related to weight, diet, exercise and alcohol consumption) could almost certainly reduce the number of patients receiving prolonged anti-hypertensive medication and improve their health.

REFERENCES

1 Pooling Project Research Group 1978 Relation of blood pressure, serum cholesterol, smoking habit, relative weight and ECG abnormalities to incidence of major coronary events: Final report of the Pooling Project. Journal of Chronic Disease 31:201–306

2 MacMahon S, Cutler JA, Stamler J 1989 Antihypertensive drug treatment: potential, expected, and observed effects on stroke and on coronary heart disease. Hypertension 13(suppl I):I-45–I-50

3 Kasl SV 1984 Stress and health. Annual Review of Public Health 5:319–41

4 LeMaire V, Mormede P 1995 Telemetered recording of blood pressure and heart rate in different strains of rats during chronic social stress. Physiology and Behavior 58:1181–8

5 Folkow B 1982 Physiological aspects of primary hypertension. Psychological Reviews 62:347–504

6 Forsyth RP 1971 Regional blood flow changes during 72 hour avoidance. Science 173:546–8

7 Lund-Johansen P 1977 Central haemodynamics in early essential hypertension. Acta Medica Scandinavia Suppl 606:35–42

8 Henry JP, Stephens PM, Santisteban GA 1975 A model of psychosocial hypertension showing reversibility and progression of cardiovascular complications. Circulation Research 36:156–64

9 Lawler JE, Barker GF, Hubbard JW, Allen MT 1980 The effects of conflict on tonic levels of blood pressure in the genetically borderline hypertension rat. Psychophysiology 17:363–70

10 Lawler JE, Barker GF, Hubbard JW, Schaub RG 1981 Effects of stress on blood pressure and cardiac pathology in rats with borderline hypertension. Hypertension 3:496–505

11 Lawler JE, Sanders BJ, Cox RH, O'Connor BF 1991 Baroreflex function in chronically stressed borderline hypertensive rats. Physiology and Behavior 49:539–42

12 Anderson DE, Kearns WD, Better WE 1983 Progressive hypertension in dogs by avoidance conditioning and saline infusion. Hypertension 5:286–91

13 Lawler JE, Naylor SK, Abel MM, Baldwin DR 1993 A chronic high-salt diet fails, to enhance blood pressure reactivity to a tone associated with footshock in SHR, BHR, and WKY rats. Physiology and Behavior 54:941–6

14 Gelsema AJM, Schoemaker RG, Ruzicka M, Copeland NE 1994 Cardiovascular effects of social stress in borderline hypertensive rats. Journal of Hypertension 12:1019–28

15 Henry JP, Stephens PM 1977 Stress, health and the social environment. Springer-Verlag, New York

16 Dampney RAL 1994 Functional organization of the cardiovascular system. Physiological Review (in press)

17 McAllen RM, Dampney RAL 1990 Vasomotor neurons in the rostral ventrolateral medulla are organized topographically with respect to type of vascular bed but not body region. Neuroscience Letters 110:91–6

18 Spyer KM 1994 Central nervous mechanisms contributing to cardiovascular control. Journal of Physiology 474:1–19

19 Roozendaal B, Schoorlemmer GH, Koolhaas JM, Bohus B 1993 Cardiac, neuroendocrine, and behavioral effects of central amygdaloid vasopressinergic and oxytocinergic mechanisms under stress-free conditions in rats. Brain Research Bulletin 32:573–9

20 Falls WA, Davis M 1995 Lesions of the central nucleus of the amygdala block conditioned excitation, but not conditioned inhibition of fear as measured with the fear-potentiated startle effect. Behavioral Neuroscience 109:379–87

21 Hauger RL, Irwin MR, Lorang M, Aguilera G, Brown MR 1993 High intracerebral levels of CRH result in CRH receptor downregulation in the amygdala and neuroimmune desensitization. Brain Research 616:283–92

22 Brod J, Fencl V, Hejl Z, Jirka J 1959 Circulatory changes underlying blood pressure elevation during acute emotional stress (mental arithmetic) in normotensive and hypertensive subjects. Clinical Science 18:269–79

23 Obrist PA 1981 Cardiovascular psychophysiology. Academic Press, New York

24 Obrist PA, Gaebelein CJ, Teller ES, Langer AW, Grignolo A, Light KC, McCubbin JA 1978 The relationship among heart rate, carotid dP/dt and blood pressure in humans as a function of the type of stress. Psychophysiology 15:102–15

25 Turner JR, Caroll D 1985 Heart rate and oxygen consumption during mental arithmetic, a video game and graded exercise: further evidence of metabolically – exaggerated cardiac adjustments? Psycophysiology 22:261–7

26 Fredrikson M, Matthews KA 1990 Cardiovascular responses to behavioral stress and hypertension: a meta-analytic review. Annals of Behavioral Medicine 12:30–9

27 Turner JR, Ward MM, Gellman MD, Johnston DW, Light KC, Van Doornen LPJ 1994 The relationship between laboratory and ambulatory cardiovascular activity: current evidence and future directions. Annals of Behavioral Medicine 16:12–23

28 Floras JS, Hassan MO, Jones JV, Sleight P 1987 Pressor responses to laboratory stresses and daytime blood pressure variability. Journal of Hypertension 5:715–19

29 Parati G, Pomidossi G, Casadei R, Ravogli A, Gropelli A, Cesana B, Mancia G 1988 Comparison of the cardiovascular effects of different laboratory stressors and their relationship with blood pressure. Journal of Hypertension 6:481–8

30 Johnston DW, Anastasiades P, Wood C 1990 The relationship between cardiovascular responses in the laboratory and in the field. Psychophysiology, 27:34–44

31 Johnston DW, Schmidt T, Vagt S, McSorley K, Albus C, Klingmann I, Bethge H 1994 The relationship between cardiovascular reactivity in the laboratory and heart rate responsiveness in real life: active coping and β blockade. Psychosomatic Medicine 56:369–76

32 Imholz BPM, Langewouters GJ, Van Montfrans GA, Parati G, Van Goudoever JV, Wesseling KH, Wieling W, Mancia G 1993 Feasibility of ambulatory, continuous 24-hour finger arterial pressure recording. Hypertension 21:65–73

33 Jain A 1995 Kardiovaskulare reaktivitat im labor und im feld. Waxmann, Munster

34 Jain A, Schmidt T, Johnston DW, Mutz G 1993 Cardiovascular reactivity in the laboratory and in the field: comparing different methods to assess reactivity in real life. Paper at the Conference on Psychophysiological Methodology of the German Psychophysiology Society, Wurzburg, June 9–12

35 Vogele A, Steptoe A 1992 Emotional coping and tonic blood pressure as determinants of cardiovascular responses to mental stress. Journal of Hypertension 10:1079–87

36 Vogele C, Steptoe A 1993 Anger inhibition and family history as modulators of cardiovascular responses to mental stress in adolescent boys. Journal of Psychosomatic Research 37:503–14

37 Menkes MS, Matthews KA, Krantz DS, Lundberg U, Mead LA, Qaquish B, Liang KY, Thomas CB, Pearson TA 1989 Cardiovascular reactivity to the cold pressor test as a predictor of hypertension. Hypertension 14:524–30

38 Light KC, Dolan CA, Davis MR, Sherwood A 1992 Cardiovascular responses to an active coping challenge as predictors of blood pressure patterns 10 to 15 years later. Psychosomatic Medicine 54:217–30

39 Carroll D, Davey Smith G, Sheffield D, Shipley MJ, Marmot MG 1995 Pressor reactions to psychological stress and prediction of future blood pressure: data from the Whitehall II study. British Medical Journal 310:771–6

40 Mann A 1986 The psychological aspects of essential hypertension. Journal of Psychosomatic Research 30:527–41

41 Gold AE, Johnston DW 1990 Anger, hypertension and heart disease. In: Bennett P, Weinman J, Spurgeon P (eds) Current developments in health psychology. Harwood, London, pp 105–27

42 Kahn HA, Medalie JH, Neufeld HN, Riff E, Goldbourt U 1972 The incidence of hypertension and associated factors: the Israeli ischemic heart disease study. American Heart Journal 84:171–82

43 Harburg E, Erfurt JC, Hauenstein LS, Chape C, Schull

WJ, Schork MA 1973 Socio-ecological stress, suppressed hostility, skin color, and black-white male blood pressure: Detroit. Psychosomatic Medicine 35:276–96

44 Julius M, Harburg E, Cottington E, Johnson EH 1986 Anger-coping types, blood pressure and all-cause mortality: a follow-up in Tecumesh, Michigan (1971–1983). American Journal of Epidemiology 124:220–33

45 Kasl SV, Cobb S 1970 Blood pressure changes in men undergoing job loss: a preliminary report. Psychosomatic Medicine 32:18–38

46 Cobb S, Rose RM 1973 Hypertension: peptic ulcer and diabetes in air traffic controllers. Journal of American Medical Association 224:489–92

47 DeFrank RS, Jenkins CD, Rose RM 1987 A longitudinal investigation of the relationships among alcohol consumption, psychosocial factors, and blood pressure. Psychosomatic Medicine 49:236–49

48 Shaper AG, Walker M, Cohen NM, Wale CJ, Thomson AG 1981 British Regional Heart Study: cardiovascular risk factors in middle-aged men in 24 towns. British Medical Journal 283:179–86

49 Whincup PH, Cook DG, Shaper AG, Macfarlane DJ, Walker M 1988 Blood pressure in British children: associations with adult blood pressure and cardiovascular mortality. Lancet ii:890–3

50 Winkleby MA, Ragland DR, Syme SL 1988 Self-reported stressors and hypertension: evidence of an inverse association. American Journal of Epidemiology 127:124–34

51 Randich A, Maixner W 1984 Interactions between cardiovascular and pain regulatory systems. Neuroscience and Behavioral Review 8:343–69

52 Bruehl S, Carlson CR, McCubbin JA 1992 The relationship between pain sensitivity and blood pressure in normotensives. Pain 48:463–7

53 Dworkin BR, Filewich R, Miller N, Craigmyle N, Pickering T 1979 Baroreceptor activation reduces reactivity to noxious stimulation: implications for hypertension. Science 205:1299–301

54 Johnston DW 1992 The management of stress in the prevention of coronary heart disease. International Research of Health Psychology 1:57–83

55 Jacob RG, Chesney MA, Williams DM, Ding Y, Shapiro AP 1991 Relaxation therapy for hypertension: design effects and treatment effects. Annals of Behavioral Medicine 13:5–17

56 Johnston DW 1991 Stress management in the treatment of mild primary hypertension. Hypertension 17 (suppl III):III-63–III-68

57 Patel C, Marmot M 1988 Can general practitioners use training in relaxation and management of stress to reduce mild hypertension? British Medical Journal 296:21–4

58 Patel C, Marmot MG, Terry DJ 1981 Controlled trial of biofeedback-aided behavioural methods in reducing mild hypertension. British Medical Journal 282:2005–8

59 Patel C, Marmot MG, Terry DJ, Carruthers M, Hunt B, Patel M 1985 Trial of relaxation in reducing coronary risk: four year follow-up. British Medical Journal 290:1103–6

60 Patel C, North WRS 1975 Randomised controlled trial of yoga and biofeedback in the management of hypertension. Lancet ii:93–5

61 Brauer A, Horlick LF, Nelson B, Farquhar JU, Agras WS 1979 Relaxation therapy for essential hypertension: a veterans administration out patients study. Journal of Behavioral Medicine 2:21–9

62 Taylor CB, Farquhar JW, Nelson E, Agras WS 1977 Relaxation therapy and high blood pressure. Archives of General Psychiatry 34:339–42

63 Bali LR 1979 Long term effect of relaxation on blood pressure and anxiety levels in essential hypertensive males: a controlled study. Psychosomatic Medicine 41:637–46

64 Irvine J, Johnston DW, Jenner D, Marie GV 1986 Relaxation and stress management in the treatment of essential hypertension. Journal of Psychosomatic Research 30:437–50

65 Southam MA, Agras WS, Taylor CB, Kraemer HC 1982 Relaxation training: blood pressure during the working day. Archives of General Psychiatry 39:715–17

66 Frankel BL, Patel DJ, Horwitz D, Friedwald MT, Gaardner KP 1978 Treatment of hypertension with biofeedback and relaxation techniques. Psychosomatic Medicine 40:276–93

67 Agras WS, Taylor CB, Kraemer HC, Southam MA, Schneider JA 1987 Relaxation training for essential hypertension at the worksite II. The poorly controlled hypertensive. Psychosomatic Medicine 49:264–73

68 Chesney MA, Black GW, Swan GE, Ward MM 1987 Relaxation training for essential hypertension at the worksite. I. The untreated mild hypertensive. Psychosomatic Medicine 49:250–63

69 Van Montfrans GA, Karemaker JM, Weiling W, Dunning AJ 1990 Relaxation therapy and continuous ambulatory blood pressure in mild hypertension: a controlled study. British Medical Journal 300:1368–72

70 Irvine MJ, Logan AG 1991 Relaxation behavior therapy as sole treatment for mild hypertension. Psychosomatic Medicine 53:587–97

71 Johnston DW, Gold A, Kentish J, Smith D, Vallance P, Shah D, Leach G, Robinson B 1993 Effect of stress management on blood pressure in mild primary hypertension. British Medical Journal 306:963–6

72 Bennett P, Wallace L, Carroll D, Smiths N 1990 Treating Type A behaviors and mild hypertension in middle-aged men. Journal of Psychosomatic Research 35:209–33

73 Davison GC, Williams ME, Nezami E, Bice TL, DeQuattro VL 1991 Relaxation, reductions in anger articulated thoughts, and improvements in borderline hypertension and heart rate. Journal of Behavioral Medicine 14:453–68

74 Schneider RA, Staggers F, Alexander CN, Sheppard W, Rainforth M, Kondwani K, Smith S, King CG 1995 A randomized controlled trial of stress reduction for hypertension in older African Americans. Hypertension 26:820–7

75 Eisenberg DM, Delbanco TL, Berkey CS, Kaptchuk TJ, Kupelnick B, Kuhl J, Chalmers TC 1993 Cognitive behavioral techniques for hypertension: are they effective? Annals of Internal Medicine 118:964–72

76 Jacob RG, Shapiro AP 1994 Is the effect of stress management on blood-pressure just regression to the mean. Homeostasis in Health and Disease 35:113–19

CHAPTER CONTENTS

5

Cancer

Ruth Cohn Bolletino
With a Summary and Overview by Lawrence L. LeShan

THE ROOTS OF MIND–BODY TREATMENT FOR CANCER PATIENTS

Cancer is no more a disease of cells than a traffic jam is a disease of automobiles. Both traffic jams and cancer are problems of the ecology — of an entire organism, in the case of the city, of the whole person, in the case of cancer.

R D Smithers, former President of the British Cancer Council, 1979

In recent years, the medical profession has regarded cancer solely as a mechanical process requiring physical intervention. Studies indicating that psychological and psychosocial factors are involved in the development of cancer have been ignored or rejected. The message is that cancer is strictly a physiological disease, and that emotions and attitudes have no bearing on illness or recovery. Many clinicians believe that assigning a role to the mind is not only erroneous, anti-scientific, and anti-intellectual, but potentially destructive as well. They believe that this idea produces guilt in the cancer patient because it suggests that the patient is somehow responsible for causing the disease[1].

Yet for centuries physicians and scientists have tried to link psychological and behavioral factors to the appearance and course of neoplastic disease. The idea that the mind and emotions play a part in the onset and progression of cancer can be traced back at least as early as the second Century AD, when Galen observed that breast cancer occurred more often in women with a 'melancholic' rather than a 'sanguine' temperament.

In 1759, surgeon Richard Guy wrote that women with breast cancer were 'of a sedentary, melancholic disposition of mind, (who) meet with such disasters in Life as occasion much trouble and grief' (p.6)[2].

In 1846 physician Walter Hoyle Walshe wrote, 'Much has been written on the influence of mental misery, sudden reverses in fortune, and habitual gloominess of temper on the deposition of carcinomatous matter ... I myself have met with cases in which the connection appeared so clear that I decided questioning its reality would seem a struggle against reason'[3].

In 1870 Sir James Paget, Queen Victoria's physician and surgeon, made a similar observation: 'The cases are so frequent in which deep anxiety, deferred hope and disappointment are quickly followed by the growth and increase of cancer that we can hardly doubt that mental depression is a weighty addition to the other influences favoring the development of a cancerous constitution' (p.91)[4].

In 1871 Sir Thomas Watson said, 'Great mental stress has been assigned an influence in hastening the development of cancerous disease in persons already predisposed... I have often so noticed this sequence that I cannot but think the imputation is true' (p.10)[2].

New York surgeon Willard Parker, who operated on breast cancer patients, declared in 1885 that 'There are the strongest physiological reasons for believing that great mental depression, particularly grief, induces a predisposition to such diseases as cancer, or becomes an exciting cause under circumstances where the predisposition has already been acquired' (p.137)[5].

In 1893 Herbert Snow, working at the London Cancer Hospital, reported that of 250 women with uterine or breast cancer studied, 156 had experienced a major loss, often the death of a loved one, shortly before their diagnosis of cancer, and that 'the number of instances in which a malignant disease of the breast and uterus follows immediately [upon] antecedent emotion of a depressing character is too large to be set down to chance' (p.10)[2].

Although observations of this kind have been recorded throughout western medical history and accepted in medical circles, as medicine approached the 20th Century the idea that cancer is linked to the patient's emotional life history began to disappear rapidly.

THE BIOMEDICAL MODEL

Lawrence LeShan observed that there were several reasons for this change. The psychosomatic viewpoint was fading out of fashion. In addition, new techniques of antiseptic and painless surgery were developed that were regarded as the best ways to treat cancer. 'Surgery focuses our attention on cancer as a local disease of a specific part of the body and not one aspect of a total human being's functioning, which is the essence of the psychosomatic view'[2]. Radiation therapy, developed shortly afterward, reinforced this concept of cancer as a local body problem. Another reason for the change was that a psychosomatic theory was useless at the time, for psychiatry had no methods to explore the matter or to intervene. There were no methods of applying the concept of the mind–body relationship in cancer, no techniques available to make the concept useful. Gradually, the idea that cancer was related to the total person began to disappear from medical textbooks and journals[2].

Larry Dossey observed that when the distinguished Irish physician Robert James Graves advised that patients' pulses be timed by a watch, it seemed logical that the human body, like all physical matter, be viewed as a machine. The Industrial Revolution had already influenced medical thought. Physicians of England and Europe 'saw machines everywhere. The heart was a pump, the lungs were bellows, the limbs were pulleys and levers, the circulation was a sophisticated hydraulic system replete with valves, locks and dams' (p.11)[1]. In this they were following the lead of Cabanis and the French Encyclopedists.

The biomedical model from which western medical theory and practice derive can be stated in terms of nine central premises[6]. Box 5.1 lists these underlying assumptions.

Box 5.1 Nine central premises of biomedicine

1. The human body is a mechanism that can be analyzed in terms of its component parts.
2. The fundamental origin of illness and disease is biological.
3. The focus of medicine is on pathology.
4. Cancer, like any disease, is an organic entity that invades the body and attacks a particular part of the body.
5. The physician's role is to select an intervention aimed at the afflicted part or at the whole body, to remove or destroy the malignancy.
6. Such interventions can be validly performed without considering the patient's body as a whole or the patient's state of mind.
7. Since human bodies are essentially the same and personal consciousness does not play a significant role in the body's functioning, the same interventions can be applied for different patients with the same organic symptoms.
8. The knowledge needed to determine treatment is complex, known only to the specialist.
9. The patient is a passive recipient of the intervention, since the patient differs only in complexity from a disabled machine requiring repair.

SEEDS OF HOLISM

Seeds of holistic thought were planted by Louis Pasteur and Claude Bernard, who argued whether the most important factor in disease was the terrain (the human body) or the germ (the disease). Bernard put forth the concept that the body always works to maintain a delicate balance in the chemistry and functioning of its many parts. When this balance is disturbed, sickness and death can result. Bernard said, 'Diseases hover constantly about us, their seeds are blown by the wind, but they take root only when the terrain is ready to receive them.' Pasteur's last words were reported to be, 'Bernard was right. The germ is little, the terrain all' (p.57)[7].

Bernard's concept of balance was restated in the 1930s and 1940s by Walter Cannon, seeking to bridge the gap between the biological and psychological approaches to medicine. As early as 1935, studying the ways the body regulates itself, Cannon suggested that an organism maintains a balance, which he called 'homeostasis', that keeps the internal environment stable. In his view, homeostasis involves not only the nervous system and biochemical system working in harmony with one another, but also involves normal life experiences which have physical effects on the body[8]. He thus identified the natural self-healing processes of an organism which enable it to return to a normal state after a disturbance. Cannon also described what he called the 'fight-or-flight' mechanism, whereby in situations of emotional stress and anxiety, the blood chemistry changes so as to provide extra energy for fighting the source of emotional stress or fleeing the scene.

One system vital to homeostasis is the immune system. Since the 1930s researchers have begun to learn more about how this biochemical defense system functions and how it is affected by psychological factors.

THE NEW FIELD OF MIND–BODY MEDICINE

Several reviews of the early literature on the relationships between personality and cancer (Kowall[9], Merloo[10], and LeShan[11]) indicate the intensivity and extensivity of the literature. These reviews covered early studies involving statistical and psychoanalytical explorations, as well as the clinical observations of oncologists.

In the early 1950s Hans Selye demonstrated that stress is a factor in disease processes. In the 1960s research in mind–body medicine burgeoned, with much of its focus on the physical effects of stress. Neal Miller's experiments showed that physical functions presumed to be involuntary could be manipulated. Other researchers studied ways to control stress in the body.

EVIDENCE FOR THE MIND–BODY VIEW

Stress and immunosuppression

Hans Selye defined stress as 'a non-specific response of the body to any demand made on it.' In other words, stress is a subjective experience. What is stressful differs from one individual to another. It can result from any situation that exceeds the individual's capacity to cope. As Jerome Frank put it, 'stress comes mainly from the patient's interpretation of events.'

Numerous researchers documented the immunosuppressive effects of stress in both humoral and cell-mediated immunity in animal studies. Animal studies, although not definitive, provided suggestive evidence and support for the relationship between psychological and immunological factors in human beings.

Animal studies

A number of researchers in various centers investigated the effects of stress on the appearance and progression of tumors. For example, in the late 1960s psychiatrist George Solomon and immunologist Alfred Amkraut induced stress in rats by shocking them and housing them in crowded cages. They then implanted tumors in the animals and compared the results with a non-stressed control group. Tumors in most of the stressed rats grew far more rapidly, indicating that environmental stress encouraged the tumor progression. Clearly stress was directly influencing immunity, but it was not clear how. A clue was provided by previous Soviet researchers, who had discovered that after they destroyed the hypothalamus in rabbits, the rabbits' immune systems became depressed. Solomon and Amkraut repeated this experiment with the same result[8].

In the 1970s, when Robert Ader conditioned rats to suppress their immune system, he showed that the model of the immune system as an automatic, autonomous system no longer applied. By demonstrating that the immune system is influenced by what the organism has been conditioned to expect, he proved that the immune response is sensitive to psychological perceptions.

Vernon Riley found that a group of mice which were genetically predisposed to cancer did not develop tumors when kept in a stress-free environment. Ninety-two per cent of those exposed to stress grew tumors, as compared with only 7% of the protected group. Riley also showed that the stressed mice exhibited a release of adrenal corticosteroids, which in turn injured their immune systems. To underline the point, Riley was able to restore the immune function of the stressed mice by injecting them with a corticosteroid antagonist[8].

Human studies

In the 1980s Janice Kiecolt-Glaser demonstrated that the tension and anxiety induced by such 'routine' stress as taking a university examination had a distinct effect on the immune system. Two blood samples, one taken from medical students a month before final examinations and a second on the first day of examination week, showed decreased proliferation of a type of lymphocyte, the 'natural killer' ('NK') cells, which are thought to play a role in tumor surveillance.

In a similar study psychiatrist Steven Locke examined a group of Harvard undergraduate students to determine the effect of stress on their immune status. He used a standard psychological test to measure stress levels, and also conducted brief interviews in which he questioned the students about their feelings of depression and anxiety. Students who reported experiencing intense anxiety and depression were found to have more depressed NK cell activity than those claiming to feel little or no distress[8].

Numerous studies have shown that the adverse effects of stress can be lessened and immunity increased by mental and emotional coping strategies.

For example, Kiecolt-Glaser and Ronald Glaser have also shown that reduction of stress results in increased immunity. In studying a group of elderly people over a period of a month, they found that relaxation training three times weekly significantly increased NK and T cell activity, with corresponding decreases in antibodies for the herpes simplex virus and in self-reported intensity of symptoms of stress[12].

The Glasers also measured the effects of relaxation training on medical students experiencing the stress of final examinations. Although students in both the relaxation and non-relaxation groups showed declines in some immune functions, the relaxation group exhibited an increase in helper T cells. Students in the non-relaxation group, unlike those in the relaxation group, reported increased anxiety and other symptoms of stress[12]. Similarly, Fawzy I Fawzy, working with Norman Cousins in the 1980s, found significant evidence showing that freeing cancer patients from depression actually increases the wide array of natural killer cells.

Helplessness and immunosuppression

In both animal and human research, the importance of one specific form of stress emerged repeatedly. That form is helplessness. While immunosuppression occurs as a result of various forms of stress, it occurs more markedly in situations of helplessness, in which there is no possibility of controlling the stressor.

Animal studies

The concept of 'learned helplessness' was first put forward in the 1960s by Martin Seligman and his colleagues. They found that when dogs were administered unavoidable shocks, eventually they just seemed to give up. Even when given a chance to escape, they acted helpless and continued to accept the shocks. In other experiments, when animals were exposed to shocks but from the start had a chance to escape, they did not learn to give up and become helpless[5].

Early in the 1970s Jay Weiss conducted a series of experiments in which two rats were exposed to the same stress, a mild shock to the tail. Only one of the rats could control the shocks. A third rat, serving as a control, was not shocked at all. The first rat learned that by rotating a wheel, he could stop the shocks for both himself and for the second rat. In this way, both rats received the same amount of stress, but one could control the situation while the other was helpless. The helpless rats developed ulcers twice as large as those of the rats with control. The work of Mark Laudenslager and Steven Maier showed similar results[13].

Human studies

Such learned helplessness is also seen in humans. In 1971 George L Engel, a pioneer in mind–body interaction, became interested in 'emotional sudden death.' To study the effects of strong emotions on health, he collected reports of sudden deaths. Most occurred within an hour of events that provoked a response of overwhelming despair, excitement or both. He suggested that one of the most frequent situations preceding emotional sudden death is a sense of impasse. When the individuals believe they can neither fight nor escape, they feel trapped and can die[1].

Further research by Martin Seligman showed that when people habitually respond to their problems with an attitude of helplessness, this attitude seems to be channeled into the body, creating physiological changes that set the stage for poor health. Seligman and his associates rated 172 undergraduates for the presence or absence of a helpless attitude. They then accurately predicted which would be sick the most. The predictions held, both 1 month later and 1 year later[1].

Studies on the impact of bereavement on the immune system suggest that the feelings of grief and helplessness that characterize bereavement may inhibit immune activity.

The first scientific study of this kind appeared in 1969. C Murray Parkes and his colleagues published a study on widowers. The researchers followed the health of 4448 widowers, all 55 years or older, for 9 years after the spouse's death. One of their most striking findings was that the widowers were dying at an unusually high rate within 6 months of their wives' deaths[8]. This was completely consistent with data picked up by insurance companies between 1900 and 1920.

Later, in a classic study of this kind on the microscopic level, Australian researcher T W Bartrop and his associates found that bereaved spouses had lower lymphocyte proliferation 8 weeks after their spouse's death, as compared with a control group[8]. Another study by Marvin Stein in New York City showed diminished lymphocyte proliferation after bereavement in husbands of women who had terminal breast cancer[8]. Women who lost unborn children showed different immune system profiles depending on the way they dealt with the loss. Those who did not accept their loss had more feeble T cell strength than those who accepted[8].

Steven J Schleifer and his colleagues found that despair during bereavement weakens immune function. Studying 15 men whose wives had terminal breast cancer, they found that prior to the wives' deaths, the men's main immune cells, the T and B lymphocytes, functioned normally. Shortly after the death and for many months, though normal in number, the cells actually stopped working. They could not be made to work even when extracted from the blood of the men and exposed in test tubes to chemicals that ordinarily activate them[1].

Studies by Kiecolt-Glaser and Glaser showed that spousal death, divorce, and separation resulted in suppression of NK activity, a lowered immune responsiveness, and higher antibody titers to latent viruses in men and women[12].

It has become increasingly clear that helplessness, a lack of control, is itself a stressor causing immunosuppression.

Helplessness and neoplastic disease

Some studies focused on the effects of the stress of helplessness on the growth of cancer cells.

Animal studies

Two Canadian psychologists, Lawrence Sklar and Hymie Anisman, implanted cancer cells in two groups of mice, then gave both groups identical electric shocks. One group could control the shocks and the other could not. The group with no control had faster growing tumors and shorter lifespans. The animals' helplessness, Sklar and Anisman said, helped bring on neurochemical, hormonal and immunological changes that facilitated the tumor growth.

More recent studies by Seligman, Madeline Visintainer and Joseph Volticelli demonstrated that cancer cells injected into rats that had helplessness-inducing shocks produced tumors twice as often as in rats that could control the identical shocks[8].

Human studies

In the mid-1950s Lawrence LeShan, an experimental and clinical psychologist, began his pioneering studies in emotional factors involved in cancer. After conducting interviews and examining projective personality tests of cancer patients, he discovered that many of these patients had experienced a form of helplessness and, as a result, despair. A year or two before their diagnosis, they had all suffered some kind of traumatic personal loss, such as the death of a loved one, a divorce, or a loss of meaningful work.

These findings were validated by projective studies described later in this chapter.

CANCER AS IMMUNE SYSTEM FAILURE

Research findings about the connection between immune system functioning and the growth of cancer cells has led to a theory widely held today about the origins of cancer.

Cell division constantly occurs in our bodies, but at any given moment some cells undergo malignant transformation. They disregard all of the regulatory signals they had previously obeyed. They do not die, do not remain in place, and do not regulate their growth in relation to the total organism as they invade adjoining parts of the body. Any normal body cell can become a renegade, either as the result of an inherited gene or from a spontaneous mutation triggered by some outside force such as a virus, a carcinogen, radiation or chance. Why cells should become cancerous is not understood. It appears to be natural for the body to develop cancer cells without the appearance of clinically recognizable tumors. Ernest Rossi pointed out that the occurrence of neuroblastomas is much higher even in babies than in the clinical incidence of the disease. Similarly, autopsies on almost all males over the age of 50 show evidence of prostatic cancer cells, yet actual clinical cancer is evident in only a minority of them[14].

Lewis Thomas said that the reason most people do not develop cancer is that 'we are equipped with an immunological apparatus sufficiently agile and sensitive for the first clone of neoplastic cells to be quickly recognized and gotten rid of'. What needs clarification, Thomas continued, is the reason for the failure of immune reactivity in those people who do develop cancer[15].

Most people do not develop cancer, even though cancer cells are continually produced, because the body's natural immunological surveillance system finds and destroys the single cancer cells before they grow into clinically observable tumors[14]. The defective cells grow slowly, and because they frequently express surface antigens, they are highly vulnerable to destruction by T lymphocytes. In this way, the seeds of a malignant neoplasia are sown constantly, but the immune system destroys them just as constantly.

A variety of immune system processes protect against tumor formation. These include cytotoxic T lymphocytes (CTL), B lymphocytes and NK (natural killer) cells. When the cellular and humoral functions of the immune system are depressed or underactive, cancer cells can escape normal surveillance mechanisms and initiate tumor development. However, the continued growth of that tumor requires further deficiencies in immune surveillance. Depression of immune surveillance can be brought about by a variety of environmental factors including stress, which promotes adrenocorticosteroid production. For a transformed cell to give rise to a detectable tumor, it must have escaped immune surveillance and destruction, undergone numerous divisions, and produced countless generations of cells, all without interference[8]. Andrew Weil wrote, 'The presence of cancer in the body, even in its earliest stages, already represents significant failure of the immune system' (p.268)[16].

George F Solomon, a pioneer on the negative results of excessive levels of stress on immune response, suggested that even minimal weakening of T cells' ability to recognize new carcinomatous antigens on the surface of mutant cells allows cancer cells to develop. 'Marginal suppression of either central or efferent activity by stress-associated events ... would aid in the progress of the tumor'[17].

More recent studies have confirmed Solomon's observation that only a slight depression of the natural immunological surveillance system is needed to greatly increase an individual's susceptibility to pathogens, particularly those that are constantly present[5].

Bernie Siegel pointed out that since immune system function is controlled by the brain, as demonstrated by Robert Ader, it follows that whatever upsets the brain's control of the immune system can foster malignancy[18]. While this neural regulation of immunity is clearly affected by genetic and enviromental factors, it can also be affected by means of the chronic stress syndrome first described by Walter Cannon half a century ago.

STUDIES ON PSYCHOLOGICAL FACTORS IN CANCER

One of the most controversial areas in mind–body research is the role of personality, life style and attitude in neoplastic disease. Various studies indicate that emotional, behavioral and psychological factors may influence neurophysiological functioning and depress immune response. This in turn creates conditions in which growth of cancerous tumors and mutant cells can proceed unchecked by the body's normal defense[5].

The research literature includes a number of different tracks. One has to do with 'cancer-prone personalities', personality traits that are believed to make people more vulnerable to cancer. Other tracks focus on improving outcome rather than on etiology. They have to do with psychosocial and 'psychoeducation' group interventions, the use of imagery, and individual psychotherapeutic interventions.

Theory of 'cancer-prone personalities'

Some researchers have studied the possibility that certain personality types are particularly vulnerable to cancer. A wide variety of personality traits, emotional styles, and life history factors have been consistently associated with the appearance and progression of neoplastic disease.

Cancer has been linked with such specific factors as depression, loneliness and repressed emotions. Thus one series of studies concluded that women with breast cancer are significantly more likely to repress anger and hostility toward others than cancer-free women[15]. Other recent studies correlated cancer susceptibility with non-expression of emotion and with passive coping styles.

However, these kinds of specific relationships appear to have been dictated more by the design of the study and the orientation of the investigator than by objective criteria. Such retrospective studies involve many variables, and are subject to distortion based on the patient's current state of mind. After digesting several decades of work on the subject of cancer and emotions, Bernard Fox, a cancer expert and behavioral epidemiologist, pointed out that it is hard to find an emotion not related to cancer in one study or another[8].

At present the field seems to be redirecting its focus. The interest in finding specific factors associated with etiology has shifted to stimulating the individual's self-healing abilities. Thus, for example, David Spiegel's study demonstrating that his support group enabled members to live longer, was not directed at factors relating to etiology of the cancer. The shift in focus is also reflected in the work of Lawrence LeShan's two books, printed 20 years apart, on the psychological aspects of malignancy. The first book involves much discussion of etiology in terms of personality traits. At that time he reported that people who repress angry, hostile feelings and who demonstrate low self-worth had a higher than average incidence of cancer. These findings, he maintains, did not stand the test of time. His second book is concerned with strategies for mobilizing the immune system.

H Stephen Greer, referring to recent studies suggesting a link between certain personality traits (such as suppression of anger, compliance, and unassertiveness) and cancer, wrote:

> These findings are of considerable interest and suggest the possibility that these psychological attributes may contribute to the development of cancer. But the case should not be overstated. It must be stressed that what has been discovered so far is a statistical link. To establish whether there is a causal link requires further research (p.xix)[19].

Psychosocial studies and interventions

Recent studies suggest that support group therapy, which provides emotional support, information about cancer and treatments, and training in stress management and coping skills, improves survival for people with certain kinds of cancer. The best known are those by David Speigel and psychiatrist Fawzy I Fawzy.

In the mid-1970s Spiegel tried to determine whether group therapy could help cancer patients cope more effectively with the fear and isolation they so often experience. He recruited 86 women with advanced metastatic breast cancer who were similar in average age at the time of diagnosis and at the time of entering the study. They were also matched for marital status and the kind of medical treatment they received. Two-thirds were randomly assigned to groups meeting for 1.5 hours a week for a year. The other third was a 'control' group, not participating in group sessions and receiving medical care only.

The weekly groups discussed their experiences with treatments and expressed feelings about their illness, including their fears of dying. They were encouraged to enhance their family support and communicate with their doctors, and they were taught relaxation and pain control techniques. Group members formed strong bonds of caring and support.

Patients who attended the group did indeed deal better with their illness and reported less pain than those in the control group.

In 1985, 10 years later, when the influence of psychological factors on cancer had become better known, Spiegel went back to determine whether support group members had lived longer than those in the control group. Skeptical that mental and emotional factors can influence the course of cancer, he expected to find no differences in survival time. Instead, he was 'shocked' to find that patients who had received group treatment had lived twice as long as those who received only medical care. Support group members survived for an average of 37 months from the beginning of the study, while the control group lived for a mean of 19 months. Three women who survived after 10 years were all support group members[20].

Although Spiegel's study has been questioned in terms of the negative emotional effects on survival time on women in the control group, who knew they were being excluded from an available form of treatment, his data have led to greatly increased interest in the possibility that psychosocial support is a valuable adjunct to medical treatment.

In a similar study, Fawzy studied immune system changes in 34 patients after short-term group treatment. The study was not designed to assess survival as an outcome, but only to study 'changes over time in methods of coping and affective disturbance'. All the patients had undergone surgery for malignant melanoma and had no current signs of cancer. A control group of similar patients was given medical treatment only. Those in the intervention group received psychological counseling, information about melanoma, and training in stress management and coping skills. The intervention was minimal, consisting of only six 1.5-hour sessions. Fawzy concluded that as a result of this brief intervention, these patients exhibited less fatigue, less depression, less mood disturbance, and greater vigor. They not only showed a greater psychological ability to cope with the stress of their illness, but also higher counts of natural killer cells and other immune system cells. These effects became stronger over the course of 1 year from the onset of the study[21,22].

In 1993, 6 years later, Fawzy went back to examine the longer-term effects on survival and time of recurrence in both groups. His recently reported findings suggest that group therapy did improve survival. In the control group, ten of the original 34 patients with stage one disease died, and three others had local recurrences. In the intervention group, three of the original 34 had died, and four had recurrences. Those who participated in the intervention group also experienced longer disease-free intervals than those in the control group[23].

Other studies demonstrated the value of psychosocial support for enhancing immune function and potentially extending life span. One of these was done by psychologist Sandra Levy and her associates Ronald Haberman, Judith Rodin, and Martin Seligman. These researchers investigated patients with melanoma and colon cancer. Their intent was to determine whether psychological treatment could increase the patients' natural immunity. In addition to medical treatment, 15 patients received an 8-week course of cognitive therapy to help them deal with their depression, 'cultivate optimism, and regain control'. They also received training in relaxation techniques to help them with their stress. Fifteen other patients received medical treatment only. The researchers found that natural killer cell activity had risen sharply in the first group, and remained unaltered in the control group. The psychosocial intervention not only strongly enhanced NK cell activity, but those who had received the intervention were less depressed. This study provides preliminary evidence that interventions aimed at increasing cancer patients' optimism and teaching them to relax can strengthen their natural killer cell activity.

Imagery

The ability of visual imagery to affect physiology directly makes it a significant mind–body bridge. Although its ability to influence outcome is open to question, imagery is practiced extensively by cancer patients and used by therapists to help alleviate symptoms and promote healing.

One of its main advocates, radiation oncologist O Carl Simonton, in collaboration with psychologist Stephanie Matthews Simonton and research psychologist Jeanne Achterberg, have taught active imagery to cancer patients in the hope of physically reversing the effects of the disease. Patients are asked to imagine their own version of immune system cells attacking the cancer cells, and to see their immune cells and the cancer treatments they are receiving as strong and powerful and the cancer cells as 'weak and confused'. The imagined scene culminates with the destruction of the cancer cells, and the revitalization of the body. While there is no hard evidence that this kind of imagery improves prognosis or lessens disease activity, patients have reported such benefits as relief from anxiety and pain, increased tolerance of cancer therapy and improved ability to cope with their illness.

Howard Hall investigated the effects of visual imagery on immunity. He hypnotized a group of healthy people, and told them to imagine their white blood cells as strong and powerful sharks attacking any destructive organisms that might be around. When he compared blood samples he had taken before and after the sessions, he found that a number of the subjects had a much stronger immune response after the session[24].

Martin Rossman, one of the most respected imagery trainers in the USA, has pointed out that there is little carefully controlled, scientific evidence regarding the medical benefits of imagery. Such studies are difficult to design and carry out because, as in Hall's study described above, imagery is usually used in conjunction with other techniques, such as hypnosis and relaxation exercises. In addition, effective imagery is so individualized that it is difficult to quantify its effects[25].

There is no definite evidence that imagery helps the immune system, although an increasing number of studies suggest that it can. It is even more difficult to prove that imagery can aid in maintaining health and preventing disease, although Hall's study strongly suggests that this possibility exists.

Psychotherapeutic studies and interventions

In the mid-1950s Lawrence LeShan, a research and clinical psychologist, began his pioneering research studies in emotional factors in cancer. He concluded that psychological conditions have an enormous influence not only on the production of cancer, but also on the disease's evolution, and even on its response to a particular treatment. Based on clinical findings and statistical observations, LeShan developed a psychotherapy approach designed to stimulate the immune system in people with cancer and to extend their lives.

Various studies of individuals with cancer showed that the loss of a person's individual ways of 'being, relating and creating', and the inability to find a satisfactory substitute, often lead to a greater chance of that person's developing cancer. These studies found not that cancer patients failed to acknowledge emotions or that they repress them, but rather that they had no targets for emotional or creative expression. For example, in the 1950s and 1960s David Kissen, a chest physician working in the mines of Scotland, assessed the psychological profiles of hundreds of patients with respiratory symptoms. He found that those who were later diagnosed as having lung cancer seemed to have what he called 'poor outlets for emotional discharge', compared with patients with other diagnoses. Later studies which Kissen and Hans Eysenck did bore out these results[4].

Other statistical studies of relative mortality rates showed that widows and widowers of all ages were found to be at higher cancer risk than the still-married of the same ages. (Bereavement studies are described in the previous section on Helplessness and Immunosuppression.) Similarly, studies investigating the impact of retirement revealed that men aged from 35 to 70 years who were forced to retire were at a much higher risk of cancer over the next 5 years than those who continued to work. LeShan found that many cancer patients had experienced a profound loss of hope and of 'a reason for being' before being diagnosed. The traumatic loss of a crucial relationship (for example, death of a spouse, divorce, children leaving the home, or loss of meaningful work) resulted in a 'barren and hopeless' outlook. Their despair came from a loss of hope that they could ever achieve meaning, purpose and fulfillment in their lives.

Viktor Frankl, who survived Nazi extermination camps, understood very well the lifesaving effects of a sense of meaning and purpose. In his work *Man's Search for Meaning*, he wrote:

> Those who know how close the connection is between the state of mind of a man — his courage and hope, or lack of them — and the state of immunity of his body will understand that the sudden loss of hope and courage can have a deadly effect[26].

Carl Jung wrote, 'Meaninglessness ... is ... equivalent to illness'[27].

Initially LeShan's conclusions about the role of hopelessness in the development of malignancy were based on interviews and projective personality tests. He tested his conclusions in a prospective study in which he tried to predict the presence of cancer on the basis of emotional characteristics. In a blinded manner, he obtained personal history records of 28 new patients attending an out-patient medical clinic. Some had malignancies. All clues revealing the diagnosis were removed.

Of the 28 patients, 15 had a variety of malignancies and 13 did not. Five of the control group had no known disease, and the others had a variety of other diagnoses. Based solely on his previous findings about psychological factors in malignancy, LeShan correctly identified 24 out of the 28 cases[4].

His findings and statistical observations, coupled with psychotherapy with numerous cancer patients, led LeShan to the development of a new strategy of psychotherapy. It differs from the classic, Freudian approach, which asks the basic questions, 'What is wrong with this person?', 'How did he or she get that way?' and 'How, given the reality of their situation, can they move in this direction?' This approach, LeShan had learned, was ineffectual for extending survival time for people with catastrophic illness. His new approach stresses the individuality of each person, encouraging them to find their best ways of being, relating and creating. Its basic questions are, 'What is right with this person?', 'What is their best way to live?' and 'How, given the reality of their situation, can they move in this direction?' The therapy focuses on encouraging people to find a way of being that brings zest and enthusiasm to their daily life. Results of this approach with cancer patients are far superior in survival time to psychotherapies based on the classic strategy[2].

Since 1991 LeShan and this writer have worked with cancer patients using a new model of individual psychotherapy: a brief, intensive 'marathon'[28]. Typically, each marathon takes place over 6 consecutive days, each involving 2 to 5 hours of psychotherapy. After an initial 1 hour session with LeShan, the client meets with me for 2 to 5 hours daily for 6 consecutive days. On the last day the client meets with both of us for a 1-hour closing session.

I use a variety of therapeutic methods that lend themselves to an intensive application, including symbolic work with drawings and dreams, Gestalt work, 'inner child' work and psychodynamic therapy. All methods are applied within the framework of LeShan's strategy. They are aimed at mobilizing the client's immune system by encouraging the client to find a way of living that brings zest and enthusiasm to his or her daily life.

All marathon clients have made significant changes in lifestyle as well as corresponding psychological changes. It is too soon to analyze the long-term physical effects. In any case the total number of clients seen is not yet statistically significant.

LeShan's early prospective study was later replicated by Arthur Schmale, Jr and Howard Iker. They studied 51 women admitted to the hospital for biopsies because of an abnormal cervical smear test. A number of these women would have normal cervical biopsy results, and Schmale and Iker attempted to predict which of the women actually had carcinoma-in-situ prior to learning the biopsy results. They administered psychological tests to determine whether the women had recently sustained a loss or another event that evoked feelings of hopelessness. Some of the women had indeed experienced profound feelings of doom. Those women felt that they had no hope of happiness. On the basis of their psychological findings, the researchers correctly predicted the biopsy result in 36 of the 51 cases, with a 73% degree of accuracy.

Bernie Siegel described the relationship between hopelessness and cancer:

> One of the most common precursors of cancer is a traumatic loss or a feeling of emptiness in one's life ... When a salamander loses a limb, it grows a new one. In an analogous way, when a human suffers an emotional loss not properly dealt with, the body often responds by developing a new growth...[18]

The idea that a patient's coping ability and attitude may promote healing has been pursued by Steven H Greer of London's Royal Marsden Hospital. In 1977, Greer, in collaboration with Keith W Pettingale and Tina Morris, studied psychological characteristics of women 3 months after mastectomy for early-stage breast cancer.

The researchers defined four categories of psychological responses to diagnosis: 'fighting spirit', 'denial', 'stoic acceptance', and 'helplessness/ hopelessness'. The women in the study were matched for clinical stage, size of the tumor, its cancerous grade, its appearance on a mammogram, and hormonal and immunological profiles. The patients were interviewed, and assessments were made of how each woman was dealing with her diagnosis.

At the 5-year follow-up, 80% of the patients who exhibited fighting spirit and 70% of those in denial were alive with no disease recurrence. By contrast, only 35% of those who showed stoic acceptance and 20% of the helplessness/hopelessness group had survived. Taken together, the fighting spirit and denial groups were more than twice as likely to be alive and well 5 years later. After 10 years and again after 15 years, Greer and his colleague found that although a number of the patients had died, the same 2:1 survival ratio remained.

As a result, Greer has developed a program designed to engender a fighting spirit among patients who feel hopeless, helpless, or otherwise lack a sense of control in their fight with cancer, designed to give patients tools to work through depression, grief and anger.

Many psychotherapists have recently become interested in what they can do to activate their cancer patients' self-healing abilities. More and more experimentation is going on in this field. Serious treatment centers, which help the patient to complete physical, psychological and spiritual healing programs incorporating main-line oncology, are growing up all over the western world. Outstanding among these are the Bristol Health Centre in Bristol, England, and the Helen Dowling Institute for Biopsychosocial Medicine in Rotterdam.

In this short overview of a rich and diverse field, many important studies and researchers have been omitted. For example, I have omitted the research work of William Greene and his team in the 1950s on the psychological context in which cancer tends to appear. The work of Elida Evans and Claus Bahnson has also not been described[29]. Nor has the 35-year predictive study of Caroline Thomas. In particular, it is important to mention H J F Baltrusch in Germany. Since 1950 he has worked full-time in psychotherapy with cancer patients and in theory development[30-33]. His contributions to the field, while crucial and seminal, have received little recognition. He was also the co-founder of the international organization of those working in the field, and his tireless efforts have kept it the major cross-fertilization center for 35 years*.

PREMISES OF HOLISTIC MEDICINE AND IMPLICATIONS FOR PRACTICE

Premises

A growing body of scientific mind–body research has demonstrated that cancer is not simply a physical disease of cells 'gone awry.' Psychological, emotional and psychosocial factors play a significant role in cancer's onset and course; any purely physical approach to treatment is incomplete. The traditional model of mind–body separation no longer stands up to scientific scrutiny (Geffen Cancer Center 1994, unpublished).

Traditional western medicine has relied on the belief that mind and body are, for the most part, unrelated and independent. Abraham Myerson, writing in 1950 about historical views

*The European working group for psychosomatic cancer research is EUPSYCA, c/o Dr HJF Baltrusch, Bergstasse 10, D-16122, Oldenberg, Germany.

of the mind–body relationship, put it this way:

Very great scientists declared that there was no way in which mental activities, especially consciousness, could be linked up with the molecular physical structure of the brain. Thus they fathered the parallelistic theory by which mind processes and brain processes ran side by side, parallel to each other, and, Euclidean-like, never meeting[34].

Holistic medicine rests on a different model of mind–body interaction. The individual is seen as a psychological-biological whole integrated within a specific physical and social environment. From this point of view, a disturbance in any part of this system affects the whole individual.

'Illness', said Jerome Frank, 'is a disturbance of the whole person in which pathogenic forces are greater than regenerative ones, and healing is the restoration of a healthy equilibrium, either spontaneously or through outside intervention[35].

To clarify the implications for medical practice of recent mind–body research, it is helpful first to contrast the assumptions of the western biomedical model with those underlying mind–body medicine. Premises of the western biomedical model are listed in Box 5.1.

Not all present-day physicians agree with the biomedical model. Andrew Weil, for example, wrote:

The biomedical model ... makes it difficult to present a view of the healing systems to doctors in training. It [emphasizes] form rather than function. The healing system is a functional system, not an assemblage of structures that can be neatly diagrammed like the digestive or circulatory systems ... Worse, the biomedical model discounts or entirely writes off the importance of the mind, looking instead for purely physical causes of changes in health and illness[16].

And Larry Dossey wrote:

I ... have been trained to believe ... that it is only the blind play of the atoms and molecules in a body that is important. These entities are unfeeling and unconscious, and their behavior controlled by neutral laws of science. How could physicians have come to believe that the perceptions of our patients — their perceived meanings and significances, their thoughts, feelings, and emotions — do not matter? Every day we see the mental moving before our eyes. The will to live, for example, can forestall death by actually changing a host of physiological responses. In the placebo response, where a fake medication means the real drug to the patient, meaning moves matter dramatically. And, as every physician knows, heart attacks or sudden death can be brought on by emotional shock...[1]

One reason that medicine has largely denied mind and meaning as important factors in illness, Dossey added, is the belief that it is 'scientific' to do so. As he put it, 'Physicians and medical researchers have expressed a genuine "physics envy" for over a century'.[1]

The holistic view, for purposes of this discussion, can be stated in the form of seven underlying premises that shape mind–body practice. They are listed in Box 5.2, and will be discussed in terms of their implications for practice[2,6,16].

Implications for practice

The first two premises are the most fundamental and are the basis for the others:

1. Mind and body are simply two aspects of the whole individual. The mind is no less medically real and significant than the body.
2. Every person has self-healing abilities.

Box 5.2 Premises of mind–body medicine

1. Mind and body are simply two aspects of a whole individual. The mind is no less medically real and significant than the body.
2. Every person has self-healing abilities.
3. Each person is unique, and must be responded to as such. To be most effective, the treatment program must be individualized for each person.
4. Each person is an integration of physical, psychological, intellectual and spiritual aspects. All aspects are equally important. All must be addressed in the approach to health.
5. Patients' healing abilities are strongly affected by their expectations and beliefs. The expectations, attitudes, beliefs and words of practitioners strongly influence the expectations of their patients.
6. Mainline medicine does not have a monopoly on the search for health.
7. Patients need to be actively involved in their own healing and in the decision-making concerning their treatments.

Self-healing powers were well known to the early Greeks. The Greek God of healing, Asclepius, had two daughters. One, Panakeia, was knowledgeable about the use of medication to treat disease. She is embodied today in the search for panaceas, drugs or treatments. The other daughter, Hygeia, was knowledgeable about how to live in concert with nature to prevent disease. She is embodied today in the search for ways to mobilize the natural defense abilities that are the indispensable agents for healing and recovery.

Hippocrates spoke of these abilities. 'First, do no harm' (primum non nocere), he told physicians; and, 'Honor the healing power of Nature' (vis medicatrix naturae).

LeShan has pointed out the conflict at the heart of current medical practice. The issue is whether the physician should focus primarily on actively intervening in disease or on helping the patient's self-healing systems to work more effectively[7].

The growing body of mind–body research has demonstrated that physicians can help their cancer patients by learning to combine these two views.

Apparently, cancer cells grow because of conditions favorable to them, such as toxic substances, malnutrition, genetic factors, and immune suppression. Whether or not the immune system is at fault when cancer develops, it now seems certain that bolstering the immune system can help fight malignancy.

The next five premises taken together define the ground of mind–body medical practice:

3. Each person is unique, and must be responded to as such. To be most effective, the treatment program must be individualized for each person.
4. Each person is an integration of physical, psychological, intellectual and spiritual aspects. All aspects are equally important. All must be addressed in the approach to health.

'It is more important to find out what patient has the disease than what disease the patient has', wrote physician Sir William Osler early in the 20th Century. Later, in the 1970s, physician George Engel and his colleagues echoed this focus on the context of a patient's illness. Instead of asking, 'What is the cause of this illness?' they asked, 'Why does *this* patient have *this* disease now[7]?'

Since then, research has verified that the onset and progression of cancer have to do not only with aberrant cancer cells, but at least as much with the terrain, the total unique person in which the malignancy grows. Purely physical causes do not explain why some people become ill and others do not. Marc Barasch, discussing the idea of a single physical cause of illness, wrote:

> If a woman smokes to relieve the stress of a miserable marriage, what is the 'cause' of her lung cancer? A genetic predisposition? The histology of oat-cell carcinoma? The smoking itself? Her relationship? How thorough is her cure if she has a lung removed but does not change her marital circumstances, let alone enquire into the personality patterns that permitted her to cling to her longtime unhappiness[36]?

Carcinogens are a real threat to the body's defense system, but they do not affect all persons who are equally exposed in the same ways. When carcinogens enter the terrain they can either be eliminated or start the malignant process. LeShan pointed out that injecting cancer-free volunteers with live cancer cells, as has been done in some studies, does not always produce cancer. In nearly all individuals, it produces instead a local irritation which soon heals by itself. To produce cancer in animals for such studies, it is necessary either to use carefully bred animals with a genetically weakened cancer defense mechanism, or to first treat the animals with total body irradiation or in other ways weaken the animals' defense[7].

The course of cancer, as well as its onset, differs in different individuals. Patients of the same age, gender, physical condition and the same type of cancer who undergo the same treatment often fare very differently. Some cancer patients far outlive medical expectations, while others die far sooner than predicted.

Both doctors and patients have assumed that doctors treat cancer. In fact, they treat people who have cancer. When they lose sight of this, doctors lose sight of the people. It is the whole, unique person that needs to be treated, not the disease. The disease is not a separate 'thing', but rather part of the total life process of the person. It grows in a context, the 'terrain'.

The strength of the terrain depends on many unique factors, including genetic heritage, general health, diet, psychological make-up, emotions and attitudes, and the strength of the cancer defense mechanism. Any or all of these factors might facilitate illness or recovery. In terms of psychological make-up alone, individuals differ dramatically. 'We differ tremendously from one another ... in our childhood and adult experiences of the world, in the degree and ways we have nurtured or repressed our different needs, in the amount and ways we have directed our energies inward and outward, in our fears of ourselves and others, and in the meaning we have found in our lives' (p.137)[2].

Barasch wrote:

> Most conventional diagnosis still tends to discard personhood in a misguided attempt to boil a case down to its bare, manipulable variables. The patient's life history and personality — as well as the living bodily context of the disease — becomes secondary to laboratory specimens and instrument read-outs. The individual is evaluated, but scarcely encountered ... This one-dimensional sketch — drawn up in the service of time-and-cost efficiency as much as science — tends to supplant other ways of knowing (p.141)[36].

There are other ways as well to 'boil down a case to its bare manipulable variables'. One is to reduce an individual to a 'stage'. ('This patient is a Stage 2 Hodgkins Disease.') Larry Dossey said that doctors hide behind the metaphor of the 'stage' instead of confronting the unique person to whom these terms apply[1].

Viewing a patient in terms of survival statistics is yet another way to avoid acknowledging the unique person. Statistics apply only to groups, not to any one individual. Many people surpass their prognosis and experience remissions unrelated to medical expectations. A growing number of studies are being done of such survivors. Barasch, who interviewed a number of them, wrote:

> What, if anything, did these people have in common? Certainly there was no pattern in their choice of medicines, which might have included carrot juice and chemo, psychotherapy and psychic healing, visualization and vincristine. Or in their methods — some had conventional treatment, some used 'complementary therapies', and some had explored the further shores of shamanic or spiritual 'healing' (p.53)[36].

Kenneth Pelletier is one of many physicians who have observed that the physician's attitude toward the patient is critically important, for the relationship between a doctor and patient exerts a powerful influence on the course and outcome of the disease.

> This relationship might directly affect underlying biochemical processes through the psychophysiological mechanisms involved in stress and its alleviation. It is also likely that the doctor–patient relationship is responsible for the placebo effect (p.35)[6].

A patient needs to be seen and responded to as a person. Today a new generation of humanistic physicians is beginning to reject their legacy of reducing a patient to a machine, a test result, a statistic, a stage, or a member of any classification. They are becoming aware that viewing a patient in this way is anti-therapeutic. They are also learning that there is no single right treatment for all cancer patients. Each patient must be regarded as a unique individual, and treatment determined accordingly.

The holistic view was first expressed by Jan Christian Smuts in his 1926 book, *Holism and Evolution*[37], and later by the psychiatrist Kurt Goldstein in his 1934 book, *The Organism: A Holistic Approach to Biology*[38]. It involves the perception that each individual is a unique integration of body, mind and spirit, all equally important. Confronting the patient as a person rather than as a medical case entails acknowledging and responding to all these aspects. All must be considered in a total treatment program.

5. Patients' healing abilities are strongly affected by their expectations and beliefs. Practitioners' expectations, attitudes, beliefs and words strongly influence the expectations of their patients.

Most cancer patients have clear expectations about the likelihood of recovery. Their expectations arise less from their medical prognosis than from their long-standing metaphysical expectations about life. Those who learned early that life can bring them good things generally expect to recover. Those who learned early that life disappoints them generally expect to die. Expectations can mobilize or weaken the powers of self-healing.

The power of expectation is illustrated clearly by the famous case documented by Bruno Klopfer in 1957. His patient, 'Mr Wright', had advanced widespread lymphosarcoma. His body was riddled with tumors, some the size of oranges. All standard treatments had failed, and he was expected to live no more than a few weeks. A new drug, Krebiozen, touted as a potential cancer cure, was being tested at the clinic where Klopfer worked. At Wright's pleading, Klopfer included him in the trial. Shortly after he administered one injection of the drug, the patient's tumor masses, Klopfer wrote, melted like snowballs on a hot stove, and in only these few days were half their original size. Wright was soon released from the hospital, apparently free of malignancy. Two months later, when newspapers printed reports of the worthlessness of Krebiozen, his tumors quickly returned. Suspecting that this was due to Wright's expectations, Klopfer decided to use him as a control patient. He told Wright that he would give him a double-strength dosage of a new, more active form of the drug — and treated him with distilled water. Again the tumors melted away, and for the next 2 months, Wright lived without symptoms. Then the newspapers published a report from the American Medical Association stating beyond doubt that Krebiozen was worthless. Wright appeared at the hospital a few days later. His tumors had reappeared, and he died within 2 days[18].

A more common example of the powerful effects of expectation is found in patients treated with chemotherapy. They feel sick just before receiving the drugs, the evening before, on the way to the hospital, or when they enter the place of treatment. They involuntarily learn to get sick as a conditioned response to their anticipated experiences of the chemotherapy situation. That patients' healing abilities are affected by their expectations is shown also in studies on the effects of placebos. Clearly, one reason for the efficacy of placebos is the belief or faith in the treatment. LeShan wrote:

> The physician's attitude and beliefs and the patient's conscious and unconscious perception of them strongly affect the results of his medications and procedures. The patient's belief systems about the effectiveness of medical procedures affect how well they work. Since the physician perceives this, the medications tend to work much better at first than they do later (p.96)[7].

Jerome Frank said:

> Physicians have also known that their ability to inspire expectant trust in a patient partially determines the success of that treatment (p.133)[35].

Bernie Siegel also affirmed that the efficacy of a placebo depends on the patient's trust in the physician:

> I've become convinced that this relationship is more important, in the long run, than any medicine or procedure ... A patient's confidence in a certain treatment can be negated by the doctor's unspoken rejection of it (p.37)[18].

Siegel told an illustrative story about the chemotherapy drug cisplatinum. When it was first used, it was received with great excitement, and doctors reported its rates of effectiveness as high as 75%. Over time, however, the new drug's success rate dropped to 30% or less. Why? Siegel speculated that at first the physicians believed they had a miracle drug, and their expectations activated the patients' healing response. Later, when the drug was administered by technicians in a routine way without the fanfare, its effects might have diminished[36].

The power of expectation extends far beyond the effects of medication. Walter Cannon, who identified the 'fight-or-flight' response to fear and danger, wrote of the wide-ranging effects that fear can impose on our bodies. Fascinated by voodoo medicine, he wondered how it is possible that one human being can point at another human being and say that at a specific time that person will die — and the prediction is fulfilled. Cannon studied people in hospitals who had been hexed, and watched them die of no cause he could determine. He discovered that what happens is that the individual accepts the truth of the witch doctor's prediction. That 'truth' can lead to death. As Norman Cousins put it, 'The will to die replaces the will to live, and the individual accepts an appointment with death'[39]. In voodoo death, as Cousins put it, 'belief becomes biology'.

Similarly, when a diagnostician paints a graphic worst case picture, appropriately reinforced with statistics, or when a physician says, 'There is nothing more we can do' or predicts how short a time the patient is likely to live, the patient may well accept the practitioner's 'truth' so that it becomes a prediction which the patient fulfills. As Jeanne Achterberg wrote, 'Images are so readily translated into physical change that dying from having been given a feared diagnosis by a credible physician is just as feasible as a hex death by a cursed Haitian' (p.78)[40].

Larry Dossey pointed out that when a physician gives a patient a diagnosis of cancer, even simply citing statistics can function as a modern-day curse:

> Even though the physician dutifully describes the prognosis as 'survival' statistics, the curse frequently has already done its work. Even though patients may be told they have a 50% chance of living another 5 years, their interpretation is frequently that they have a 50% chance of dying. Like the accursed individual in voodoo societies, they may cooperate by succumbing 'on time' (p.90)[1].

George Melton, an AIDS patient, wrote, 'When I got my diagnosis, I sentenced myself to death.'

The conclusion is clear. If we can sentence ourselves to death and keep that appointment, we can keep an appointment with life. 'If the mind can program the body to die, it can program the body to live' (p.39)[12]. The physician can help.

Physicians' words or even unspoken attitudes have enormous power to affect the lives of the human beings in their care. A patient of mine was fortunate to find an oncologist who apparently knows the power of his words. A year earlier she had completed treatment for ovarian cancer. Now, after a routine blood test indicated a recurrence, a laparoscopy revealed numerous widespread small tumors as well as a larger inoperable tumor. Her surgeon, who could not deal with delivering bad news to an already terrified patient, minimized these findings to her. It was up to the oncologist to tell her the whole truth. He said, 'We found small cancer cells in your peritoneal area, as well as a two-centimeter tumor on your spleen. None of these can be removed surgically. I know this sounds frightening, but I want you to know that I'm not about to dig a hole and bury you. No one is giving up hope. There are treatments that can be used that have been effective. Here is what I propose we do...' While giving a complete report, this physician acknowledged his patient's fear and also conveyed hope. With his word 'we', he let her know that she was not alone, and that there were people working for her health. As she left his office, for the first time in weeks she was optimistic and ready to do everything she could to fight for her life.

How could any patient have hope if her own doctor conveys hopelessness? It would be helpful to all cancer patients if their physicians did not allow statistics to determine their attitude and their behavior. 'Statistics are important when one is choosing the best therapy for a specific situation, but once that choice is made, they no longer apply to the individual' (p.39)[18].

Physicians are concerned not to give 'false hope'. However, if nine out of ten people with a certain form of cancer have died of it, giving 'false hope' means no more than encouraging a patient to believe that she might be the tenth who survives. Remissions, inexplicable from a medical viewpoint, occur that defy the statistics. The reality is that no one knows for certain how long any patient will live. LeShan, referring to physicians' predictions of survival time to patients, said, 'Physicians often play God, but so few of them have the qualifications.' And Carl Simonton said, 'In the face of uncertainty, there is nothing wrong with hope.'

Siegel observed, 'All patients [who want to live] must be accorded the conviction that they can get well, no matter what the odds' (p.68)[18]. Hope comes about largely as a result of the patient's confidence and trust in the healer.

Physicians tend to be more logical, statistical, and rigid, and less inclined to have hope than their patients. When physicians run out of remedies, they're likely to give up. They must realize, however, that lack of faith in the patient's ability to heal can severely limit that ability. 'We should never say, "There's nothing more I can do for you." There's always something more we can do, even if it's only to sit down, talk, and help the patient hope and pray' (p.38)[18].

6. Mainline medicine does not have a monopoly on the search for health.

Medical practitioners can expand their thinking beyond standard treatment methods. Typically, oncologists advise no treatment other than surgery, chemotherapy and radiation. Now, to be sure, there are new medical options: bone marrow transplants, stem cell transplants, and the use of growth factors as part of the chemotherapy regimen. However, when medical treatment is not indicated or when it is finished, physicians usually say that there is nothing more that can or needs to be done for the patient.

There is much more that can be done, both during and after medical treatment, to bolster the 'terrain' in which the cancer grew.

It has been estimated that 10 to 50% of all cancer patients in the USA use at least one form of complementary or alternative treatment — and do not confide in their medical oncologists[41]. Their reluctance to discuss this matter with their physician reflects their lack of trust that the physician is open to non-conventional treatment. This reluctance and lack of trust are not helpful to the patient–doctor relationship.

The physician can help by encouraging the patient to seek complementary therapies, and in particular, encouraging those who cannot be treated with surgery, chemotherapy, radiation or transplants to become informed about alternative therapies. (Informal estimates suggest that the overall long-term remission rate of patients treated with alternative therapies is 10%.) Also, patients can be made aware of psychosocial support groups, and encouraged to learn about healthy diets and nutritional supports. They can be made aware of such complementary modalities as exercise programs, stress reduction techniques, herbal remedies, acupuncture, meditation, and visualization.

These are not treatments for cancer, but they can supplement and support medical treatment by aiding in the healing process.

Typically, patients interested in adjunctive and alternative modalities need to spend a great deal of time and energy researching what is available. Physicians can help by suggesting books or offering information about non-standard therapies, and by providing lists of competent alternative and complementary practitioners.

Cancer creates an emotional, as well as a physical, crisis for any patient. The physician, recognizing the debilitating effects of stress, can encourage patients to consider seeing a psychotherapist trained in working with people with cancer. The physician is not a trained psychotherapist, and should not be expected to function as one. However, it would be enormously helpful to patients if their physicians asked, 'How are you dealing with all this?' — and took the time to listen carefully to the patient's answer.

LeShan observed that a patient, experiencing anxiety, fear, physical discomfort, and the pain of living with cancer, wakes up each morning to a nightmare, with a nightmare's 'special ego-weakening and emotionally and physically exhausting effects'. As in any nightmare, terrible things are happening, and perhaps worse are threatened; there is nothing the person can do; and there is no time limit[2].

While emotions do not cause cancer, they can affect the course of cancer. Norman Cousins graphically described the psychology of seriously ill patients[42]. Patients, he wrote, experience feelings of helplessness — a serious disease in itself. They fear they will die, or that they will never function normally again, and they feel a wall of separation between themselves 'and the world of open movement, open sounds, open expectations.' Often reluctant to be regarded as complainers, they do not wish to add to the already great burden of apprehension felt by their family. This increases their isolation. They are trapped between the terror of loneliness and the desire to be left alone. They feel a lack of self-esteem, fearing that their illness might be a manifestation of some inadequacy. They fear that decisions are being made behind their backs. They fear intrusive treatments and encounters with intimidating technology. 'Most of all,' Cousins wrote, 'there is the utter void created by the longing — ineradicable, unremitting, pervasive — for warmth of human contact.'

Barasch, a former cancer patient, wrote, 'Patients [diagnosed with cancer]... face the challenge of affirming their own individuality precisely at a time when everything — their disease, their clinicians, the world at large — seems intent on eroding it' (p.198)[36].

Besides the difficulties in dealing with their diagnosis, illness and treatment, many cancer patients have experienced a loss in their lives prior to diagnosis that left them feeling hopeless about creating a life that they would find meaningful and fulfilling.

In addition to helping the patient to deal with the diagnosis, illness and treatment, psychotherapy can help to enrich the patient's life by clarifying why the patient wants to live. Its relevant questions are, 'What do you want to do with the time remaining to you in your life, whether it be 3 months or 30 years?', 'What has stopped you in the past from living the kind of life that reflects who you are?', and 'How can you develop a realistic plan to enable you to change yourself and your life in this direction?'

In the disease-oriented approach to medicine, both patients and physicians assume that the purpose of medical treatment is to restore patients to the state they were in before their symptoms appeared. Yet it was while they were in that state that the cancer developed. So something must be different; something must change. All aspects of the person must be evaluated in terms of the possibility of positive change. At the same time, the best possible care must be given to the body. As Andrew Weil put it:

> Because it represents failure of the healing system, cancer, even in its early and localized stages, is a systemic disease. Patients must work to improve general health and resistance by making changes on all levels: physical, mental/emotional, and spiritual (p.274)[16].

7. Patients are helped by becoming actively involved in their illness and treatment.

In early animal experiments, the rats who were powerless to control stressful stimuli were less able to defend themselves against implanted tumors. In studies with human beings, individuals in situations where they felt helpless, hopeless and with no control experienced chronic stress and weakened immune function. Cancer, wrote Barasch, is:

> a fundamental loss of control, a form of possession by bodily forces we cannot contain, and by social forces — doctors, hospitals, even family and well-meaning friends — that threaten to contain us. Gears whose existence we never suspected whir into motion, oiled by decades of cultural consensus. Suddenly, ordinary coping mechanisms are rendered null and void, our identity is subsumed under the badge "patient". We are dispossessed of ourselves (p.197)[36].

He continued:

> From patients' point of view, modern medicine may represent an invasion not just of the body but of the renascent sense of self ... they are struggling to reclaim. The predominant style of medicine too often runs counter to patients' own healing requirements. They need to develop autonomy, but are instead infantilized, kept in the dark. They need to actively affirm their uniqueness, but are reduced to passive recipients of normative "protocols"; they need time but are rushed onto a virtual conveyor belt ... They need a hopeful vision of the future, and are instead provided with often pessimistic ("realistic") prognoses... (p.201)[36]

All individuals, ill or well, need to assert their autonomy. When they actively engage in decisions, and take steps to deal with their fears, blocks, or feelings of powerlessness and despair, they are moving away from helplessness.

Numerous studies have demonstrated that medical results are far better when patients are involved in decisions about their treatment and care than when they surrender to the authority of others. Patients are the leading authorities on how they feel, including their experience of symptoms and their response to treatment. Physicians are the authorities on medical diagnosis and care. Together as a team with mutual respect, they can collaborate to work effectively.

Physicians can affect the health of their patients by the ways they interact with them. One way they can encourage patients to collaborate with them is by listening to what the patients say. 'Very often the patients' verbal account of their illnesses is ignored,' wrote James Pelletier, 'and physicians rely almost entirely upon laboratory assessments'[6].

When patients are diagnosed, they have urgent questions which require clear, accurate answers. To participate actively in their own well-being, they need as much information as they ask for and can accept. A lack of understanding about their illness or treatment can lead to unnecessary fear and suffering. Only when adequate answers are given to their questions can patients relax sufficiently to allow healing to occur (Geffen Cancer Center 1994, unpublished).

Physicians can encourage patients to become involved in making decisions about medical treatment instead of passively accepting treatment — and allow them time to do so. To whatever extent is appropriate, patients need to participate in decisions about their treatment. They also need to know that they can refuse treatment.

Often physicians with incurable or terminally ill patients feel frustrated or impotent. As a result they avoid discussing the illness with the patient, or avoid the patient altogether. Two physicians, Richard Gorlin and Howard Zucker, who taught a course in humanistic medicine at the Mount Sinai Medical School, tried to make their students aware of their feelings about patients and the ways those feelings affect the care they provide. In an article in the *New England Journal of Medicine*, Gorlin and Zucker pointed out:

> It is critical to realize that even when there is no further specific therapy available, there are constructive things that can and should be done to help the patient and the family endure the experience (p.185)[8].

Patients who can be treated need to know what they can do to recover their health, and to prevent recurrences. The physician's job can go far beyond 'repair'. When patients are well, the physician can encourage them to collaborate by teaching them how to remain healthy.

ALTERNATIVE THERAPIES

There are a wide variety of promising alternative approaches to cancer. Many of them are in need of further study to determine their potential. 'Alternative' treatments include both those that are adjunctive or complementary to conventional treatment and those that are used in place of them.

Alternative treatments are relatively nontoxic. While they vary greatly, they are all aimed at cleansing the body or stimulating its natural defense systems.

In addition to psychological and behavioral treatments discussed earlier, alternative medicine includes: nutritional therapies, acupuncture, herbal treatments, and a variety of pharmacologic and biologic treatments. Success rates vary widely. What works for one patient may be ineffective for another with the same or different malignancy. Researchers who have investigated alternative health clinics and interviewed patients report that success rates average approximately 4–10%, which includes terminal cases[43].

Dietary therapies

A preponderance of scientific and clinical evidence shows beneficial effects for many cancer patients from a nutritional component in cancer care. Nutrition can help not only to prevent cancer by creating an oxygen-rich bodily environment that is hostile to cancer cells and beneficial to existing healthy cells, but also to strengthen patients during debilitating treatments. Many anticancer diets are largely vegetarian or low-fat, limiting or avoiding animal products, and emphasizing vegetables, fruits and whole grains, particularly organically grown foods. An example is the Bristol Cancer Help Centre diet, which is strictly vegetarian. Another example is the anticancer dietary system developed by the Dutch physician Cornelis Moerman, consisting of a meatless, high-fiber diet rich in vitamins and minerals, combined with eight supplements found to be vital to ideal health: citric acid, iodine, iron, sulfur, and vitamins A, B-complex, C and E.

In a study released by the German Cancer Research Center in Heidelberg, vegetarians were found to have a more active immune system. Their white blood cells were twice as effective against tumor cells as those of meat eaters.

The use of vitamin and mineral supplements has been found to be therapeutic. For example, vitamins C and E are said to block the formation of cancer-causing agents and the conversion of some carcinogens into 'active form'. Vitamin A and beta carotene block the action of tumor-causing agents. Vitamins A, C and E may be active in reversing the entire process of free radicals, and may also act to aid in the destruction of newly formed cancer cells. Numerous other supplements — notably zinc, magnesium, B vitamins and chromium — are being studied in terms of their usefulness against malignancy[44].

Clearly no-one diet and supplement program is appropriate for every cancer patient. Any nutritional regimen needs to be tailored to each individual's needs. Some dietary programs are part of a multi-faceted approach that includes conventional cancer treatment, stress reduction, exercise and psychological support.

Besides diets and supplements recommended for people with cancer, there are a number of alternative, unconventional nutritional therapies which attempt to eliminate physiological or biochemical factors supporting the growth of cancer cells[43].

For example, macrobiotics, popularized by Michio Kuchi, consists largely of cooked vegetables and whole grains along with a spiritual philosophy incorporating many aspects of daily life.

The Gerson regimen, developed by the late physician Max Gerson, consists of a low sodium, high potassium vegetarian diet, various pharmacological agents and coffee enemas. Gerson believed that his treatment regimen aids in the elimination of 'toxins'. The regimen of William Donald Kelley, currently practiced by Nicholas Gonzalez, MD, in New York, involves dietary guidelines, vitamin and enzyme supplements and computerized metabolic typing. Wheatgrass therapy, developed by Ann Wigmore, combines the use of wheatgrass juice with a diet of organic raw fruits and vegetables, sprouted grains, nuts and seeds, fermented foods (to prevent harmful bacteria from growing in the intestinal tract), and greens such as buckwheat and sunflower.

Acupuncture

Acupuncture has been used to manage chronic pain, either to replace conventional analgesia or to minimize its needed dosages. Studies have shown that acupuncture, acupressure and moxibustion (the application of heat to acupuncture points) can have a variety of beneficial effects. These include: significantly reducing the nausea and vomiting produced by chemotherapy; controlling or alleviating certain kinds of cancer-related or treatment-related pain; alleviating side effects of radiation, most notably edema; and, according to animal studies, possibly contributing to life extension[23].

Herbal treatments

Herbs are the sources of much of the mainstream pharmacopeia, and are also used in many unconventional cancer treatments.

These include mixtures of herbal products, such as essiac, an herbal tea developed by a nurse, Rene Caisse, and currently offered in Canada. Essiac consists of Indian rhubarb, sheepshead sorrel, slippery elm and burdock root.

The Hoxey treatment, developed by the late Harry Hoxey and currently offered in Tiajuana, consists of several preparations, all made from herbs combined with inorganic compounds.

Iscador, made from mistletoe, became prominent through the work of Rudolph Steiner, and is used mainly in the context of Anthroposophic medicine in Europe.

Besides proprietary herbal mixtures, there are single-agent treatments, such as chaparral tea, made from the leaves and twigs of the creosote bush, and pau d'arco, a substance derived from the inner bark of trees in South America[45].

There is no question that the ingredients of many traditional Chinese herbal remedies are pharmacologically active against cancer. Chinese herbal therapies have already produced a significant number of anticancer drugs, including Indirubin, Irisquinn and Zhuyline Polysaccharide[23]. Other Chinese herbs, such as Astragalus membranaceus and ginseng, are undergoing clinical trials. Western cancer patients widely report that traditional Chinese medicine, which includes herbal remedies, offers considerable relief from the side effects of chemotherapy and radiation, as well as being a method of pain control[23].

Pharmacological and biological approaches

A large and diverse group of cancer treatments have as their central component a pharmacological or biological substance, such as biochemical agents, vaccines, blood products and synthetic chemicals. They are intended to extend survival time, with or without affecting the tumor directly[45].

One such treatment, developed by the late Virginia Livingston in San Diego, has as its main component a vaccine designed to treat and prevent infection with the microbe which Livingston believed to cause cancer. The treatment also includes other components aimed at bolstering immune responses and counteracting effects of microbial infection, including antibiotics, nutritional supplements and a special diet.

Stanislaw Burzynski, MD, PhD in Texas offers what he calls 'Antineoplastons,' substances described as peptides or amino acid derivatives isolated from urine or synthesized in the laboratory.

In New York, Emanuel Revici, MD, offers what is described as 'biologically guided chemotherapy', consisting of a variety of minerals, lipids and lipid-based substances.

'Eumetabolic' treatment, offered by Hans Nieper, MD in Germany, consists of a combination of conventional and unconventional agents (including pharmaceutical drugs, vitamins, minerals, and animal and plant extracts) along with a special diet. Nieper also recommends that his patients avoid particular foods, agents and physical locations that he believes to be damaging.

Gaston Naessens, a French biologist now in Canada, developed a non-toxic cancer treatment called 714-X, an aqueous solution of nitrogen-enriched camphor molecules. The camphor-nitrogen compound is injected into the body's lymphatic system, and is said to strengthen the immune system.

Hydrazine sulfate, undergoing clinical trials as an anticancer drug, is said to cause malignant tumors to stop growing or to reduce in size. Other pharmacological or biological agents used singly or in combination include vitamin C, popularized by Linus Pauling; dimethyl sulfoxide (DMSO), an industrial solvent often used with laetrile and vitamin C; cellular treatment involving processed tissue from animal embryos or fetuses; shark cartilage; and various substances containing oxygen, including hydrogen peroxide and ozone, taken orally, rectally or through blood infusion.

Ozone therapy, combining ozone and oxygen, has been found to shrink tumors, as well as destroy viruses and bacteria in the bloodstream. In treating cancer ozone is usually an adjunctive therapy, but sometimes a primary therapy. A number of studies indicate that when ozone is used with radiation or chemotherapy, lower dosages of the conventional agents will achieve either the same or a better effect[43].

Immunological therapies

In addition to the orthodox forms of immunotherapy currently being explored in clinics and cancer centers as adjuncts to standard medical treatments (BCG, interferon, interleukin-2, TNF and monoclonal antibodies) there are a number of alternative immunological therapies. One is the Livingston treatment described earlier.

Another alternative immunological therapy is that of the late Lawrence Burton of the Grand Bahamas, who offered 'immunoaugmentative therapy', consisting of daily injections of dilute serum fractions made from pooled blood samples.

In Germany Josef Issels has achieved remissions through a combination of therapies designed to reduce tumors and rebuild the immune system. Among other methods, his 'whole body' approach includes anticancer vaccines, a low-protein organic diet, and fever therapy to stimulate immune function.

CONCLUSION

The scope of mind–body medicine is wider than that of traditional medicine. It includes maintenance of health and prevention of illness, therapies to restore natural healing abilities, psychotherapy or counseling, lifestyle change, and support of the patient as a unique, autonomous, responsible, capable individual. Jeremy Geffen, a medical oncologist who combines traditional and complementary treatments in his cancer center, urges that a new paradigm of medicine is needed, one that cares for the mind, heart and spirit as much as for the body (Geffen J, personal communication).

Comprehensive cancer treatment is holistic, involving the use of medical technology to reduce or remove tumors as well as restorative therapies to build up the terrain of the cancer patient.

Rene Dubos wrote:

> The only trouble with scientific medicine is that it is not scientific enough. Modern medicine will become really scientific only when physicians and their patients have learned to manage the forces of the body and the mind that operate in vis medicatrix naturae [in reality, self healing] (p. 23)[46].

SUMMARY AND OVERVIEW OF THE FIELD OF THE PSYCHOSOMATIC ASPECTS OF CANCER

Lawrence LeShan

In the late 1940s and early 1950s the study of the psychological aspects of neoplastic disease, a field which had lain nearly dormant since the studies of Herbert Snow around 1900, suddenly sprang into large-scale activity. All over the western world individuals and small teams, largely unknown to one another, began to work in this area. Serious research started at the Karolinskaya in Sweden, at the Kiev Oncological Institute, at Roswell Park in New York State, Oldenberg in Germany, Australia, in the mines of Scotland, and at a dozen or so other places. Although it was difficult to publish at the time since most journal editors went along with the prevailing medical opinion that this area was the purview of charlatans only, the situation gradually changed. The first major conference in the area was held at MD Anderson Hospital in 1953[47]. An international organization of workers in the field was formed in 1956 by H J F Baltrusch and this writer, and has continued to meet every 2 years since then (see footnote, p.98). An 18 page review of the literature appeared in the prestigious *Journal of the National Cancer Institute* in 1959[3]. The field developed to a point where the New York Academy of Sciences held two 3-day symposia on the subject in the 1960s[48,49].

From 1950 to the 1970s most of the work was correlational without much attempt to study intervention variables. Thus Gotthard Booth related development and 'spontaneous' regression of tumors to psychological and Rorschach variables[50]. A study at Walter Reed Hospital showed that Hodgkin's Disease tended to be selective in terms of intelligence — that is, it was statistically more likely to appear in persons of higher intelligence than the norm[51]. In the still valid words of Sidney Peller who had shown years earlier that widows and widowers have a higher cancer rate than their non-widowed peers, 'the circumstances in the carcinorelevant mechanism remains to be clarified'[52].

After the 1970s, studies more and more began to relate psychological variables to measures believed related to the immune system. These included T cell counts and similar factors. In the 1980s the field as a whole became much more widely known to the general public through the work of Bernie Siegel and his best-selling book[18].

Such landmark studies as those of Ronald Greer et al.[53], of Grossarth-Matticek[54] and of Sandra Levy[55] have now demonstrated clearly that psychological factors do affect the development of tumors. The data are now so strong that they can no longer be ignored by those wishing to sustain a scientific attitude towards the cancer field.

Slowly and with much experimentation, this knowledge is being put to use. Various centers for cancer patients, such as the Bristol Cancer Help Centre (in Bristol, England), Commonweal (Bolinas, California), Life After Cancer (Asheville, North Carolina) and the Helen Dowling Institute (Rotterdam), are attempting, through psychological means, to help patients mobilize their self-healing abilities (immune system) and bring them to the aid of the medical program. Increasing numbers of serious psychotherapists are attempting to define the best therapeutic strategies for this purpose. One such strategy has been devised by the present author and is being used increasingly widely[2].

The field at this time is in very rapid expansion on all fronts. It is a rare month that goes by without the appearance of new publications on the subject. The relatively new journal *Advances* continues to publish a large number of studies and reviews in the field. The future is, as in any scientific area, unpredictable, but it is now extremely likely that cancer will increasingly be viewed as a systemic rather than as a local disease, and that treatment will more and more focus on the whole person and not just on a collection of cells.

REFERENCES

1 Dossey L 1992 Medicine and meaning. Bantam, New York

2 LeShan L 1994 Cancer as a turning point. Plume, New York

3 LeShan L 1959 Psychological states as factors in the development of malignant disease: a critical review. Journal of the National Cancer Institute 22:1–18

4 LeShan L 1977 You can fight for your life. M. Evans, New York

5 Pelletier J 1992 Mind as healer, mind as slayer. Delta, New York

6 Pelletier K 1979 Holistic medicine. Dell, New York

7 LeShan L 1982 The mechanic and the gardener: how to use the holistic revolution in medicine. Holt, Rinehart & Winston, New York

8 Locke S, Colligan D 1987 The healer within: the new medicine of mind and body. New American Library, New York

9 Kowal SJ 1955 Emotions as a cause of cancer: 18th and 19th century contributions. Psychoanalytic Review 42:217–27

10 Meerloo J 1954 Psychological implications of malignant growth: survey of hypotheses. British Journal of Medical Psychology 27:210–15

11 LeShan L, Worthington R 1956 Personality as a factor in the pathogenesis of cancer: a review of the literature. British Journal of Medical Psychology 29:49–56

12 Cousins N 1989 Head first. Dutton, New York

13 Borysenko J 1988 Minding the body, mending the mind. Bantam, New York

14 Rossi EL 1988 The psychobiology of mind–body healing. W W Norton, New York

15 Temochek L, Dreher H 1992 The type C connection. Random House, New York

16 Weil A 1995 Spontaneous healing. Alfred Knopf, New York

17 Amkraut A, Solomon G F 1975 From the symbolic stimulus to the pathophysiological response: immune mechanism. International Journal of Psychiatry in Medicine 5(4):541–63

18 Siegel B 1986 Love, medicine and miracles. Harper & Row, New York

19 Greer S 1994 Introduction. In: Dryer H Your defense against cancer. Harper Collins, New York

20 Spiegel D 1991 A psychosocial intervention and survival time of patients with metastatic breast cancer. Advances 7(3):10–19

21 Fawzy F I, Cousins N, Fawzy N W et al 1990 A structured psychiatric intervention for cancer patients: I Changes over time in methods of copying and affective disturbance. Archives of General Psychiatry 47:720-5

22 Fawzy F I, Kemeny M E, Fawzy N W et al 1990 A structured psychiatric intervention for cancer patients: II Changes over time in immunological measures. Archive of General Psychiatry 47:729–35

23 Lerner M 1994 Choices in healing. MIT Press, Cambridge, Massachusetts

24 Dreher H 1994 Your defense against cancer. Harper Collins, New York

25 Rossman M L 1993 Imagery: learning to use the mind's eye. In: Goleman D, Gurin J (eds) Mind–body medicine. Consumer Reports Books, New York

26 Frankl V E 1984 Man's search for meaning. Simon &

Schuster, New York
27 Jung C G 1965 Memories, dreams and reflections. Jaffe A (ed.), Winston C (trans.). Vintage, New York
28 Bolletino R, LeShan L 1995 Cancer patients and 'marathon' psychotherapy: a new model. Advances 11(4):19–35
29 Bahnson C B 1980 Stress and cancer: state of the art. Psychosomatics 27
30 Baltrusch H J F, Walter M B 1988 Stress and cancer: a psychobiological approach. Current Advances 2
31 Baltrusch H J F 1978 Psychosomatic cancer research: present status and future perspectives. Psychologie et Cancer, Masson, Paris
32 Baltrusch H J F 1977 Psychotherapy with cancer patients. In: Antonelli F (ed) Therapy in psychosomatic medicine. Pozzi, Rome
33 Baltrusch H J F 1975 Results of clinical psychosomatic cancer research. Psychosomatic Medicine 5:175–208
34 Myerson A 1950 Speaking of man. Alfred Knopf, New York
35 Frank JD, Frank JB 1991 Persuasion and healing. Johns Hopkins University Press
36 Barasch M I 1995 The healing path. Penguin, New York
37 Smuts J C 1973 Holism and evolution. Greenwood, Westport, Connecticut
38 Goldstein K 1939 The organism: a holistic approach to biology. American Book Company, New York
39 Cousins N 1989 Overcoming fear. Advances 6(2):33–5
40 Achterberg J 1985 Imagery in healing. Shambala, Boston
41 Utne Reader 1995 Sept-Oct, 71:51
42 Cousins N 1981 Anatomy of an illness. Bantam, New York
43 Walters R 1993 Options: the alternative cancer therapy book. Avery, New York
44 Lewith G T, Kenyon JN, Lewis P S 1996 Complementary medicine: an integrated approach. Oxford University Press, Oxford
45 USA Congress, Office of Technological Assessment 1990 Non-conventional cancer treatments. US Government Printing Office, Washington DC
46 Dubos R 1981 Introduction. In: Cousins N Anatomy of an illness. Bantam, New York
47 Gengerelli J A, Kiker P I (eds) 1954 The psychobiological variables in human cancer. University of California Press, Berkeley, California
48 New York Academy of Science 1966 Conference on psychological aspects of cancer. Annals of the New York Academy of Science 125
49 New York Academy of Science 1968 Conference on psychological aspects of cancer. Annals of the New York Academy of Science 164
50 Booth G 1973 Psychological aspects of 'spontaneous' remission of cancer. Journal of the American Academy of Psychoanalysis 3
51 LeShan L, Marvin S, Lyerly O 1959 Some evidence of a relationship between Hodgkin's disease and intelligence. American Medical Association Archives of General Psychiatry I:447–9
52 Peller S 1962 Cancer in man. International University Press, New York
53 Pettingale K W, Philithis S, Greer R S 1981 The biological correlates of psychological response to breast cancer. Journal of Psychosomatic Research 25
54 Grossarth-Matticek R 1980 Social psychotherapy and the course of cancer. Psychotherapy and Psychosomatics 33
55 Levy S M, Lee J, Bagley C, Lippman M 1988 Survival hazards analysis in first recurrent breast cancer patients: seven year follow-up. Psychosomatic Medicine 50:520–8

6

HIV disease: Psychological well-being, health and immunity

Gail H. Ironson
Teresa E. Woods
Michael H. Antoni

CHAPTER CONTENTS

INTRODUCTION

Does psychological state bear any relationship to physical health in HIV disease? There are two bodies of literature which may shed some light on this question. The first examines whether psychosocial interventions, which are designed to ameliorate stress, have any impact either on disease progression or immunological markers of health in HIV disease. The second examines whether psychological factors predict disease progression in HIV. This chapter reviews both areas of inquiry and discusses them in relation to psychoneuroimmunology (PNI), a rapidly expanding field of research that provides the scientific background for asking why stress would be expected to impact the immune system in HIV.

The importance of an individual's psychological state in determining their immunity was demonstrated in an early study showing that immunosuppression could be psychologically conditioned[1]. Subsequent research has shown that the central nervous system and the immune system are linked via the autonomic nervous system and neuroendocrine circuits[2,3]. The importance of PNI is supported by a growing body of studies showing that a wide variety of stressors and negative affective states can have a significant immunosuppressive effect[4].

During stressful situations catecholamines, cortisol, prolactin, and the natural opiates beta-endorphin and enkephalin are all released. Each has a powerful impact on immunity. However, the effects are complex with each hormone having different effects on immunity. While these hormones surge through the body the immune cells are hampered in their ability to function well[3]. Stress suppresses immune resistance, at least temporarily, and this may be a survival mechanism to attempt to conserve energy, with the body giving priority to the emergency at hand. However, if the stress is constant and intense, the immunosuppression may become long lasting[3,5].

Given the growing body of evidence that the mind and the immune system are linked via the autonomic and neuroendocrine systems, and that stress affects immunity, it would seem reasonable to suggest that psychosocial factors could play an important role in an illness, such as HIV, that is associated with many stressors.

PATHOPHYSIOLOGY OF HUMAN IMMUNODEFICIENCY VIRUS (HIV)

HIV is a progressive debilitating disease caused by infection with the HIV-1 virus. The disease progresses through several stages, the last of which is known as Acquired Immune Deficiency Syndrome (AIDS)[6]. Primary infection with HIV is followed by an acute mononucleosis-like syndrome with increased B cell activation in 50–70% of infected individuals. This occurs approximately 3 to 6 weeks after initial infection[7]. Within 4 to 12 weeks there is usually a detectable antibody response to HIV[8]. During this time there is viral replication and dissemination, particularly in the lymphoid organs. Following primary infection, the majority of patients enter a clinical remission which typically lasts for 10 years[9]. During this time lymphadenopathy may be evident, but there are few, if any other symptoms. During this latent period, although the patient may appear to be healthy, there is often a significant drop in peripheral CD4+ cells, and viral replication continues in the lymphoid organs. There is often little evidence of HIV in the peripheral blood at this time[10]. This is currently classified as Centers for Disease Control (CDC) Category A[11]. Eventually, most, if not all infected persons become symptomatic. As CD4+ cell counts drop below 500, the symptoms of thrush, night sweats, viral and fungal infections occur with greater frequency[6], although these symptoms can be present even in individuals with higher T cell counts. Symptomatic presentations meet the definition for CDC Clinical Category B[11]. AIDS occurs when the person has a CD4+ count of 200 or less, or less than 14% of total lymphocyte count (whether symptomatic or not), or the occurrence of opportunistic infections such as *Pneumocystis carinii* pneumonia, cryptococcal meningitis, or neoplasms such as Kaposi's sarcoma[7, 12].

MIND–BODY INTERVENTIONS IN PATIENTS WITH HIV/AIDS

Numerous studies have looked at stress management interventions in HIV populations and have included immune measures as well as psychological well-being as dependent variables. Although several have looked at disease progression as measured by changes in CD4 counts, few have looked at symptom development. Many reasons may exist for this gap in the literature, the most obvious being that the disease has been identified for a much shorter period of time than other diseases, such as cancer and cardiovascular disease.

Seroconversion

At the University of Miami a series of studies has been conducted to examine psychological interventions at various time points within the course of HIV. The first protocol focused on whether stress management would buffer the impact on gay men of finding out their HIV serostatus. The 65 gay men (who did not know their serostatus at entry into the study) were randomly assigned to either a cognitive behavioral stress management (CBSM) intervention, an exercise intervention, or a control group.

Five weeks later (after the men in the intervention group had a chance to learn some of the stress management skills), in the middle of the intervention, blood was drawn for serostatus testing. The men received news of their serostatus within 3 days and then received another 5 weeks of the intervention (10 weeks total). This allowed follow-up through the initial adjustment period. Topics included in the CBSM intervention included awareness of stress and negative thoughts, cognitive restructuring techniques, relaxation techniques, education (about safer sex, HIV, and the immune system), handling anger, assertiveness, and social support.

The results of this study supported the buffering effects of the CBSM intervention. HIV positive men in the intervention group showed no significant change in anxiety or depression scores pre to post notification whereas the HIV positive men in the control group showed significant increases in anxiety and depression[13]. In addition, the same buffering effect was present for the HIV positive men who had been assigned to the exercise intervention[14]. Social support was probably a key element in the buffering effect of the CBSM intervention; men in the control group experienced a significant decrease in social support during the notification period, whereas those in the CBSM group maintained their social support levels[15]. In fact, subsequent studies have demonstrated the mediating effect of both coping and social support[16].

In addition, the HIV positive subjects in the CBSM group had significant increases in CD4+ numbers and natural killer (CD56) cell counts and slight increases in phytohemagglutinin (PHA) responsivity and natural killer cell cytotoxicity (NKCC) over the pre- to post-notification period[13]. In contrast, the HIV positive controls showed slight decrements in responsivity to PHA, and reduced NKCC and CD56+ (natural killer) cell counts following notification of seropositivity, with no change in CD4+ counts. Exercise had a similar buffering effect on several immune measures. Seropositive exercisers had no significant change (or non-significant increases) in CD4+, NK cell counts or NKCC[14], whereas the control seropositives showed a significant decline in NK cells. The stress management intervention was also associated with consistent immune changes after the notification period, not just during the notification period. Antibody titers to Epstein–Barr Virus (EBV) and to human herpes virus type-6 (HHV-6) decreased significantly in both the CBSM and exercise intervention groups, indicating better control of these latent ubiquitous viruses, whereas the antibody titers in the assessment-only controls remained constant over the 10-week intervention period[17].

Symptomatic and asymptomatic HIV positive men

The second study conducted at the University of Miami included men who already knew their serostatus, were all verified as being HIV positive, but had no symptoms. The men in the CBSM group showed significant decreases in maladaptive coping strategies (i.e. behavioral disengagement, denial) over the 10 weeks[18].

The third group we focused on were HIV positive men whose disease had progressed to a symptomatic stage (category B of the 1993 CDC definition), but who did not have an AIDS defining illness. Across the 10 weeks the CBSM group showed a significant decrease in depression and anxiety and a significant decrease in IgG antibody titers to herpes simplex virus-2[19], whereas the control group showed no change in either mood or antibody titers. The intervention group also showed significant improvements in certain coping styles such as acceptance and reframing as well as increases in social attachment[16]. Preliminary data from an exercise intervention with the same target population showed no effect on CD4 counts in either the exercise or control groups. However, when those assigned to exercise were divided into compliant subjects (attending more than 50% of the exercise sessions) and non-compliant (attending less than 50%) there were marked differences in results: the compliant participants had an increase in CD4 cell counts approaching significance ($P<0.10$), whereas the non-compliant exercise subjects showed slight immunosuppression[20].

Disease progression

Following the subjects in the first protocol over 2 years, we found that distress at diagnosis, denial of HIV-positivity, and low treatment adherence were all significant predictors of faster disease progression, with denial and low treatment adherence remaining significant even after controlling for initial disease severity[21]. In addition, change in denial and relaxation practice correlated with several immune measures at 1-year follow-up, suggesting a link between psychological strategy and immune status. However, being assigned to an intervention group alone was not related to having fewer symptoms or greater survival at 2-year follow-up. Thus, health benefits seemed to be limited to those who attended regularly, broke through denial, and practiced relaxation techniques outside of group.

Another study carried out by Mulder and colleagues[22] compared the effects of two 15-week long group interventions, cognitive-behavioral therapy (CBT), and experiential therapy (ET) on the rate of decline of immunologic parameters relevant to disease progression in gay men infected with HIV. Both interventions were aimed at reducing stress, improving coping and social support, and encouraging the expression of emotions. The CBT intervention included training in cognitive restructuring, exercise and relaxation, behavior change, assertiveness skills, coping skills, and information on stress responses. The ET focused on increasing awareness of the here and now and of the patient's inner experiential process. Because subjects were recruited from a larger longitudinal study, there was a comparison group from the parent study that could be used for determining differences in rapidity of immune changes in the two intervention groups and the natural longitudinal course of the disease. Data from the parent study were also used to determine whether the speed of changes in immune parameters occurred before, during, or after the interventions. The rate of decline in CD4+ cells was significantly less after both interventions. However, a similar reduction in the rate of decline in T cell response was observed in the comparison group indicating that the psychosocial intervention programs did not appear to be causing these changes[22]. Psychological benefits of both CBT and ET interventions included a significant decrease in distress compared to a wait list control group, but there were no changes in coping style, social support or emotional expression[23]. Follow-up results showed that greater reductions in distress, from entry into an intervention to the 9-month follow-up, predicted immune (CD4) changes over 2 years.

Sexual behavior

Coates et al.[24] tested the effectiveness of stress reduction training, which included teaching systematic relaxation, health habit changes (i.e. diet, rest, exercise), and skills for managing stress, to HIV positive gay men. The 64 men were randomized to the stress reduction training group which met for eight 2-hour sessions once per week and one all-day retreat, or to a control group[24]. There was no impact of the intervention on immune function, but stress management training did have an impact on sexual behavior with men in the intervention group having significantly fewer sexual partners. No psychological changes in the intervention or control groups were reported.

The lack of immune changes may indicate that stress reduction has no effect on immune function in HIV positive men. However, a number of alternative explanations should be considered. First, the authors note that confronting issues related to AIDS may have induced stress in the intervention group rather than reduced it. Alternatively, the intervention may not have been psychologically potent enough to impact immunity: measuring psychological distress before and after the intervention would have provided some evidence in that regard. Finally, the inclusion of an HIV negative control group might have helped answer the question of whether the lack of effect may be specific to the HIV positive group.

Grief counseling

Goodkin has examined the effects of a support group intervention focused on helping gay men through the grieving process[25,26]. Loss of a partner or one or more friends is a stressor many gay men face as a result of the AIDS epidemic. There are several studies showing that bereavement is associated with immune suppression[27,28,29]. Thus, an intervention addressing bereavement concerns has both the potential to reduce the distress associated with loss and to counteract the negative effects of bereavement on the immune system. In the Goodkin study[25] 93 gay men (56 HIV positive men who were either asymptomatic or mildly symptomatic, and 37 HIV negative men) were randomly assigned to a 10-week bereavement support group (36 HIV positive, 27 HIV negative) or a control condition.

The support group included such topics as grieving and bereavement, relationship with the care provider, interacting with the family, death and loss, surviving, examining one's own spirituality and mortality, social support and moving on. Psychological findings showed the intervention was associated with a reduction in distress, as measured by the Profile of Mood States (POMS), and grief, as measured by the Texas Inventory of Grief. Immune findings were different for the HIV negative and positive groups. The HIV positive control group showed a decline in CD4 over time whereas the HIV positive intervention group did not ($P<0.01$). In contrast, the HIV negative intervention group showed an increase in CD4 number over time. Finally, the HIV positive intervention group did demonstrate a significant increase in NK cells.

Thus there are now two studies which demonstrate that psychosocial interventions addressing either the stress of seroconversion[13] or bereavement[25] buffer or help protect immune function in addition to psychological function.

Depression and coping

A more recent study focused on HIV positive gay men (n=128) who had some symptoms of depression (CESD scores of 10 or more) and had a CD4 count in the 200 to 600 range. This randomized controlled study compared the efficacy of coping effectiveness training (CET), a cognitive behavioral stress management group approach (n=51), to an HIV educational, information control group (n=53) and to a wait list control group (n=24)[30,31]. The CET intervention is based, in part, on a theory developed by Folkman et al.[32] which suggests that stressful situations can be divided into those aspects which are changeable and those which are not changeable[32]. The coping approach should then be matched to the situation. For example, problem-focused coping is more appropriate for situations that have aspects that are changeable such as problems with the insurance company. In contrast, emotion-focused coping is more appropriate for situations that are not changeable such as the sadness of visiting a friend with HIV in hospital. The skills taught in the group encompass both the problem-focused approaches, including decision making, communication skills, negotiation skills, as well as the emotion-focused approaches such as relaxation, distancing, and cognitive restructuring.

Results indicated a significant increase in self-efficacy, decrease in perceived stress, and decrease in burnout in the CET intervention group compared with either the HIV information or wait list control groups. In addition, the changes in coping efficacy were strongly related to the changes in psychological distress. In contrast, there were no differences in symptoms or changes in CD4 counts between the groups. Thus CET was effective in improving psychological outcomes, but had no effect on the disease over the short 3-month period of the study[30,31].

Several other studies have shown psychosocial group interventions with HIV positive patients to be successful in reducing distress and depression[33,34]. Kelly and colleagues[34] found that both a social support group intervention and a cognitive behavioral group intervention were effective in reducing not only depression, but also hostility and somatization in depressed men (CESD≥16) with HIV as compared with a control (no intervention) group condition. Interestingly, the social support intervention seemed to be particularly effective in reducing unprotected anal intercourse, psychiatric symptoms and somatization, whereas the cognitive-behavioral intervention was associated with less frequent drug use.

Thus the results of several studies[16,30,31,33,34] suggest that psychosocial interventions can be effective in reducing distress and depression in HIV seropositive men and that this change may be related to changes in coping skills and social support[16,30,31,34], although one intervention study showed effects on depression but not coping or social support[23].

Relaxation and massage

Two other related studies which focused more on the relaxation aspect of interventions rather than the cognitive, talking and sharing aspects of stress management have been done. In the first, 26 symptomatic seropositive gay men were randomly assigned to an 8-week intervention consisting of training in thermal biofeedback, guided imagery, and hypnosis, or to a wait list control group[35]. Relaxation training was associated with reduced self-reported symptoms of HIV such as fever, fatigue, pain, headache, nausea, and insomnia and was also associated with increased vigor and hardiness, relative to control subjects. However, there were no changes in anxiety, depression, or CD4 counts. The authors speculated that if they had selected a depressed HIV positive population they may have obtained changes in immunity and depression measures.

Ironson investigated the effects of a passive relaxation technique, massage, in gay men[36]. In contrast to other relaxation techniques massage does not require effort on the part of the participant and the amount of time the participant spends with the technique can be determined exactly. The study included 29 gay men (20 HIV positive, nine HIV negative) who received a daily 45-minute massage each weekday for a month. A subset of 11 HIV positive subjects were also observed for a month-long period without any massages and thus served as a within-subject control group. Compared with the control period, the massage period was associated with a significant increase in NK cell numbers, Natural Killer Cell Cytotoxicity (NKCC), soluble CD8 receptor levels, and the cytoxic subset of CD8 cells (CD8+ S6F1+). There was no change in HIV disease progression markers (CD4+, CD4/CD8 ratio, beta-2 microglobulin, neopterin). Cortisol levels also decreased significantly over the course of the month for those receiving massage, suggesting a possible mechanism for the immune modulation. Finally, there were significant decreases in anxiety and increases in relaxation which correlated with increases in the NK cell counts. Thus, massage seems to have a significant impact on both psychological and several immune parameters relevant to cytotoxic capacity.

Summary of results of mind–body interventions in HIV disease

In summary, the research in HIV disease suggests that mind–body interventions consistently produce an impact on psychological well-being, but their impact on either the immune system or general health is more mixed. While no studies were associated with sustained significant increases in the critical disease progression marker, the CD4 count, in HIV positive individuals, three interventions, stress management[13], exercise[14], and bereavement support[15], prevented the decline in CD4 numbers that was observed in the control groups. In contrast, two intervention studies produced an increase in CD4 count in HIV negative individuals[25,36]. This suggests psychosocial interventions may have a role to play in protecting or buffering the decline in immunity that inevitably occurs in HIV disease, but one should not expect a sustained increase in CD4 counts as a result of psychosocial interventions in HIV positive gay men.

However, two studies, one examining the effects of massage[36], and the other a bereavement support intervention[25], produced increases in NK cell numbers which may be important in the control of viral replication. Studies examining the effects of mind–body interventions on the control of other viruses in HIV men, namely EBV, HHV-6[17] and HSV-2[19] demonstrated that mind–body interventions produced lower antibody titers and thus better control of latent viruses. However, more studies are needed to clarify whether this is a consistent effect of mind–body interventions. Unfortunately, the follow-up period of most studies was insufficient to determine whether interventions associated with psychological and immunological changes impacted health outcomes. The only study which found that intervention-associated variables, such as adherence and decreases in denial, were associated with slower disease progression[21] was based on just a 2-year follow-up and a small sample size. Because long-term follow-up of HIV positive men is fraught with difficulty, studies have tended to use surrogate markers of disease progression. While many studies have used CD4 count, future studies should incorporate viral load, which has now been shown to be a more sensitive predictor of disease progression.

PSYCHOSOCIAL PREDICTORS OF DISEASE PROGRESSION IN HIV/AIDS

Several psychological factors have been explored as possible predictors of immune changes and disease progression in HIV. These studies may be particularly useful as the results can help guide health care professionals in deciding what factors to focus on in designing future interventions.

Depression

Depression has been examined in several relatively large studies, and the results are mixed. In one study the CD4 cell count declined faster in depressed HIV positive men compared with non-depressed men during the 5.5-year follow-up period[38]. In contrast, Lyketsos found that depressive symptoms did not predict a faster rate of decline in CD4 cell counts in HIV positive men over an 8-year follow-up period[39]. Neither study was able to demonstrate a relationship between depression and mortality or the subsequent diagnosis of AIDS. In contrast, while Rabkin and colleagues found no relation between depression, distress, stress and changes in the CD4 or CD8 cell counts over a 6-month follow-up period they did find a relationship between depression and symptoms[40].

Perry and colleagues also found no association between a variety of psychological states and the CD4 cell count 6 months and 1-year later, but they did find that hopelessness, which is often a component of depression, was a significant predictor of the decline in CD4 counts[41]. Work by Kemeny suggests that a sustained severely depressed mood may be the critical variable since HIV positive men with chronic major depression over a 2-year period had a significantly steeper rate of decline in their CD4 cells over the subsequent 5-year follow-up period compared with non-chronically depressed men, matched for age and baseline CD4 counts[42]. In a series of studies Kemeny attempted to disentangle grief during bereavement and depressed mood unrelated to bereavement. She found that depressed mood was related to CD4 cell counts and other indicators of HIV progression only in the non-bereaved group[43,44]. Thus a high depression score may represent different psychological processes in the bereaved and non-bereaved groups.

In summary, these studies suggest that chronic, more severe depression, unrelated to bereavement, may predict the decline in CD4 cell counts. In addition, there is evidence to suggest that depressed individuals with a high CD4 count on entry to a study showed a faster decline in CD4 counts than those with low CD4 counts on entry[38]. However, a reanalysis of the Lyketsos data showed no such relationship[39]. The evidence suggesting that depression may predict the development of symptoms or mortality appears to be even weaker.

Coping strategies

Several studies have reported that active coping is associated with improvements in immunity and health outcomes while denial or withdrawal is associated with poorer immunity and health outcomes. For example, in a group of gay men receiving news of an HIV positive diagnosis, the use of denial or behavioral disengagement to cope predicted lower CD4 counts at 1-year follow-up, irrespective of CD4 counts at entry[45]. In addition, denial and behavioral disengagement predicted a greater likelihood of progression to HIV-related symptoms and AIDS at the 2-year follow-up[21]. Similarly, other studies in HIV positive gay men have found that passive coping strategies, which involve denial and disengagement, are inversely related to long-term CD4 cell counts[46], and denial or repression predicts the emergence of symptoms[47]. In addition, gay men using avoidance to process the emotional news that they were HIV positive showed greater levels of depression and anxiety and poorer immune responses when measured 10 weeks later[48].

In contrast to the negative impact of passive coping, active coping was positively related to both improved NKCC and blastogenic response to PHA in a sample of bereaved HIV positive gay men[25]. Similarly, self-oriented, active, optimistic coping behavior was associated with prolonged survival in HIV positive hemophiliac men[49], and active confrontational coping with HIV infection was predictive of decreased clinical progression over a 1-year period.[50]

Not only does denial predict survival time but 'realistic acceptance' has also been reported to be a significant predictor of decreased survival in gay men diagnosed with AIDS[51]. One possible explanation for these seemingly contradictory results may be that both rigid denial or fatalistic acceptance may disable the individual from developing a 'fighting spirit'. Kemeny, in her discussion suggests that 'realistic acceptance' is fatalism masquerading as realism and notes that 'fatalistic men survived a significantly shorter period of time when compared with their less fatalistic counterparts'. Mulder reported that individuals who used distraction as a coping strategy had a slower rate of decline in their CD4 counts, less appearance of syncytium-inducing HIV variants, and less progression to immunologically defined AIDS (<200 CD4/mm^3) over a 7-year follow-up period[52]. However the use of distraction had no impact on the development of symptoms.

Therefore it seems that the most effective coping strategy for gay men with HIV may be to avoid obsessive rumination with a healthy dose of distraction, while avoiding the extremes of denial or acceptance to the point where fatalism occurs.

Negative expectations and optimism

The effects of negative expectations and fatalism have been explored in three longitudinal studies.[44] Reid found that negative expectations and fatalism were associated with poorer health outcomes in HIV especially when combined with bereavement. In the first study, fatalistic gay men with a diagnosis of AIDS had significantly shorter survival times, 9 months on average, as compared with less fatalistic men[53], irrespective of AZT use or initial CD4 count. The shortest survival time was found for men who were both fatalistic and bereaved within the past year. In a second study the steepest declines in CD4 cell counts and the poorest proliferative responses to PHA were seen in those with negative expectancies and a loss due to AIDS in the previous year. These subjects also had a more rapid increase in markers of disease progression including neopterin and beta$_2$-microglobulin[54]. In the third study asymptomatic HIV positive men who had negative expectancies and were bereaved were more likely to develop HIV related symptoms over the next 2.5 to 3.5 years[55].

In contrast to the deleterious effect of negative expectations, optimism or optimistic behavior has been associated with improved survival. Temoshok found that an optimistic attitude may protect HIV infected individuals, slowing the progression to AIDS[56]. Similarly Blomkvist found in a group of HIV infected hemophiliacs one's own psychosocial prognosis, i.e. one's ability to see a future for oneself and a number of future social activities, was related to prolonged survival, regardless of age and baseline

CD4 levels[49]. The authors have subsequently referred to this factor as 'self-oriented active-optimistic coping behavior'[57].

Social support and loss

Only a few studies have examined social support and its longitudinal relationship with health in HIV. Theorell and colleagues[57] asked a cohort of HIV-infected hemophiliacs in Sweden questions about the sources of emotional support in their lives in 1985 and than followed their health until 1990. Those scoring low in 'availability of attachment' (AVAT), had a significantly more rapid deterioration in CD4+ count than those with high AVAT scores, although AVAT scores were not significantly associated with mortality. Another support measure, a rating of problem-solving help used (i.e. someone who seeks advice about how to solve a problem) distinguished those who were still alive from those who had died in a group of AIDS-PCP subjects studied by Solomon et al.[58]

More recent studies have examined the impact of the loss of social support due to bereavement. Following the death of a partner Kemeny and colleagues[54] found a decrease in the lymphocyte proliferative response to PHA and an increase in immune activation in HIV seropositive bereaved men as compared with non-bereaved controls. In another study AIDS specific bereavement was a predictor of CD4 decline in a group of 85 HIV positive men in New York City[29]. Goodkin et al.[25] assessed 79 HIV seropositive gay men at two time points 6 months apart and found that among the bereaved, NKCC was decreased at both time points, and lymphocyte response to PHA was decreased at the second time point. These findings are also consistent with the negative impact of bereavement on the immune system in non-HIV populations[27,28].

Other psychosocial variables

The role of a number of other psychosocial variables including disclosure, adherence and hardiness have been examined longitudinally for relationships with disease progression in HIV. For example, Cole followed 80 HIV positive gay men for 9 years and found that gay men who concealed their sexual orientation had a faster course of HIV infection[59]. The authors point out that concealment of homosexuality (vs. disclosure) was associated with a difference in HIV progression times of about 1.5 to 2 years which is similar to that associated with major biobehavioral variables such as anti-retroviral use and age.

Ironson found a constellation of activities including the practice of relaxation techniques, doing homework, and attending cognitive behavioral stress management intervention group sessions were significantly related to slower disease progression to AIDS at a 2-year follow-up period[21]. One possible explanation may be that the improvement in health was a direct effect of absorbing and practicing the intervention, with decreased sympathetic activity as a result of the relaxation techniques, less distress following the cognitive restructuring and reframing and improved self-care as a result of enhanced coping abilities. Alternately the improvements in health seen in this study may be due to a factor totally unrelated to the intervention, such as conscientiousness. Thus, conscientious individuals may come to the group sessions and do all the homework, keep all their doctors appointments and diligently follow their advice. More research is needed to determine why health outcomes improved. Finally, Solomon demonstrated that hardy individuals, those with a sense of commitment and control, and with an ability to see change as a challenge, were more likely to be alive at follow-up than less hardy individuals[58].

Spirituality and religiosity in HIV/AIDS

The role of spirituality and religion in chronic diseases is attracting increasing scientific interest and although there have been no longitudinal studies assessing its impact in AIDS its potential importance warrants discussion here. Historically, religion and medicine have both played a part in the management of illness and death in society. Indeed, in western civilization, many of the most prestigious medical schools and hospitals were founded by and receive substantial support from established major religions.

In a 1989 survey of 160 family doctors and general practitioners, a significant proportion of those surveyed felt doctors should address religious issues if the patient feels they are important. Nearly 65% of the doctors surveyed went so far as to state that prayer with patients was an appropriate therapeutic tool[60]. While the literature regarding the impact of religion on physical and mental health is vast, little exists examining the direct relationship between religion and HIV or AIDS. Most studies that do exist are anecdotal in nature, and even those publications offer disparate views of religion's role in the progression of the disease. Carson presented one of the first empirical studies examining the role of religion in HIV disease[61]. To determine whether there was quantitative support for the anecdotal evidence of long-term survivors with AIDS, she studied 100 subjects who were either HIV positive or had been diagnosed with AIDS. Her results demonstrated a positive relationship between physical hardiness and self-perceived spiritual health, participation in prayer, and participation in meditation.

In a similar study Hall investigated the experience of eight men and two women with AIDS[62]. Interviews were analyzed to determine how individuals interpreted their illness and how they maintained hope while coping with the disease. There were four major ways in which individuals maintained as sense of hope: through a belief in miracles, through religious belief, by involvement with work or hobbies, and through the support of family and friends.

Woods examined the association between religiosity, immunity and affective state in mildly symptomatic HIV-infected gay men[63]. Analysis of the subjects' responses to a series of religious-based questions revealed that a subject's religious behavior and their religious coping style were associated with affective state and immunity. Those subjects in whom religion formed part of their coping strategy reported significantly lower symptoms of depression and anxiety than subjects for whom religion played no part. In addition, subjects engaging in a high degree of religious activity, such as praying, reading spiritual material and attending religious services, had significantly higher CD4 cell counts and percentages than subjects not engaging in regular religious activity.

In contrast, existential loneliness was found to be a prominent feature in a study of eight male outpatients with AIDS[64]. The authors suggested that this loneliness was related to problems of faith and religion, living in the face of death, and the nature of the search for meaning. Religious issues may present particular problems for HIV positive gay men. A recent study which examined the relationship between religious faith and homosexuality, discovered that of the 45 HIV positive gay men in the study, nearly 50% felt compelled to abandon the religious faith of their childhood and no longer endorsed a formal religion[65].

ALTERNATIVE ORGANIC TREATMENTS FOR HIV/AIDS

Since the beginning of the AIDS pandemic, a variety of alternative organic and herbal treatments have been used, in addition to the psychosocial interventions, in the treatment of HIV and AIDS. Since these therapies, which vary substantially in philosophy, modality and cost, also fall under the rubric 'alternative' they are addressed briefly in this chapter. Greenberg[66] reported the AIDS community as tending to fall into two separate camps regarding alternative therapies. Some dismiss all alternative treatments, regardless of evidence demonstrating efficacy, and others defend all alternative treatments, regardless of evidence demonstrating toxicity or lack of efficacy. He further suggests that the reality of most alternative therapies probably lies somewhere between these two extremes. Some alternative therapies may be effective, some are clearly ineffective, and most possess some degree of toxicity. A number of the more commonly used organic therapies are discussed below.

Artemisia

'Artemisia' or Qing Hao (Artemisia annua) has been used as an anti-malarial herb in China since before 340 AD. More recently, an extract of the herb, artemisnin or qinghaosu (QHS) has shown efficacy against malaria[67]. In the test tube, concentrations of QHS (0.4 micrograms/ml for 5 days) inhibited *Toxoplasma gondii* in human fibroblast cells. At a dose of 1.3 micrograms/ml for 14 days, *T. gondii* was completely eliminated. Cells exposed to this dose for up to 27 days showed no toxic effects[67].

Astragalus

'Astragalus' (Astragalus membranaceous) is a herb used in China, reportedly for the purpose of boosting the immune system and preventing chemotherapy-related bone marrow suppression and nausea. In the former Soviet Union and Japan, it is used to treat heart attacks and strokes[68]. It has been reported that an extract of Astragalus, Fraction 3 (F3), has stimulated immune responses in vitro and in animal studies. In one study, injections of F3 into rats treated with the immunosuppressive drug cyclophosphamide resulted in the rats rejecting grafts of foreign tissue[69]. In vitro, F3 improved the antitumor activity of interleukin-2 (IL-2) in human lymphokine-activated killer cells[70]. In another in vitro study[71], an Astragalus decoction, obtained by boiling the ground root in water, increased the proliferation of lymphocytes taken from healthy individuals and patients with cancer. A team at Loma Linda University used a similar method to obtain an extract that increased the activity of human macrophages in vitro[72]. Both studies reported that the observed effects decreased at higher doses[71,72].

Bitter Melon

'Bitter Melon' (Momordica charantia) is the fruit of a vine-type climbing plant and is a relative of the Chinese Cucumber. Scientists have identified several active proteins extracted from Bitter Melon, including MAP-30, alpha-momorcharin, and beta-momorcharin[73]. In vitro, MAP-30 inhibited the ability of HIV to infect cells and to replicate, as assessed by expression of the HIV core protein p24 and by levels of reverse transcriptase in certain cell cultures[74].

Blue-green algae

'Blue-green algae' (Cyanobacteria) is a generic name for algae found in most wet places. In 1989, scientists at the National Cancer Institute (NCI) reported that extracts from L. lagerheimmi and P. tenue, two specific types of blue-green algae found only off the islands of Hawaii and Palau, contained sulfolipids which inhibited the cytotoxic effects of HIV and reduced HIV replication in vitro[75].

Echinacea

The leaves and root of 'Echinacea' (Echinacea angustifolia or E. purpurea) have been used by Native Americans for a broad range of pains and illnesses. Broad immunostimulatory effects have been attributed to the herb. Advocates of Echinacea have pointed to in vitro and animal studies to support these claims[76]. In vitro studies conducted in Germany showed that purified extracts from Echinacea stimulate T cells and macrophages[76] and may have anti-viral properties[77].

Germanium-132

'Germanium-132' (Ge-132) is a mineral composed of the elements hermanium, oxygen, carbon, and hydrogen. High levels of the mineral are found in ginseng, and high levels of the element germanium are found in garlic, comfrey and watercress. In an animal study, oral administration of Ge-132 stimulated production of gamma-interferon (gamma-IFN) and activation of macrophages and natural killer cells[78]. In humans, Ge-132 has been shown to enhance T and B cell function and natural killer cell proliferation[79]. An abstract at the Ninth International Conference on AIDS in Berlin reported that germanium may act synergistically with alpha interferon in inhibiting HIV replication in vitro[80].

Prunellin

'Prunellin' is the isolated active component of Prunella vulgaris, a herb of the family Labiatae, which is commonly known as 'self-heal' and was once used to treat cuts and wounds[81]. In vitro studies with prunellin blocked cell-to-cell transmission of HIV. Polymerase chain reaction (PCR) showed, in vitro, that cells exposed to HIV in the presence of prunellin remained completely uninfected[79]. Researchers from Lady Davis Institute for Medical Research suggested that prunellin exerted an anti-HIV effect by preventing the virus from binding to cells[66].

RECOMMENDED STRATEGIES FOR LONGEVITY

In reviewing the literature from studies of long-term survivors of AIDS[40,58,82,83] and the longitudinal studies reviewed in this chapter Ironson[84] suggests there are four psychosocial adjustment strategies which might predict long-term survival of individuals with HIV/AIDS.

Healthy self-care

Self-care encompasses three components: good medical care, maintaining a healthy lifestyle, and recognition of the personal dimension. Good medical care requires that the patient establishes a collaborative relationship with their doctor and takes personal responsibility for their own health. Maintaining a healthy lifestyle involves discontinuing negative habits and undertaking health promoting habits, including learning to manage individual mental and emotional responses to stress. The third component of self-care is the personal dimension. This requires that the individual have an awareness of their own psychological and physical needs and be able to act on them.

Maintain connectedness

This strategy recognizes the importance of maintaining a social support structure. Having at least one confidant is crucial to maintaining connectedness. In addition, being able to disclose a gay lifestyle and communicate openly about important concerns is vital. Thus, social connectedness may be related to emotional expression. Finding supportive relationships with people who accept and understand the situation is helpful. For some, having HIV creates a new support system. Becoming active in helping others with HIV, and becoming active in the community of people with AIDS is a new form of connectedness which can be beneficial.

Maintain a sense of meaning and purpose

Maintaining a sense of meaning and purpose provides the individual with something to live for and can underpin the actual will to live. Having a sense of meaning and something to live for provides an attitudinal and cognitive focus. Maintaining a positive, optimistic outlook is an important component of a healthy attitude. Some long-term survivors find new meaning as a result of being HIV positive. Others find meaning in their relationship with a higher power. Still others find their purpose in relationship to someone who needs them or someone they want to spend time with.

Maintain perspective

This strategy is built on attitudinal and cognitive approaches which have emotional consequences. A failure to maintain perspective can result in depression, negative affect, and hopelessness. Accepting the reality of an AIDS diagnosis without seeing it as an imminent death sentence is a key factor in maintaining perspective, as is believing one can live with AIDS. Distraction as a coping strategy is important and not allowing AIDS to become the sole focus of one's life helps in maintaining a healthy, positive outlook, taking each day as it comes. Maintaining perspective is very similar to the idea of balance. Extremes in anything mental, emotional, physical, social or spiritual are to be avoided. Behaviorally, balance involves maintaining a daily routine, keeping life as normal as possible, and not disengaging socially or emotionally.

SUMMARY AND RECOMMENDATIONS

Numerous studies have demonstrated that psychological factors are related to disease progression in HIV. Furthermore, several studies have indicated that psychosocial interventions can buffer the impact of stressful events such as bereavement or HIV notification on the emotional distress and immune impairment seen in HIV. Thus there appears to be a clear role for mind–body medicine in HIV disease. This chapter has reviewed the studies which can be used to identify those who may be at risk, such as the recently bereaved or the clinically depressed, and those with poor coping strategies which may handicap their health. Interventions could be tailored to those individuals who need help. For example, fatalistic or depressed people could receive training in cognitive restructuring; those who are anxious could be taught relaxation techniques; those who are socially isolated or bereaved could be treated in a group format with opportunities to share their grief, connect with others, and learn skills for widening and maintaining strong social connections. More work needs to be done to determine the ultimate impact of psychological factors and mind–body interventions on health and quality of life in HIV and where such approaches fit in with standard medical care. The importance of psychosocial factors should be recognized, but they should complement rather than replace standard medical and pharmaceutical approaches.

REFERENCES

1 Ader R, Cohen N 1975 Behaviorally conditioned immunosuppression. Psychosomatic Medicine 37:333–40

2 Felton D et al. 1985 Noradrenergic sympathetic innervation of lymphoid tissue. Journal of Immunology: 135

3 Rabin B et al. 1989 Bidirectional interaction between the central nervous system and the immune system. Critical Reviews in Immunology 9(4):279–312

4 Herbert TB, Cohen, S 1993 Stress and immunity in humans: a meta-analytic review. Psychosomatic Medicine 55:364–79

5 Ironson G, Wynings C, Schneiderman N, Baum A, Rodriguez M, Greenwood D, Benight C, Antoni M, LaPerriere A, Huang H S, Klimas N, Fletcher M 1997 Post traumatic stress symptoms, intrusive thoughts, loss and immune function after Hurricane Andrew. Psychosomatic Medicine 59:128-141

6 Redfield R, Burke D 1988 HIV infection: the clinical picture. Scientific American 259:90–98

7 Tindall B, Cooper D 1991 Primary HIV infection: Host responses and intervention strategies. AIDS 5:1–14

8 Clerici M, Berzofsky JA, Shearer GM, Tacket CO 1991 Exposure to HIV-1-specific T helper cell responses before detection of infection by polymerase chain reaction and serum antibodies. Journal of Infectious Disease 164:178–84

9 Stine GJ 1996 AIDS update. Prentice Hall, Upper Saddle River, New Jersey

10 Pantaleo G, Graziosi C, Fauci A 1993 The immunopathogenesis of human immunodeficiency virus infection. The New England Journal of Medicine 328:327–35

11 Centers for Disease Control (CDC) 1992 1993 Revised classification system for HIV infection and expanded surveillance case definition for AIDS among adolescents and adults. Morbidity and Mortality Weekly Report 41(RR-8):1–17

12 Kaplan LD, Wofsky CB, Volberding PA 1987 Treatment of patients with AIDS and associated manifestations. JAMA 257:1367–76

13 Antoni M, Baggett L, Ironson G et al. 1991 Cognitive-behavioral stress management intervention buffers distress responses and immunologic changes following notification of HIV-1 seropositivity. Journal of Consulting and Clinical Psychology 59(6):906–15

14 LaPerriere A, Antoni M, Schneiderman N et al. 1990 Exercise intervention attenuates emotional distress and natural killer cell decrements following notification of positive serologic status for HIV-1. Biofeedback Self Regulation 15:229–42

15 Friedman A, Antoni M, Ironson G et al. 1991 Behavioral interventions, changes in perceived social support, and depression following notification of HIV-1 seropositivity. Presented at the Annual Meeting of the Society of Behavioral Medicine, Washington D C, March, 1991

16 Lutgendorf S, Antoni M, Ironson G, Klimas N, Starr K, Schneiderman N, Fletcher MA 1997 How acceptance and social support mediate distress outcomes in

symptomatic HIV seropositive gay men during a cognitive behavioral stress management intervention. Psychosomatic Medicine (in press)

17 Esterling B, Antoni M, Schneiderman N. et al. 1992 Psychosocial modulation of antibody to Epstein-Barr viral capsid antigen and human herpes virus type-6 in HIV-1 infected and at-risk gay men. Psychosomatic Medicine 52:397–410

18 Antoni M, Ironson G, Helder L, Lutgendorf S, Friedman, A, LaPerriere A, Fletcher MA, Schneiderman N 1992 Stress management intervention reduces social isolation and maladaptive coping behaviors in gay men adjusting to an HIV seropositive diagnosis. Presented at the annual meeting of the Society of Behavioral Medicine, New York, March 25–28

19 Lutgendorf S, Antoni M, Ironson G, Klimas N, Kumar M, Starr K, Schneiderman N, McCabe P, Cleven K, Fletcher M A 1997 Cognitive behavioral stress management decreases dysphoric mood and herpes simplex virus-Type 2 antibody titers in symptomatic HIV-seropositive gay men. Journal of Consulting and Clinical Psychology 65(1):31–43

20 LaPerriere A, Klimas N, Fletcher M A, Perry A, Ironson G, Perna F, Schneiderman N 1995 Exercise Immunology and HIV Disease. Paper presented at the Second International Society of Exercise and Immunology Congress. Brussels, Belgium

21 Ironson G, Friedman A, Klimas N, Antoni M, Fletcher M, LaPerriere A, Simoneau J, Schneiderman N 1994 Distress, denial and low adherence to behavioral interventions predict faster disease progression in gay men infected with Human Immunodeficiency Virus. International Journal of Behavioral Medicine 1:90–105

22 Mulder CL, Antoni M, Emmelkamp P et al. 1995 Psychosocial group intervention and the rate of decline in immunologic parameters in symptomatic HIV-infected homosexual men. Psychotherapy and Psychosomatics 63:185–92

23 Mulder CL, Emmelkamp P, Antoni MH et al. 1994 Cognitive-behavioral and experiential group psychotherapy for HIV-infected homosexual men: A comparative study. Psychosomatic Medicine 56:423–31

24 Coates T, McKusic L, Kuno R, Stites D 1989 Stress reduction training changed number of sexual partners but not immune function in men with HIV. American Journal of Public Health 79:885–7

25 Goodkin K, Tuttle R, Blaney NT, Feaster D, Shapshak P, Burkhalter J, Leeds B, Baldewicz T, Kumar M, Fletcher MA 1996 A bereavement support group intervention is associated with immunological changes in HIV-1+ and HIV-1-homosexual men. Paper presented at the annual meeting of the American Psychosomatic Society, Williamsburg, VA, March. Abstract in Psychosomatic Medicine 58:83

26 Goodkin K, Feaster D, Tuttle R, Blaney NT, Kumar M, Baum M, Shapshak P, Fletcher MA 1996 Bereavement is associated with time-dependent decrements in cellular immune function in asymptomatic human immunodeficiency virus type 1 seropositive homosexual men. Clinical and Diagnostic Laboratory Immunology 109–118

27 Bartrop R, Lazarus L, Luckhurst E et al. 1977 Depressed lymphocyte function after bereavement. Lancet 1:834–6

28 Irwin M, Daniels M, Smith T L et al. 1987 Impaired natural killer cell activity during bereavement. Brain Behavior and Immunology 1:98–104

29 Kemeny ME, Dean L 1995 Effects of AIDS-related bereavement on HIV progression among New York City gay men. AIDS Education Prevention 7 (Suppl): 36–47

30 Chesney MA, Folkman S, Chambers D 1996 The impact of a cognitive-behavioral intervention for coping with HIV disease. Paper presented at the annual meeting of the American Psychosomatic Society, Williamsburg, VA, March. Abstract in Psychosomatic Medicine 58:86

31 Chesney MA, Folkman S, Chambers D 1996 Coping effectiveness training for men living with HIV: preliminary findings. International Journal of STD and AIDS 7(Suppl. 2):75–82

32 Folkman S, Chesney M, McKusick L, Ironson G, Johnson DS, Coates TJ 1991 Translating coping theory into intervention. In: Eckenrode J (ed) The social context of stress. Plenum, New York, pp 239–60

33 Fawzy I, Namir S, Wolcott D 1989 Group intervention with newly diagnosed AIDS patients. Psychiatric Medicine 7:35–46

34 Kelly JA, Murphy DA, Bahr GR et al. 1993 Outcome of cognitive-behavioral and support group brief therapies for depressed, HIV-infected persons. American Journal of Psychiatry; 150:1679–86

35 Auerbach J, Oleson T, Solomon G 1992 A behavioral medicine intervention as an adjunctive treatment for HIV-related illness. Psychology and Health 6:325–34

36 Ironson G, Field T, Scafidi F, Hashimoto M, Kumar M, Kumar A, Price A, Goncalves A, Burman I, Tatenman C, Patarca R, Fletcher M A 1996 Massage therapy is associated with enhancement of the immune system's cytotoxic capacity. International Journal of Neuroscience 84:205–17

37 LaPerriere A, Fletcher MA, Antoni MH et al. 1991 Aerobic exercise training in an AIDS risk group. International Journal of Sports Medicine 12:S53–7

38 Burack JH, Barrett DC, Stall RD, Chesney MA, Ekstrand ML, Coates TJ 1993 Depressive symptoms and CD4 lymphocyte decline among HIV-infected men. JAMA 270:2567–73

39 Lyketsos C, Hoover D, Guccione M, Senterfitt W, Dew M, Wesch J, Van Raden M, Treisman G, Morganstem H 1993 Depressive symptoms as predictors of medical outcomes in HIV infection. Journal of the American Medical Association 270:2563–7

40 Rabkin J, Remien R, Katoff L, Williams J 1993 Resilience in adversity among AIDS long term survivors. Hospital and Community Psychiatry 44(2):162–7

41 Perry S, Fishman B, Jacobsberg L, Frances A 1992 Relationships over 1 year between lymphocyte subsets and psychosocial variables among adults with infection by Human Immunodeficiency Virus. Archives of General Psychiatry 49:396–401

42 Kemeny M, Duran R, Taylor S, Weiner H, Visscher B, Fahey J 1990 Chronic depression predicts CD4 decline over a five year period in HIV seropositive men. Paper presented at the Sixth International Conference on AIDS, San Francisco CA

43 Kemeny M, Weiner H, Taylor S, Schneider S, Visscher

B, Fahey JL 1994 Repeated bereavement, depressed mood, and immune parameters in HIV seropositive and seronegative gay men. Health Psychology 13:144

44 Kemeny M 1994 Stressful events, psychological responses and progression of HIV infection. In: Glaser R, Kiecolt–Glaser J (eds) Handbook on stress and immunity. New York: Academic Press pp 245–266

45 Antoni MH, Goldstein D, Ironson G, LaPerriere A, Fletcher MA, Schneiderman N 1995 Coping responses to HIV-1 serostatus notification predict concurrent and prospective immunologic status. Clinical Psychology and Psychotherapy 2:234–48

46 Goodkin K, Blaney N, Feaster D, Klimas NG, Baum M, Fletcher MA 1993 Psychosocial changes predict long term changes in psychological distress and laboratory progression markers of HIV-1 infection. In: IXth International Conference on AIDS. Abstract Book. V. II. Berlin, Germany PO-D22-4074, p 897

47 Solano L, Costa M, Salvati S, Coda R, Aiuta F, Mezzaroma I, Bertini M 1993 Psychosocial factors and clinical evolution in HIV-1 infection: A longitudinal study. Journal of Psychosomatic Research 37(1):39–51

48 Lutgendorf S, Antoni M, Ironson G, Kumar M, Klimas N, Schneiderman N, Fletcher M 1995 Cognitive processing of stressful emotional material predicts changes in mood and immune functioning. Psychosomatic Medicine 57:60

49 Blomkvist V, Theorell T, Jonsson H, Schulman S, Berntorp E, Stiegendal L 1994 Psychosocial self-prognosis in relation to mortality and morbidity in hemophiliacs with HIV infection. Psychotherapy and Psychosomatics 62:185–92

50 Mulder C L, Antoni M, Duivenvoorden H, Kaufman R, Goodkin K 1995 Active confrontational coping predicts decreased clinical progression over a one year period in HIV-infected homosexual men. Journal of Psychosomatic Research 39(8):957

51 Reed GM, Kemeny ME, Taylor SE, Wang HJ, Visscher BR 1994 Realistic acceptance as a predictor of decreased survival time in gay men with AIDS. Health Psychology 13(4):249–307

52 Mulder CL, deVroome EM, van Griensen G, Antoni M 1995 Distraction as a predictor of the biological course of HIV-1 infection over a 7 year period in gay men. Psychosomatic Medicine 57:67 (Abstract)

53 Reed G, Kemeny M, Taylor S, Visscher B, Fahey J 1994 Negative HIV-specific expectancies and health outcomes in HIV-related disease. Invited Symposium presented at the 52nd Annual Scientific Meeting of the American Psychosomatic Society. Boston, MA

54 Kemeny M, Weiner H, Duran R, Taylor S, Visscher B, Fahey J L 1995. Immune system changes following the death of a partner in HIV+ gay men. Psychosomatic Medicine 57:547–554

55 Reed GM, Kemeny ME, Taylor SE, Vischer BR (in Press) Negative HIV-specific expectancies and AIDS-related bereavement as predictors of symptom onset in asymptomatic HIV seropositive gay men. Health Psychology

56 Temoshok L, O'Leary A, Jenkins S 1990 Survival time in men with AIDS: Relationships with psychological coping and autonomic arousal (Abstract). International Conference on AIDS 6:435

57 Theorell T, Blomkvist V, Jonsson H, Schulman S, Berntorp E, Stigendal L 1995 Social support and the development of immune function in human immunodeficiency virus infection. Psychosomatic Medicine 57:32–6

58 Solomon G, Temoshok L, O'Leary A, Zich J 1987 An intensive psychoimmunologic study of long-surviving persons with AIDS. Pilot work, background studies, hypotheses, and methods. Annals of the New York Academy of Sciences 496: 647–55

59 Cole S, Kemeny M, Taylor S, Visscher B, Fahey J 1996 Accelerated course of HIV infection in gay men who conceal their homosexuality. Psychosomatic Medicine 58:219–231

60 Koenig H, Bearson L, Dayringer R 1989 Physician perspectives on the role of religion in the physician-older patient relationship. Journal of Family Practice 28(4):441–8

61 Carson V 1993 Prayer, meditation, exercise, and special diets: behaviors of the hardy person with HIV/AIDS. Journal of the Association of Nurses in AIDS Care 4(3):18–28

62 Hall B 1994 Ways of maintaining hope in HIV disease. Resource of Nursing and Health 17(4):283–93

63 Woods T, Antoni M, Ironson G, Kling D 1996 Religiosity and its relationship to affective and immune measures in HIV-infected gay men. Paper presented to the American Psychosomatic Society 1996 Annual Meeting

64 Cherry K, Smith D 1993 Sometimes I cry: The experience of loneliness for men with AIDS. Health Communication 5(3):181–208

65 Wagner G, Serafini J, Rabkin J, Remein R 1994 Integration of one's religion and homosexuality: A weapon against internalized homophobia? Journal of Homosexuality 26(4):91–110

66 Greenberg J 1993 An alternative treatment activist manifesto. Gay Men's Health Center Treatment Issues, Winter:2–12

67 Ou-Yang K et al. 1990 Antimicrobial Agents and Chemotherapy 34:1961–5

68 McCaleb R 1990 Better Nutrition, October:22–32

69 Chu D T et al. 1988a Journal of Clinical Laboratory Immunology 25:125–9

70 Chu D T et al. 1988b Journal of Clinical Laboratory Immunology 26:183–7

71 Sun Y et al. 1983 Journal of Biological Response Modifiers 2:227–37

72 Lau B H et al. 1990 International Clinical Nutrition Review 10:430–4

73 Cunnick J et al. 1993 Journal of Naturopathic Medicine 4:16–21

74 Lee-Huang S et al. 1990 Journal of the Federation of European Biochemical Society 272:12–18

75 Gustafson K R et al. 1989 Journal of the National Cancer Institute 81:1254–8

76 Foster S 1990 Echinacea: Nature's immune enhancer. Healing Arts Press Rochester, VT

77 Wacker A et al. 1978 Planta Medica 33:89–102

78 Green CJ 1995 Nutritional support in HIV infection and AIDS. Clinical Nutrition 14(4):197–212

79 Henderson C W 1993 AIDS therapies

80 Narovlyansky A et al. 1993 Abstract PO-A13-0240. Ninth International Conference on AIDS. Berlin. June, 1993

81 Tabba H D et al. 1989 Antiviral Research 989 (11):263–73
82 Remien RH, Rabkin JG, Williams JBW 1992 Coping Strategies and health beliefs of AIDS longterm survivors. Psychology and Health 6:335–45
83 Barroso J 1993 Reconstructing a life: a nursing study of long term survivors of AIDS. Unpublished dissertation, University of Texas at Austin
84 Ironson G, Solomon G, Cruess D, Barroso J, Stivers M 1995 Psychosocial factors related to long-term survival with HIV/AIDS. Journal of Clinical Psychology and Psychotherapy 2(4):249–66

CHAPTER CONTENTS

7

Abdominal symptoms and the mind

Michael J.G. Farthing
Jennifer Gomborone

INTRODUCTION

The idea that the abdominal organs are the seat of the soul and a focus for our emotions has been with us for many centuries. *Gut reactions* are spontaneous feelings not filtered by a sophisticated cerebral cortex. Most of us are quite accustomed to the sensation of 'butterflies' or urgency and bowel frequency when faced with a stressful event such as a 'blind date' or an important professional examination. These and other abdominal symptoms, particularly those due to changes in intestinal motility, are thought to be mediated by the autonomic nervous system, indicating a clear connection between the brain and the gut.

History shows us that beliefs about changes in mood were also focused on the abdomen. Melancholia, that is *black bile*, the predecessor of depression, was thought to emanate from an abnormality of alimentary functions. Many early remedies for mood disorder focused on the alimentary tract which seemed to be an approachable target for the herbal remedies of early medicine.

The importance of abdominal symptoms that are not related to any defined organic disease is no longer contested. *Functional abdominal symptoms* as they have become to be known, are extremely common. They have entered and sometimes dominated the lives of many highly successful individuals. Charles Darwin was racked with abdominal pain which in later life restricted his movements away from home, as did the abdominal symptoms of Thomas Carlisle. Sigmund Freud clearly recognized the importance of the gastrointestinal tract as a mirror of the mind and our emotions, and based some aspects of his analytical theories of personality development on the beginning and end of the gastrointestinal tract, namely the mouth and the anus. The gastrointestinal tract and its disorders have never been the subject of cocktail party debate, but perhaps now is the time for these previously indelicate issues to emerge from the closet.

FUNCTIONAL ABDOMINAL DISORDERS: DEFINITIONS

There is an extensive consortium of symptoms that collectively can be included under the umbrella term 'functional gastrointestinal disorder' (Box 7.1)[1]. Within this definition, symptoms not explained by structural or biochemical abnormalities in the gastrointestinal tract may be attributable to the upper or lower gastrointestinal tract. The definition of a *functional bowel disorder* focuses on symptoms attributable to the mid- or lower intestinal tract and usually include abdominal pain, distension and disordered defecation. The *irritable bowel syndrome,* the most common of all of the functional bowel disorders, has an even more restricted definition in which abdominal pain is associated with defecation or a change in bowel habit, with other additional features of disordered defecation and abdominal distension[2,3]. The insistence that both abdominal pain and disordered bowel habit must be present may be too restrictive, and many gastroenterologists would make a positive clinical diagnosis of the condition even if abdominal pain is only a minor, infrequent symptom or is absent, providing that the other characteristic features are present. Currently accepted definitions of *functional gastrointestinal disorder, functional bowel disorder* and the *irritable bowel syndrome* are shown in Box 7.1. Although different symptom complexes clearly form the basis of a symptom-based classification, there is no pathophysiological evidence that differentiates many of these conditions in terms of cause and development. However, a classification system is vital for patients enrolled in research studies to maximize the potential for comparability between different centers[4,5]. Within the broad definition of a *functional gastrointestinal disorder,* many sub-classifications have been suggested emphasizing the protean nature of functional abdominal disorders (Box 7.2).

Box 7.1 Functional disorders of the gastrointestinal tract

Functional gastrointestinal disorder

A variable combination of chronic or recurrent gastrointestinal symptoms not explained by structural or biochemical abnormalities. Some symptoms may be attributable to the oropharynx, esophagus, stomach, biliary tree, small or large intestine, or anus.

Functional bowel disorder

A functional bowel gastrointestinal disorder with symptoms attributable to the middle or lower intestinal tract. The symptoms include abdominal pain, distension and disordered defecation.

Irritable bowel syndrome

A functional bowel disorder in which abdominal pain is associated with defecation or changes in bowel habit, and with features of disordered defecation and with distension.

EPIDEMIOLOGY

Several surveys have shown that functional gastrointestinal symptoms occur in up to a fifth of adults in the industrialized world[6,7]. A recent community survey found symptoms typical of the irritable bowel syndrome (IBS) in more than a fifth of women and a tenth of men, and that prevalence was similar throughout life[7]. Women seem to present more commonly with irritable bowel symptoms than men, although the prevalence of symptoms in the community is similar in men and women. The IBS is a transcultural disorder, with a similar prevalence reported in China, India, Japan and South America although the prevalence may be lower in other parts of South East Asia and in Africa[1]. In the developing world, symptoms of the IBS

Box 7.2 The functional gastrointestinal disorders

1. Functional esophageal disorders
    - Globus
    - Rumination syndrome
    - Functional chest pain or presumed esophageal origin
    - Functional heartburn
    - Unspecified functional esophageal disorder
2. Functional gastroduodenal disorders
    - Functional dyspepsia
        - Ulcer-like dyspepsia
        - Motility-like dyspepsia
        - Reflux-like dyspepsia
        - Unspecified functional dyspepsia
    - Aerophagia
3. Functional bowel disorders
    - Irritable bowel syndrome
    - Functional abdominal bloating
    - Functional constipation
    - Functional diarrhea
    - Unspecified functional bowel disorder
4. Functional abdominal pain
    - Functional abdominal pain syndrome
    - Unspecified functional abdominal pain
5. Functional biliary pain
    - Sphincter of Oddi dyskinesia
6. Functional anorectal disorders
    - Functional incontinence
    - Functional anorectal pain
        - Levator syndrome
        - Proctalgia fugax
    - Pelvic floor dyssynergia
    - Unspecified functional anorectal disorder

may be more common in cities than in rural areas. Only a minority of individuals with symptoms present to doctors. Our recent survey of 854 employers of a single business community in London showed that 16.6% had symptoms of the condition, but only a quarter of these people had consulted a doctor.

The IBS accounts for between 20–50% of referrals to gastroenterologists and thus represents a substantial workload for hospital specialists. In the USA the condition accounts for an estimated 2.4–3.5 million visits to physicians each year and 2.2 million prescriptions are issued[8]. Further financial implications result from days lost at work.

Abdominal bloating occurs in a similar proportion of the population as the IBS; in one survey it occurred in 25% of men and 30% of women[9]. In a Bristol survey bloating was more common in individuals with colonic or dyspeptic pain and was particularly associated with constipation[10].

Functional constipation occurs in up to 20% of the population and is more common in women whereas *functional diarrhea* is less common, occurring in only 4% of healthy subjects[11,12]. The prevalence of *functional abdominal pain* is not clearly defined, but appears to be much less common than classic IBS in the community and gastroenterology clinics.

The prevalences of functional disorders of the ano-rectum are poorly defined. Pain in the ano-rectum occurs either in the form of the *levator ani syndrome* (vague dull ache or pressure sensation high in the rectum) or *proctalgia fugax* (sudden severe pain in the anal area) with prevalences of up to 7 and 18% respectively, although there does appear to be considerable overlap between the two syndromes[13].

CLINICAL PATTERNS

Functional gastrointestinal symptoms often masquerade as organic disorders with similar symptom patterns that superficially resemble organic disorders. However, the symptom complex is often less well defined in functional disorders, and may be associated with other abdominal symptoms producing an overlap syndrome. An example might be an individual with epigastric pain or discomfort resembling a peptic ulcer, but associated with additional symptoms such as post-prandial bloating and intermittent lower abdominal discomfort with disordered defecation. However, there are a number of functional syndromes which have a typical constellation of symptoms.

Esophageal syndromes

One of the most commonly recognized functional esophageal symptoms is that of *globus*. Sufferers report a sensation of a lump in their throat usually combined with difficulty in swallowing at a site located high in the esophagus. The sensation can be so intense that even swallowing of saliva may be difficult. The *rumination* syndrome is less common, but is characterized by the cyclical regurgitation of food from the esophagus into the mouth which is then swallowed again. So-called *functional* or *non-cardiac chest pain* is well recognized by both cardiologists and gastroenterologists and may resemble the pain of myocardial ischemia, or esophageal spasm. The relationship to exercise however, is usually less clear than that associated with myocardial ischemia, and exercise electrocardiography and coronary angiography are by definition normal. Similarly, esophageal manometry shows a normal motor pattern in the esophagus without evidence of the intermittent high pressure waves of esophageal spasm. Some patients only experience retrosternal pain when swallowing solid food and this has been termed the *tender esophagus*. These patients have no evidence of macro- or microscopic esophagitis and esophageal manometry is normal. It is presumed to be due to visceral hyperalgesia.

Functional gastrointestinal disorders

Functional dyspepsia is the most common and clinically important disorder in this group of syndromes. Dyspepsia comes from the Greek, *dys* meaning 'bad' and *peptein* meaning 'to digest'. Dyspepsia is usually characterized by upper abdominal pain most commonly located to the epigastrium, which may or may not be related to meals[14]. Abdominal pain is usually accompanied by one or more of a consortium of other symptoms which include upper abdominal discomfort, early satiety, post-prandial fullness, nausea, retching, vomiting and upper abdominal bloating. It goes without saying that routine investigations such as barium meal examination, upper gastrointestinal endoscopy and abdominal ultrasound are all normal. Attempts have been made to classify functional dyspepsia into *ulcer-like functional dyspepsia* in which the symptoms appear to closely mimic those of a peptic ulcer and *dysmotility-like functional dyspepsia*, in which the symptoms suggest an abnormality of gastric emptying with early satiety, post-prandial fullness, nausea and bloating predominating[14]. A third group of *unspecified functional dyspepsia*, refers to patients whose symptoms do not clearly fall into the preceding two groups. The evidence however, that these symptom patterns reflect fundamental differences in pathophysiology has not been clearly established.

Functional bowel disorders

The dominant disorder in this symptom group is the *irritable bowel syndrome*. IBS is a functional bowel disorder in which abdominal pain is associated with defecation or a change in bowel habit, and there are accompanying features of disordered defecation and abdominal distension. In 1978 Manning et al. described several abdominal symptoms that were more likely to be present in IBS than in organic disease (Box 7.3)[3]. These symptoms were tested prospectively in subsequent studies and their validity confirmed. The more of these symptoms that are present, the more likely the patient is to have IBS[4]. Kruis et al. added other criteria, including a requirement for symptoms to have been present for more than 2 years and the use of symptom complexes that increase the chances of making a positive clinical diagnosis[5]. However, this system is cumbersome to use and difficult to apply. It was found that the positive symptom criteria were not well defined and the system appeared to identify organic disease better than IBS. It therefore failed to achieve acceptance. A recent report produced clear cut diagnostic criteria for IBS,

Box 7.3 Symptoms more likely to be found in the irritable bowel syndrome than organic abdominal disease

- Pain eased after bowel movement
- Looser stools at onset of pain
- More frequent bowel movements at onset of pain
- Abdominal distension
- Mucus in rectum
- Feeling of incomplete evacuation

Box 7.4 Diagnostic criteria for the abdominal bowel syndrome

At least 3 months of continuous or recurrent symptoms of:

1. Abdominal pain or discomfort which is:
   - Relieved with defecation and/or
   - Associated with change in frequency of stool and/or
   - Associated with a change in consistency of stool.
2. Two or more of the following, on at least a quarter of occasions or days:
   - Altered bowel frequency (>3 bowel movements a day or <3 bowel movements a week)
   - Altered form of stool (lumpy/hard or loose/watery stool)
   - Altered passage of stool (straining, urgency, or feeling of incomplete evacuation)
   - Passage of mucus
   - Bloating or feeling of abdominal distension.

which are particularly valuable as entry criteria for research studies (Box 7.4)[1].

The severity of irritable bowel symptoms varies widely. In its mildest form, patients may experience pre-defecatory lower abdominal pain and a modest increase in bowel frequency usually early in the morning before leaving for work. In others pain and bowel frequency may be incapacitating and render the individual house-bound. Others may only be able to venture out providing the exact location of public toilets on any particular journey is accurately known, because of the fear that severe urgency and frequency might lead to incontinence. In many the symptoms are worse during stressful life events. Abdominal bloating with or without visible abdominal distension is a particularly distressing symptom and commonly associated with pain and disordered defecation. In many patients, the bloating becomes worse as the day progresses. In some individuals this condition can be avoided by eating small amounts or by eating nothing at all.

In recent years, it has become clear that the abdominal symptoms of IBS are often associated with so-called non-colonic symptoms[15,16]. These include nausea, vomiting and early satiety. In addition there may be symptoms apparently emanating from other abdominal organs including urinary symptoms such as nocturia, frequency, urgency and the feeling of incomplete emptying of the bladder. In women, dyspareunia is also commonly associated with IBS. There is also evidence to suggest that there may be abnormalities in extra-abdominal organs such as the lungs, in which bronchial hyperreactivity has been shown to occur more frequently in IBS sufferers than in healthy control subjects[17]. These observations suggest that there is a more generalized disorder of smooth muscle or visceral hypersensitivity in IBS patients, that is not limited to the gastrointestinal tract or even the abdominal organs.

In some patients all of the diagnostic criteria for the IBS may not be present. Functional constipation or functional diarrhea may exist as isolated symptoms. In such individuals it is generally wise to pursue more active investigation to ensure that an organic cause for the diarrhea or constipation is not present. In such cases it is particularly important to exclude inflammatory bowel disease, infection or colon cancer.

Functional abdominal pain

Pain as an isolated symptom is one of the more difficult functional bowel symptoms to manage[18,19]. Pain is usually present most of the time and when long-standing can completely dominate the patient's life. Eventually most individuals undergo extensive investigation often involving several specialist centers and multiple doctors. The majority of patients with the functional abdominal pain syndrome have some form of psychiatric disorder[20]. Depression and anxiety are the most common diagnoses, although in some it may be part of a more generalized somatization disorder in which abdominal pain is one of many symptoms for which the patient may have consulted a variety of other specialists. The onset of the pain may coincide with a major life event such as separation, divorce or loss of a close relative.

Overlap syndromes

Careful evaluation of large groups of individuals with functional abdominal disorders, notably those with IBS non-ulcer dyspepsia, indicate that there is considerable overlap between the major symptom patterns. Similarly, within the sub-groups of non-ulcer dyspepsia, patients do not neatly fulfill isolated criteria for *ulcer-like* or *dysmotility-like* sub-groups there often being extensive overlap between the two despite a major symptom favoring one of the sub-divisions. Recent evidence suggests that there is also overlap with non-abdominal functional disorders, notably with low back pain (fibromyalgia) and also with chronic fatigue syndrome. Tiredness and exhaustion for instance are extremely common in patients with IBS[15]. These observations suggest that there may be some common factor(s) in the etiopathogenesis of these so-called functional syndromes, a strong candidate being the presence of psychological distress.

PHYSIOLOGICAL BASIS FOR SYMPTOM PRODUCTION

Although there is an extensive list of functional gastrointestinal disorders (Box 7.2), very few of these have been subjected to systematic evaluation with respect to the underlying pathophysiological mechanisms of symptom production. However, both non-ulcer dyspepsia and IBS have been the subject of many studies in recent years and thus a major emphasis will be placed on these two conditions.

Non-ulcer dyspepsia

Although the physiological mechanisms of symptom production in non-ulcer dyspepsia have not been clearly defined, there are a number of factors that have been implicated including gastric acid secretion, disorders of gastrointestinal motility, alteration in visceral sensation and more recently, the presence of *Helicobacter pylori* (Box 7.5). Like IBS, a possible role for the central nervous system has also been proposed.

Box 7.5 Possible factors in the development of non-ulcer dyspepsia

- Disordered gastric acid secretion
- Disordered gastrointestinal motility
  - Gastroparesis
  - Small bowel dysmotility
- Visceral hypersensitivity
  - Acid
  - Balloon distension
- Central nervous system dysfunction

Gastric acid

Several studies have measured basal and peak acid output in patients with non-ulcer dyspepsia, but there is no convincing evidence of gastric acid hypersecretion. However, in therapeutic studies in which a H_2-receptor antagonist has been compared with placebo, meta-analysis does suggest that H_2-receptor antagonists have on average a 20% advantage with regard to symptom relief[21], suggesting that while acid secretion is within normal limits, these individuals may have an increased sensitivity to gastric acid.

Gastrointestinal motility

Several studies have suggested that some patients with non-ulcer dyspepsia have a gastroparesis with impaired gastric emptying of solids. This has been observed in 40–50% of patients, but clearly cannot explain non-ulcer dyspepsia symptoms in all individuals[22–24]. Mangall et al. studied gastric emptying of liquids, but only found impaired emptying with liquids of a high fat content[25]. More recently, Troncon et al. failed to find any significant delay in gastric emptying of solids, but did notice a highly significant difference in food distribution in the stomach[26]. In healthy control subjects, food was retained in the proximal stomach before passing through the pylorus into the small intestine, whereas in non-ulcer dyspepsia, patients' gastric contents were distributed throughout the antrum and proximal stomach. The mechanism of this impaired motor function has not been clearly defined, although there is some evidence of efferent vagal dysfunction which might result in low vagal tone, antral hypomotility and abdominal discomfort.

Oro-cecal transit time is slightly increased in patients with non-ulcer dyspepsia, although in the study by Waldron et al. there was substantial overlap with healthy control subjects[27]. It seems unlikely that small intestinal hypomotility can explain the symptoms of non-ulcer dyspepsia.

Visceral sensation

As already stated, the therapeutic studies with H_2-receptor antagonists suggest that there might be increased sensitivity to gastric acid, although there is no direct evidence that this is a major pathogenetic mechanism in non-ulcer dyspepsia. However, a number of studies have used gastric distension to study pain thresholds and to measure gastric compliance; these have confirmed that patients with non-ulcer dyspepsia have lower thresholds for pain and bloating produced by balloon distension[28–30]. Mearin et al. demonstrated a highly significant difference in gastric sensation between non-ulcer dyspepsia patients and healthy controls using a gastric barostat[29]. This occurred in the absence of any abnormality of gastrointestinal motility and a cold-stress test for somatic sensation was not significantly different from healthy control subjects. These observations would support the hypothesis that some patients with non-ulcer dyspepsia have a 'gastric hypersensitivity' which need not be related to abnormalities of gastric motility.

Helicobacter pylori

On average, 50% of patients with non-ulcer dyspepsia are infected with *Helicobacter pylori* with associated antral gastritis[31]. However, *H. pylori* is not associated with any particular symptom pattern and cannot be linked to specific abnormalities of acid secretion, gastroduodenal motor abnormalities or responses to distension. On balance, short-term eradication studies do not suggest improvement in symptoms although in one study[32], patients were reviewed again 1 year following eradication and there was a significant improvement in symptoms in the group of non-ulcer dyspepsia patients who had successfully undergone eradication therapy[33]. These observations require confirmation in larger prospective studies.

Irritable bowel syndrome

Intestinal motility

The diverse symptomatology of IBS has made it difficult to propose a simple mechanistic theory of symptom production (Box 7.6). However, the variation in bowel habit suggests that there might be a primary motor disorder of the gut, predominantly involving the colon[34]. Motor activity in the human intestine can be studied either by measuring changes in the patterns of intestinal pressure or by measuring gut transit rates. Studies of colonic activity in the basal state have yielded conflicting results, but there is some agreement that the colon of patients with IBS is hyper-reactive, particularly to physiological stimuli such as eating a meal[34,35]. In the small intestine, some studies have shown an increase in 'clustered contractions' in patients with IBS[36]. Other investigators have found that these short bursts of intense activity are found with similar frequency in healthy control subjects[37]. Some studies have shown that the periodicity of the migrating motor complex is shorter in diarrhea-predominant than in constipation-predominant patients or control groups, particularly because of a shorter cycle length during the daytime. However, other studies

Box 7.6 Possible factors in the development of the irritable bowel syndrome

1. Disordered motility of the gut
   - Small intestine
   - Colon
   - Esophagus and stomach
2. Altered gut sensation
   - Increased awareness of normal gastrointestinal events
   - Reduced sensation threshold for 'pathophysiological' events
3. Involvement of the central nervous system
   - Altered central processing of end-organ motor and sensory activity
   - Effect of mood on gastrointestinal function

have failed to confirm this. Similarly, acute stress has shown to increase small bowel motility in some studies but inhibited it in others. Thus, the results of studies examining colon and small intestine in patients with IBS, indicate that there is no clearly reproducible abnormality that is present in all patients and that can be regarded as pathognomonic of the condition. All studies show a substantial overlap between the IBS and control subjects, indicating that while these tests have potential value in studying pathophysiology, they have no role in confirming or refuting the diagnosis. Despite the difficulty of interpreting studies of intestinal motility, measures of intestinal transit have produced more concordant results, particularly with respect to the reduction in oro-cecal and whole gut transit times in diarrhea-predominant IBS.

Overall, these findings suggest that while motor abnormalities may be present in some patients with IBS, the abnormalities are not consistent, can overlap significantly with a healthy control population and do not support the view that IBS is due to an easily definable primary motor disorder of the gut.

Visceral sensation

For more than 20 years, evidence has been produced to suggest that at least some of the symptoms of IBS may be due to an alteration of gut sensation, visceral hyperalgesia[30]. Hyperalgesia describes a condition in which pain threshold is reduced and/or the response to a painful stimulus is greater in magnitude and longer in duration. Since there is no obvious local cause in the gut; it has been suggested that in IBS this is due to *secondary hyperalgesia* associated with central hyperexcitability. *Allodynia*, a condition in which pain is produced by a stimulus that does not normally produce pain, may also exist in IBS which again may be of central origin. Increased sensitivity to distension of the rectum exists in some patients with IBS[38,39]. This sensitivity is not global, since somatic pain thresholds in IBS are either normal or increased[40]. Altered sensation may also be important in the production of other symptoms such as abdominal distension and the feeling of incomplete evacuation[41].

Altered visceral sensation and/or allodynia may also account for some of the non-colonic symptoms such as urinary frequency, feeling of incomplete bladder emptying, dyspareunia and possibly other gastrointestinal symptoms such as nausea and early satiety. The autonomic nervous system and smooth muscle are common factors in all of these non-colonic systems which supports the view that central control/perception rather than primary multi-end organ hyper-reactivity or hypersensitivity, is the logical hypothetical route to explain pathogenesis.

Central nervous system

In many healthy individuals, emotional factors alter gut function producing symptoms such as bowel frequency, nausea, vomiting and early satiety. Many of us can recall isolated episodes immediately prior to taking an important examination, waiting in the 'wings' before a theatrical performance or music recital, or before an interview. With experience, confidence, and time, these physiological responses, mediated at least in part by the autonomic nervous system, usually diminish in frequency and severity. However, in some individuals they remain prominent to the point when they interfere with daily life and may be triggered perhaps on a daily basis by what would be generally regarded as 'non-stressful' stimuli such as shopping or going to work. These environmental stresses can also produce non-colonic symptoms such as urinary frequency. In the experimental setting, psychological stress has been shown to produce changes in motility in the small and large intestine and some studies have suggested that responses in IBS patients are exaggerated compared with healthy controls[34]. Thus, the gastrointestinal tract can respond to emotional factors both in the research laboratory and during normal daily life; this may be a factor in the production of

IBS symptoms. To support this view several studies have shown that immediately before presenting with IBS symptoms, stress scores are increased compared with healthy individuals[42].

If emotional factors and stress are important in symptom production in IBS and other functional gastrointestinal disorders then why does the entire population not suffer from these disorders? This may relate both to local permissive factors in the gut (and possibly other organs) or perhaps more likely, to permissive factors within the psyche itself. As far as the gut is concerned, factors such as an episode of travelers' diarrhea or food poisoning may provide the trigger which disrupts the bowel function and heralds the start of functional abdominal symptoms. However, in the absence of continuing evidence of intestinal infection, it is uncertain as to why chronic dysfunction continues, despite resolution of the primary insult. This lends weight to the argument implicating central processing in symptom production. The specific importance of mental state and the appreciation and reporting of functional abdominal symptoms are discussed in more detail below.

PSYCHOLOGICAL FACTORS IN SYMPTOM PRODUCTION

It has long been recognized that functional gastrointestinal disorders are associated with psychological issues. This umbrella term incorporates such elements as psychiatric disorder, adverse life events, psychoneurotic personality traits and abnormal illness behavior. The distinction between these psychological abnormalities is not always clear, particularly in studies from the turn of the century, when psychology and psychiatry were in their infancy, and used terminology and concepts which have subsequently evolved.

The earliest pertinent references examining the relationship between gastrointestinal disorders and psychological factors are descriptive in nature and began to appear in the late 19th Century. Siredy (1869) and Da Costa (1871) attributed what was then called mucous colitis to neurasthenia, which is a syndrome of mental and physical fatigue, akin to anxiety disorder and mild depression[43,44]. White (1905) reported that most of his patients with gastrointestinal complaints were 'nervous, neurasthenic, hypochondriacal and hysterical individuals'[45], and other authors have used terms such as 'neurasthenia with catarrh of the bowel' and 'nervous dyspepsia' to emphasize a primary role for psychological influences[46,47].

One of the earliest systematic clinical studies was published by Bockus et al. (1929), in which 50 cases of mucous colitis were reported and they concluded from their observations that nervousness of some type was present in practically every case[48]. Forty-six per cent were considered to be depressed and several of these patients' episodes of depression coincided with attacks of mucous discharge, diarrhea or colic. However, the authors noted that the patients were for the most part averse to being described as nervous and minimized their considerable emotional suffering, apparently to avoid the stigma of neurosis. White and Jones (1940) studied 57 mucous colitis patients in some detail and divided them into two groups: 'less neurotic' and 'more neurotic', according to the degree of functional impairment associated with their psychoneurotic symptoms[49]. For example, tension was recorded in 96%, anxiety in 82%, depression in 74% and rigidity of thought (obsessionality) in 50%. On the basis of these symptoms all patients could be classified as having a formal psychiatric diagnosis using conventions of the time. However, a major problem with all the earlier studies is that neither the functional abdominal disorders nor the psychiatric disorders were clearly defined. Much of the earlier work was based on inferred etiological explanations which, being highly subjective, were also unreliable.

Diagnosable psychiatric illness

The more recent studies which have examined psychological abnormalities in patients with functional gastrointestinal complaints are to be commended for their use of such diagnostic criteria and structured interviews[50–53]. Studies using the more sophisticated techniques have indicated that up to 40–50% of all patients seen in medical out-patients with a functional gastrointestinal disorder have demonstrable psychiatric illness and that these patients have a worse prognosis than those who are psychologically normal[54–56]. For example, in the study by Haug et al., the relationship between psychological factors and somatic symptoms was examined in patients with functional dyspepsia and they found that this particular group reported higher levels of state/trait anxiety, depression and general psychopathology[57]. They also found that a lower level of functioning and somatic complaints originating from different organ systems were more commonly reported in these patients compared with duodenal ulcer patients or healthy controls.

There are also a number of studies that have evaluated the lifetime prevalence of psychiatric diagnoses in patients with gastrointestinal complaints. Thus, Walker et al. using a highly structured computer-based interview to arrive at DSM-III-R diagnoses in IBS patients and controls with inflammatory bowel disease found that the lifetime prevalence of psychiatric disorder was 93% in the IBS patients and 19% in the organic controls[58]. In all cases the diagnoses were affective in type, and in several cases more than one diagnosis was attributed to a single patient. Lydiard et al. obtained a similar lifetime prevalence to Walker's group of 94% in their IBS patients[59]. The rates for generalized anxiety (26%) and panic disorder (26%) were much higher than in Walker's study while the rate of depression was very similar (23%).

Creed and Guthrie reviewed the nature of the relationship between abdominal symptoms and psychiatric disorder and proposed three possibilities: (i) the patient may have developed abdominal and psychiatric symptoms simultaneously in which case treatment of the psychiatric symptoms may also relieve the bowel symptoms; (ii) psychiatric disorder may precipitate hypervigilance and increased worry about bowel symptoms, resulting in frequent visits to the doctor; and (iii) those with chronic neurotic symptoms as part of their personality may be at high risk of becoming persistent clinic attenders[60].

Studies that have addressed the question of the temporal relationship between psychiatric disorder and gastrointestinal symptoms have found that in most cases the psychiatric disorder precedes the abdominal symptoms, and that the course of these symptoms tends to conform to that of the psychiatric disorder[61]. In one of our own studies where we assessed the prevalence of gastrointestinal symptoms in a sample of psychiatric in-patients suffering from either anxiety or depression, not only were gastrointestinal symptoms found to be remarkably common, but in most of the cases, the onset of psychiatric disorder was followed by a subjective exacerbation of abdominal symptoms[62].

Personality traits

Attempts have been made to identify a comprehensive personality profile which characterizes patients with gastrointestinal disorders by comparing them with other patient groups (e.g. neurotic or general medical patients), and the general population. Chaudhary and Truelove described the personality profiles of IBS patients and compared these with ulcerative colitis patients[63]. They found IBS patients to have mainly compulsive features: meticulousness, excessive cleanliness, punctuality, meanness, stubbornness and rigidity of behavior, whereas such features were rarely encountered in patients with ulcerative colitis. Hill and Blendis assessed a consecutive series of outpatients with abdominal pain for which no organic cause could be found[64]. The patients tended to be more 'neurotic' than a normal population, and were judged to be more conscientious with high standards of personal behavior. Sjodin and Svedlund determined personality characteristics according to a Swedish version of the Edwards Personal Preference Schedule (EPPS) in patients with either IBS or non-ulcer dyspepsia (NUD) patients[65]. The EPPS is an inventory designed to measure the relative strength of 14 factors. These are achievement, deference, order, exhibition, autonomy, affiliation, introception, succorance, dominance, abasement, nurturance, change, endurance and aggression. They found no differences between the IBS and NUD patients, but both differed from the normal controls in relation to such factors as achievement and order, which is in accordance with previous findings of obsessional or compulsive features.

In summary, although the findings have not always been consistent on standardized personality assessments, patients with functional gastrointestinal disorders obtain more abnormal scores than either general medical patients or healthy controls. The sort of traits identified include elements of obsessionality and hypochondriasis.

Life events and gastrointestinal symptoms

The relationship between life events, emotions and gastrointestinal symptoms has long been recognized, and many clinicians believe and act upon the assumption that these symptoms frequently reflect either acute or chronic life stress. Attempts have been made to study this relationship in a systematic way[66]. The application of stress in experimental situations, the documentation of illness following naturally occurring stressors and studies of patient populations with a retrospective evaluation of their prior exposure to life stress have all added to the body of evidence that stress can exert significant effects on the gastrointestinal tract.

In the early days of radiology, Cannon in 1902 reported changes in the contour of and the flow of bismuth through the alimentary tract of cats exposed to situations where they apparently expressed rage or fear[67]. Other studies have looked at the effects of emotion on the stomach and duodenum in people with fistulae. For example, in the famous case of Thomas, who had a stomach fistula following a gunshot wound, Wolf and Wolff in 1943 found that emotional states such as anger, hostility and resentment were associated with increased motility of the stomach and rapid gastric emptying[68]. Abbott et al. found that increased bile appeared in the gastric contents when subjects were subjected to stressful interviews[69]. Others have shown that the motility of the sigmoid colon could be altered in association with changes in the emotional state[70,71]. For example, anger and excitement have been shown to increase the colonic motility index whereas happiness was found to reduce it. The commonly reported experience of diarrhea immediately before a stressful experience has reinforced the view that colonic motility is strongly influenced by emotion.

Another method of studying the relationship between psychological stressors and physical illness is to investigate a population of people with the same illness for evidence of antecedent stressors. This method is potentially highly informative since it relates to naturally occurring disorders. One of the early descriptive studies by Chaudhary and Truelove found that stressful life events influenced the onset and/or course of gastrointestinal symptoms in three-quarters of their patients presenting with abdominal pain and altered bowel habits[63]. Environmental stressors such as marital difficulties, problems with children or parents and worries related to business or career were found to be most common. Similarly, Waller et al. studied IBS patients prospectively over a 6-year period and they found that 84% related their gastrointestinal symptoms to stress[72].

A number of methodological problems were reported with these earlier studies however, and in an attempt to overcome these difficulties semi-structured interview schedules were devised. Pre-eminent among these is the Bedford College Life Events and Difficulty Schedule (LEDS)[73]. One of the earliest studies to apply the LEDS to groups of patients with either functional or organic bowel disease was that by Craig and Brown[74]. They found that 57% of the functional group, 23% of the organic group and 15% of a healthy comparison group had experienced a threatening life event or chronic difficulty during the preceding 38 weeks. The majority of events in the functional group involved losses and disappointments, which are the kind of events associated with the onset of depression. Further support for these findings was provided by Creed et al. in three separate studies using a modified version of the LEDS[75,76]. The study groups consisted of patients subjected to appendicectomy for acute abdominal pain, patients attending gastroenterology clinics, patients admitted after self-poisoning, and an age and sex-matched comparison group free of gastrointestinal symptoms. The results of this study showed that it was the type rather than number of life events that was important. The proportion who had experienced any kind of life event over the 38-week study period was similar in all the groups considered. However, threatening life events were experienced by a greater proportion of all the patient groups compared with the healthy comparison group, and severely threatening life events occurred more frequently in the functional abdominal pain and self-poisoning groups.

It is clear from the existing literature that life events are related to both the onset and course of functional gastrointestinal disorder and that this effect is not necessarily mediated by either concomitant psychiatric disorder or trait neuroticism.

Negative cognitions and attribution style

Complaint-related cognitions and the individual's attribution style are believed to influence the course of functional abdominal complaints[77]. Illness-related fears and beliefs about disease, somatic attributions concerning the gastrointestinal tract and catastrophic cognitions are thought to play an important part in the genesis of a physical illness and lead to differences in the way symptoms are perceived and acted upon. In one of our own studies, we identified abnormal illness attitudes in IBS patients which distinguished them from patients with organic gastrointestinal disease or depression, and healthy controls[78]. The elevated scores on bodily preoccupation, disease phobia and hypochondriacal beliefs that we found among our IBS patients indicate that they found bodily sensations worrisome and difficult to ignore, that they feared having a serious illness, and that they believed that their doctors may have failed to diagnose their condition correctly. Such a constellation of beliefs are likely to underpin illness behavior in terms of repeated consultations. Illness attitudes will also exert an influence on how severe a symptom is judged to be, which in turn, might prompt the individual to focus anxiously on physical sensations, which may actually serve to amplify those sensations. The identification and modification of these dysfunctional thoughts at an early stage in medical consultation is likely to lead to a more favorable outcome in the treatment of functional abdominal complaints.

Factors affecting consultation behavior

There is little doubt that psychological factors influence medical consultation. Most epidemiological surveys have shown that symptoms such as recurrent abdominal pain, nausea, hard or loose stools and abdominal distension are all common, but only a minority of sufferers consult a doctor[79]. Equal numbers of males and females have been found to experience gastrointestinal symptoms, whereas in hospital or general practice populations women outnumber men two to one[80]. This has generally been explained in terms of women's greater readiness to consult. This explanation is based on the conceptual model of illness behavior[81]. Essentially this is an interaction between physiological events, which are the basis of physical sensations, and a psychosocial dimension, which determines how those sensations are perceived and acted upon. We have found, as have others, that patients who had consulted about their abdominal symptoms suffered more frequent and severe bouts of abdominal pain and reported a greater disturbance in their bowel habits than those who had not consulted[62,82]. However, our extensive psychological evaluation using both self-rating inventories and structured psychiatric interviews revealed that the consulting group were more psychologically disturbed, with 64% qualifying for a formal psychiatric diagnosis compared with only 22% in the non-consulting group. We concluded from these findings that the psychiatric morbidity was exerting an influence in terms of how the individual sufferer perceived physiological events, with an emphasis on the possible sinister nature of their symptoms.

PSYCHOLOGICAL FACTORS IN ORGANIC GASTROINTESTINAL DISORDERS

Organic gastrointestinal disease is associated with pre-existing personality and emotional disturbance[83,84]. However, it is not clear to what extent psychological factors affect the onset or course of disease. Rating instruments can be used to examine and measure these interpersonal and intrapsychic processes which appear to be implicated in the development of disease[85–87].

Sixty years ago it was thought that ulcerative colitis and peptic ulcer were classical psychosomatic diseases[88]. Murray was one of the first to recognize the importance of psychogenic factors in the etiology of ulcerative colitis[89]. Research into this area of study has provided impressive evidence that psychological disturbance plays an integral part in both the etiology and the course of organic gastrointestinal disorders[90–92].

Aspects of personality

An extensive review of the literature was provided by Engel from Rochester, New York in 1955[93]. He reviewed the data on more than 700 patients with ulcerative colitis and found that a high proportion of ulcerative colitis patients had obsessive-compulsive character traits, which included neatness, orderliness, punctuality, and conscientiousness. Along with these character traits, guarding of affectivity, over-intellectualization, rigid attitudes toward morality and standards of behavior were often noted, and a prominence of the so-called 'anal characteristics' was identified. Other psychological abnormalities included dysfunctional relationships with significant others, with terms such as 'infantile dependence', 'abnormal attachment', and 'parent controlled' being used. Similar personality traits and euphemisms have also been used to describe patients with Crohn's and peptic ulcer disease[94,95]. For example, in the study by Robertson et al. (1989) it was found that patients with inflammatory bowel disease scored significantly higher on the neuroticism and introversion scales of the Eysenck Personality Inventory compared with patients with diabetes or healthy controls[96]. Other common characteristics reported included obsessive-compulsive behavior, dependency, anxiety, over-conscientiousness, aggression and perfectionism. These characteristics were found to be as prominent in their patients before diagnosis (new referrals) as in their established cases with inflammatory bowel disease. The authors concluded from this that the traits that they identified were not simply the result of long-standing illness, but were more likely to be a part of the premorbid personality. In a similar vein, Bauer and Bergmann and Magni et al. reported that in their patients with peptic ulcer, a typical personality profile was characterized by high anxiety, dependence and introversion[97,98]. Emotional lability of thought and rigidity was also found to be common.

The presence of alexithymia in gastrointestinal disorders was also of interest and was found to have some relevance in patients with inflammatory bowel disease. Sifneos introduced the term in the early seventies, and described alexithymia as an inability to express feelings in words[99]. Similarly, Marty and de M'Uzan have usefully coined the term 'pensee operatoire' to describe a state of mind characterized by pragmatic, operational thinking and the absence of fantasy life[100]. In the study by Nakagawa et al. in 1979, a high prevalence of alexithymia was found in patients with digestive diseases such as chronic pancreatitis, peptic ulcer and ulcerative colitis[101]. In this study, patients with IBS were found to be more neurotic, but characteristics of alexithymia were more prominent in patients with chronic pancreatitis and ulcerative colitis. In addition, alexithymia was found to be a feature in 50% of patients with peptic ulcer disease. The study by Weinryb et al. provided further support for these original findings by reporting a high prevalence of alexithymia in their patients with ulcerative colitis[102]. They also found that this feature as well as other personality traits such as abnormal aggression and dysmorphophobia had negative effects on adaptation after colectomy.

In summary, it is clear that no single characteristic type of personality was found in any of the patient groups with organic gastrointestinal disease, but some traits such as obsessiveness and alexithymia were found to be the most common.

Presence of psychiatric disorder

Psychopathology is also prevalent in organic gastrointestinal disease with disorders such as depression, anxiety states and panic disorder being frequent concomitants. However, it is not clear if psychiatric illness predates the onset of the disorder or whether it is intrinsic to the disease process and the suffering caused[103,104].

In 1959, Paulley reported on the histologic and psychological findings in patients with idiopathic steatorrhea[105]. In this study he gave a descriptive account of the mental peculiarities that he observed in these patients. His observations prompted other researchers to extend these findings using more stringent and methodologically sound interview-based techniques to arive at psychiatric diagnoses. Studies by Sheffield, Whybrow, and Gazzard reported prevalence rates of depression in patients with Crohn's disease of 32–38%[106–108]. High rates of obsessive features have also been found in Crohn's patients[92,109]. For example, in the collaborative study by Goldberg and Creamer, 80 patients with diseases of the small intestine were administered a standardized psychiatric assessment at each out-patient visit over a 1 year period. A total of 158 interviews were carried out and patients with idiopathic steatorrhea, Crohn's disease and alactasia were included in the study. Thirty-eight per cent were found to have a psychiatric illness with depression being the most commonly reported. They also found that the patients with a psychiatric disorder attended the out-patient department more frequently than those who were considered psychologically normal, and patients with a family history or a previous history of psychiatric illness were much more likely to become ill during the survey year. An additional finding was that a positive family history of psychiatric illness was significantly more common in idiopathic steatorrhea.

In a number of recent reports however, the association between psychiatric illness and inflammatory bowel disease appears to be confined to Crohn's disease. Helzer et al. found no association between ulcerative colitis and psychiatric disorder, whereas in Crohn's disease, the association was more robust. In the latter study high rates of both obsessive and depressive illnesses were found with an overall prevalence rate of 50%. They concluded from these findings that there is a need for early identification and treatment of psychiatric disturbance in patients with Crohn's disease[110,111].

Similarly, high rates of affective disturbance have been reported in patients with peptic ulcer disease[112,113]. In the study by Sjodin et al., 103 out-patients with chronic peptic ulcer were assessed and almost all patients reported experiencing some kind of mental symptoms. Anxiety, depression and neurasthenia were significantly more common in peptic ulcer patients when compared with healthy controls[114].

The influence of stress

It is generally accepted that stress can produce or aggravate physical symptoms although there is no consensus about its role. Human and animal studies have shown effects on vascularity, secretion and motility of the gastrointestinal tract with Beaumont being one of the first to report[115]. He observed changes in gastric activity and mucosal appearance in response to psychological and physical stimuli in a patient with a traumatic fistula. Others have shown distinct changes in gastric function as a response to different emotional states[70]. For example, fear or depression are associated with mucosal pallor and diminished activity and secretion in the stomach, whereas the opposite is found in such emotional states as intense pleasure or anger[71]. Physiological abnormalities have also been shown to occur in other areas of the gastrointestinal tract. Jacobson et al. reported that strong emotions induced esophageal spasms, and in a more recent study by Young et al. it was shown that when patients with esophageal spasm were exposed to 'white noise' or complex psychometric tests, high amplitude, high velocity esophageal contractions occurred as a response to these stimuli[116,117].

The role of acute or chronic life stress has also been studied extensively in organic gastrointestinal disease. Garrett et al. examined the effect of minor daily stressors on the primary indices of Crohn's disease and found that there was a relationship between daily stress and self-rated disease severity even after controlling for the effects of major life events[120]. Piper and Tennant reported broadly similar results in their patients with chronic peptic ulcer disease[121]. They found that there were no differences between peptic ulcer patients and matched controls on the occurrence of acute stress, whereas the occurrence of chronic difficulties (events persisting for or greater than 6 months) were shown to be twice as common in the group of ulcer patients.

In conclusion, the evidence suggests that psychopathology is intrinsic to disease of the bowel both 'functional' and 'organic'. How far psychological processes can be implicated in the etiology and maintenance of the disease is much less clear. One can only say with certainty that psyche and soma are intimately involved, and it is important that the physician approaches each individual case holistically.

IMPLICATIONS FOR MANAGEMENT OF FUNCTIONAL ABDOMINAL DISORDERS

Gastroenterologists, general practitioners and patients with functional abdominal disorders are under no illusions that no universally effective treatment exists for the condition. For example, a review of controlled clinical trials of therapeutic agents in the irritable bowel syndrome, reinforced this view and showed that most trials were flawed and even those purporting to show therapeutic benefits should be questioned. Management can be considered under three headings, namely (i) the consultation, (ii) end-organ therapy and (iii) central therapy (Box 7.7).

Box 7.7 Approaches to the management of functional abdominal disorders

- Consultation
  - 'Positive' diagnosis of functional disorder
  - Avoid overinvestigation in young (<40–45 years) patients
- End-organ therapy
  - Non-dyspepsia
    - Trial of antacids — H_2RA etc
    - Prokinetics — cisapride, domperidone
  - IBS
    - Explore dietary triggers?
    - Fiber for constipation
    - Anti-diarrheals for bowel frequency
    - Smooth muscle relaxants for pain
    - Modify visceral sensation:? $5\text{-}HT_3$ antagonists
      ? Kappa opioid agonists
- Central therapy
  - Physiological explanation of symptom production
  - Counseling
  - Psychotherapy, hypnotherapy, cognitive therapy
  - Antidepressants

Consultation

In many patients with functional abdominal disorders, it is possible to make a positive diagnosis on the basis of the clinical history and physical examination. IBS for example is not a diagnosis of exclusion in patients below the age of 45 years and providing there are no other causes for concern such as weight loss, dysphagia, rectal bleeding or iron deficiency anemia, then the general physical examination, rectal examination and sigmoidoscopy should suffice. If there are concerns about inflammatory bowel disease then it is helpful to check inflammatory markers (ESR, C-reactive protein, platelet count). Anti-endomysial antibodies now represent a sensitive and specific screening test for celiac disease. In patients over the age of 45 years, the colon should be examined either by double-contrast barium enema or colonoscopy, although the latter is preferred as it enables multiple biopsies to be taken to exclude the rarer forms of colitis such as lymphocytic or collagenous colitis, which produces persistent diarrhea without causing macroscopic abnormalities in the colon.

Similarly, in younger patients with non-ulcer dyspepsia, gastroscopy can often be avoided. However, the reassurance of a negative examination is sometimes required in patients who fail to respond to symptomatic treatment. In patients over the age of 45 years, upper gastrointestinal endoscopy is generally required to exclude organic disease. It may be particularly helpful to distinguish *true* reflux esophagitis from *reflux-like* non-ulcer dyspepsia. Patients with functional abdominal pain often present a formidable diagnostic challenge, since they are often reticent to accept that the pain does not have an organic basis. Abdominal ultrasound and sometimes abdominal CT scan may be necessary to provide this reassurance. However, it is essential to set limits as there is often a continuing desire for more and more investigations and further 'second opinions' from other clinicians.

The subsequent clinical outcome is often set at the first consultation. Time is required to explain the possible mechanisms of symptom production, to reassure about fears of serious organic disease and to explore potential social and psychological factors which may have led to the consultation with the general practitioner and hospital referral.

End-organ therapy

If there are no obvious psychosocial factors or mood disorder then it is reasonable to consider therapeutic agents that are targeted directly towards the site in the gastrointestinal tract which, on the basis of the symptom pattern, seems to be the most hopeful therapeutic target.

Non-ulcer dyspepsia

Most patients are initially treated either with antacids or an H_2-receptor antagonist and as stated previously, meta-analysis of published studies suggests that some patients respond[21]. However, this is by no means universal and many clinicians will then proceed to give a trial of a prokinetic drug such as cisapride or domperidone. Although this class of drugs can certainly make objective improvements in upper gut motility disorder, the correlation with improvement in symptoms is less impressive. However, since therapeutic options are limited it seems reasonable to give this approach a trial.

Irritable bowel syndrome

Perhaps the most attractive *end-organ therapy* for IBS sufferers and possibly those with other functional disorders, is that of dietary modification. Nanda et al. showed that 47% of patients with IBS will respond to a systematic exclusion diet and many could identify specific foods that triggered symptoms[122]. Follow-up over a year indicated that these patients remained well with dietary modifications. It is certainly reasonable to try and identify specific foods that aggravate symptoms and recommend avoidance, although highly complex exclusion diets have little to commend them in the treatment of IBS and other functional disorders and may be counterproductive. Some patients however, are particularly sensitive to caffeine and food stuffs that contain sorbitol and thus withdrawal of these can often be of great therapeutic benefit.

One of the most controversial issues in the management of IBS has been the role of dietary and other fibers. Ten years ago virtually every patient with IBS was recommended to take a high fiber diet, despite controlled clinical trial evidence which showed that its effect was not superior to placebo. Recent studies suggest that in at least 50% of patients, fiber actually makes IBS symptoms worse[123]. The main indication for fiber in IBS is when there is associated constipation. Soluble fiber seems to be more effective and has fewer adverse effects than dietary wheat fiber.

A variety of drugs are available to minimize IBS symptoms although a critical review of controlled trials in this area concluded that there is no effective medication for the treatment of IBS[124]. Cramping abdominal pain is sometimes helped by an anti-spasmodic and a recent meta-analysis confirms that at least some anti-spasmodics are effective in IBS[125]. Similarly, bowel frequency may be reduced in some patients by a standard anti-diarrheal preparation such as loperamide. Both anti-spasmodics and anti-diarrheals should be used only when symptoms are present and not on a regular basis. To obtain a clinical effect, the dose of anti-spasmodic may need to be relatively high, often to the point when adverse effects are evident.

A new group of drugs is emerging that appear to be able to modify visceral sensation. This would seem to be a productive approach in the treatment of abdominal pain in functional abdominal disorders since there is now increasing evidence that visceral hyperalgesia is an important component of the pathophysiology of these disorders[30]. 5-HT_3 receptor antagonists and Kappa opioid agonists have both been shown to be effective in altering visceral sensation in the gut in animal models. Preliminary clinical studies also suggest that they may have a pain modifying effect in functional abdominal syndromes, but further placebo controlled studies are required to confirm their efficacy.

Central therapy

Despite the paucity of effective agents for *end-organ therapy* in IBS, clinical trials of *central therapy* have been encouraging. Hypnotherapy and psychotherapy have both been shown to be of value in the management of IBS however, expertise and facilities are not available to all patients and thus, use of psychotropic drugs should be considered[126–128]. Affective disorder may not be clinically apparent and depression may be atypical. The classic somatic symptoms of depression may not be present other than sleep disturbance and fatigue. There is little to lose from a trial of an antidepressant and providing adequate explanation is given as to why the drug may be of value, the majority of patients will accept this approach. Added selling points include the correction of sleep disturbance, the increase in pain threshold and therefore possible relief of abdominal pain and the potential to correct any defecatory disorders. Our own recent studies suggest that different classes of antidepressants have contrasting effects on bowel function[129,130]. The tricyclic antidepressant imipramine, for example slows intestinal transit and therefore may be the drug of choice for diarrhea-predominant IBS patients[129], whereas paroxetine, the serotonin-reuptake inhibitor, tends to decrease intestinal transit rates and therefore may be more appropriate in constipated patients[130].

Psychological treatment

A number of uncontrolled and semi-controlled studies using psychological treatment approaches have been carried out with both functional and organic gastrointestinal disease patients[131–134]. Much of the earlier work was based on patients who were seen after several previous medical referrals, ineffective attempts at treatment, and a variety of potentially conflicting explanations of the problem. There is now a greater emphasis on liaison work, with those involved in psychological treatment working in primary and secondary medical settings. The four main types of psychological treatments that have been used include psychotherapy, hypnotherapy, behavior therapy and cognitive-behavioral therapy.

Psychotherapy

It is commonly believed that psychological treatment necessarily involves lying on a couch and talking about one's childhood, but contemporary approaches tend to emphasize dealing with problems in the here and now. This will often involve learning alternative strategies for handling stressful situations[135]. In a recent randomized controlled trial of 102 patients with

IBS, Guthrie and co-workers in Manchester showed that relaxation and brief dynamic psychotherapy was effective in up to two-thirds of their patients who did not respond to standard medical treatment alone. In this study, patients were encouraged to examine how psychological symptoms related to bowel symptoms and any other emotional problems were explored[127].

Hypnotherapy

A rather different approach involves the application of hypnosis. Again, the idea is not to delve around in the recesses of the unconscious mind, nor is it to be confused with the antics of stage hypnosis. This technique deals directly with the problem in hand, and involves what is termed gut-centered hypnosis, which enables the patient to exert some control over what their gastrointestinal tract is doing. In the first of the series of studies by Whorwell et al. (1984) the therapeutic effects of hypnotherapy were assessed and compared with the use of supportive psychotherapy in 30 patients with refractory IBS. In the group receiving hypnotherapy, seven 30-minute sessions of gut-centered hypnosis were administered to each patient. In addition, the patients were given an auto-hypnosis tape to be used at home on a daily basis. At the end of the 3 month study period, the hypnotherapy group reported a significant reduction in their IBS symptoms. In addition, an overall improvement in their general well-being was also reported. These findings differed significantly from both the psychotherapy and control group. There were however, small but significant improvements reported by the psychotherapy group and these improvements were confined to abdominal pain, abdominal distension and general well-being. At follow-up, the hypnotherapy group reported no incidences of relapses or no other new symptoms[136].

This same research group confirmed the successful effect of hypnotherapy in patients with severe intractable IBS in a much larger study in 1987. In addition, by categorizing the total group into IBS sub-groups, e.g. classic cases, atypical cases and cases exhibiting significant psychopathology, the authors found that the response rate was greatest for those with classical IBS (95%) compared with atypical cases (43%) or those with an associated psychiatric disorder (60%). They also found that patients over 50 years of age had a poorer response rate (25%) to hypnotherapy[126]. Harvey et al. (1989) also evaluated the use of hypnotherapy and found that not only was hypnotherapy an effective treatment for intractable irritable bowel sufferers, but also showed that hypnotherapy in groups of up to eight patients was as effective as individual therapy, and that only four 40-minute sessions were required. This report has important implications for treatment of IBS with hypnotherapy as it helps to answer some of the main objections to its more widespread use, namely, its lengthy time course, individual expense and necessity for specifically trained practitioners[137].

Others have demonstrated changes in rectal sensitivity after a session of hypnosis. In one study, the effect of hypnotherapy on anorectal physiology was assessed in 15 patients with IBS, and these results were compared with that of a control group. They found that significant changes in rectal sensitivity occurred in patients with diarrhea-predominant IBS both during and after a course of hypnotherapy. Patients with constipation also demonstrated a trend towards normalization of rectal sensitivity although no changes in rectal compliance or distension-induced motor activity occurred in either of the IBS sub-groups. Furthermore, it has been shown that the rate at which intestinal contents move through the gut can be influenced by these techniques, and reports on symptom reduction are encouraging[138].

Whorwell's group has extended its work on the use of hypnosis in gastrointestinal disorders and has included patients with peptic ulceration. They found that these patients also respond favorably to gut-centered hypnosis[139].

Behavior therapy

The application of behavior therapy involves teaching the patients various exercises and strategies to aid symptom control. Progressive muscle relaxation therapy and thermal biofeedback make up part of this category and have been used previously to treat patients with IBS or inflammatory bowel disease. The results of these studies showed that in both patient groups a clinically significant reduction in their gastrointestinal symptoms was achieved[140,141].

Multidimensional approach

One the most effective psychological treatments now being offered to patients is a combination of relaxation techniques and cognitive-behavioral strategies[142]. This treatment package is aimed at changing the way in which patients evaluate the meaning of their abdominal symptoms, but also changing maladaptive behaviors that the patient has developed as a response to coping with their illness such as changes in toilet use, avoidance behavior and excessive use of medication such as laxatives to help control bowel functioning.

In summary, while burgeoning research into the pathophysiology of gastrointestinal disorders may one day offer a cure, there are psychological approaches currently available which do have much to offer in the terms of the management of these distressing conditions.

Alternative therapy

The use of alternative medicine in the treatment of gastrointestinal disorders, particularly the irritable bowel syndrome, has become increasingly popular and it is estimated that over two million people in the UK alone consult practitioners of alternative medicine each year. Under this umbrella term, there are a wide variety of alternative therapies offered with yoga, meditation and herbal remedies being the most commonly used. In the study by Smart et al. (1986) an assessment was made of the use of alternative medicine in 461 patients with either irritable bowel syndrome or organic gastrointestinal disease. They found that significantly more IBS patients had consulted practitioners of alternative medicine and that the current usage of alternative remedies was significantly greater in the IBS group (11%) compared with patients with Crohn's disease or other organic GI disease (4%). In addition, IBS patients expressed a greater willingness to consult an alternative practitioner if conventional treatment failed[143].

More recently, the use of Aloe Vera for treating gastrointestinal disorders has received much publicity, although no double-blind clinical trials have been conducted to test the validity of its effectiveness on symptom reduction. Most of the supporting evidence for its effectiveness has been based on testimonials from individual sufferers with particular relevance to functional abdominal pain, spastic colon and those suffering from an altered bowel habit.

However, the use of alternative therapies in gastroenterological practice is hampered by the lack of any firm guidelines on their role and a paucity of well conducted clinical research. Furthermore, the scientific basis for many alternative approaches remains unclear and their effectiveness unproven[144].

CONCLUSION

Functional gastrointestinal disorders are not only extremely common but constitute a major burden on health care resources. For example, irritable bowel syndrome, the most prevalent of the functional bowel disorders, forms up to 50% of new referrals to gastroenterologists, and is present in 20% of adults in the industrialized world. Therefore it is incumbent on all clinicians to have a strategy for managing functional gastrointestinal disorders. Current evidence seems to suggest that perception plays a central role in the pathogenesis of these disorders rather than changes in visceromotor tone or the induction of gastrointestinal hypersensitivity. Consequently, appropriate treatment should involve psychological intervention with a focus on teaching individuals more effective coping strategies. Whether the psychological intervention should involve psychotherapy, hypnotherapy or behavioral therapy should probably be patient-driven, as all have been shown to be effective in a proportion of patients. The effectiveness of other alternative therapies remains unproven and further research is awaited before these can be widely recommended. Current opinion favors a multidimensional approach using a combination of relaxation and cognitive behavioral strategies. In short a mind–body approach is essential if the millions of individuals suffering worldwide with functional gastrointestinal symptoms are to be helped.

REFERENCES

1 Thompson WG, Creed F, Drossman DA, Heaton KW, Mazzacca G 1992 Functional bowel disease and functional abdominal pain. Gastroenterology International 5:75–91

2 Thompson WG 1993 Irritable bowel syndrome: pathogenesis and management. Lancet 341:1569–72

3 Manning AP, Thompson WG, Heaton KW, Morris AF 1978 Towards positive diagnosis of the irritable bowel. British Medical Journal 2:653–4

4 Thompson WG 1984 Gastrointestinal symptoms in the irritable bowel compared with peptic ulcer and inflammatory bowel disease. Gut 25:1089–92

5 Kruis W, Thieme CH, Weinzier M et al. 1984 A diagnostic score for the irritable bowel syndrome, its value in exclusion of organic disease. Gastroenterology 25:1089–92

6 Jones R, Lydeard S 1992 Irritable bowel syndrome in the general population. British Medical Journal 304:87–90

7 Heaton KW, O'Donnell LJD, Braddon FE, Hughes AO, Cripps PJ 1992 Symptoms of irritable bowel syndrome in a British urban community: consulters and non-consulters. Gastroenterology 102:1962–7

8 Sandler RS 1990 Epidemiology of irritable bowel syndrome in the United States. Gastroenterology 99:409–15

9 Johnsen R, Jacobsen BK, Forde OH 1986 Associations between symptoms of irritable colon and psychological and social conditions and lifestyle. British Medical Journal 292:1633–5

10 O'Donnell LJD, Heaton KW, Mountford RA, Braddon FE 1990 Prevalence of the irritable bowel syndrome in a random sample of the British population. Gut 31:A1173

11 Thompson WG, Heaton KW 1980 Functional bowel disorders in apparently healthy people. Gastroenterology 79:283–8

12 Drossman DA, Sandler RS, McKee DC, Lovitz AJ 1983 Bowel patterns among subjects not seeking health care. Gastroenterology 83:529–34

13 Harvey RF, Salih SY, Read AE 1983 Organic and functional disorders in 2000 gastroenterology outpatients. Lancet 1:632–4

14 Talley NJ, Colin-Jones D, Koch LK, Koch M, Nyren O, Stanghellini V 1991 Functional dyspepsia: a classification with guidelines for diagnosis and management. Gastroenterology International 4:145–60

15 Whorwell PJ, McCallum M, Creed FH, Roberts CT 1986 Non-colonic features of irritable bowel syndrome. Gut 27:37–40

16 Talley NJ, Phillips SF, Bruce B, Zinsmeister AR, Wiltgen C, Melton LJ 1991 Multisystem complaints in patients with the irritable bowel syndrome and functional dyspepsia. European Journal of Gastroenterology and Hepatology 3:71–7

17 White AM, Stevens WH, Upton AR, O'Byrne PM, Collins SM 1991 Airway responsiveness to inhaled methacholine in patients with irritable bowel syndrome. Gastroenterology 100:68–74

18 Drossman DA 1982 Patients with psychogenic abdominal pain: six years' observation in the medical setting. American Journal of Psychiatry 139:1549–57

19 Klein KB 1990 Chronic intractable pain. Seminars in Gastrointestinal Disease 1:43–56

20 American Psychiatric Association Somatoform Disorders 1987 In: Diagnostic and Statistical Manual of Mental Disorders — revised. American Psychiatric Association 255–67

21 Dobrilla G, Comberlata M, Steele A, Vallaperta P 1989 Drug treatment of functional dyspepsia. A meta-analysis of randomized controlled trials. Journal of Clinical Gastroenterology 11:169–77

22 Corinaldesi R, Stanghellini V, Raiti C, Rea E, Salgemini R, Barbara L 1987 Effect of chronic administration of cisapride on gastric emptying of a solid meal and on dyspeptic symptoms in patients with idiopathic gastroparesis. Gut 28:300–5

23 Jian R, Ducrot F, Ruskone A et al. 1989 Symptomatic radionuclide and therapeutic assessment of chronic idiopathic dyspepsia: a double-blind placebo-controlled evaluation of cisapride. Digestive Diseases and Sciences 34:657–64

24 Greydanus MP, Vassallo M, Camilleri M, Nelson DK, Hanson RB, Thomforde GM 1991 Neurohormonal factors in functional dyspepsia: insights on pathophysiological mechanisms. Gastroenterology 100:1311–8

25 Mangnall YF, Houghton LA, Johnson AG, Read NW 1994 Abnormal distribution of a fatty liquid test meal within the stomach of patients with non-ulcer dyspepsia. European Journal of Gastroenterology and Hepatology 6:323–7

26 Troncon LEA, Bennett RJM, Ahuluwalia NK, Thompson DG 1994 Abnormal intragastric distribution of food during gastric emptying in functional dyspepsia patients. Gut 35:327–32

27 Waldron B, Cullen PT, Kumar R et al. 1991 Evidence for hypomotility in non-ulcer dyspepsia: A prospective multi-factorial study. Gut 246–51

28 Bradette M, Pare P, Douville P, Morin A 1991 Visceral perception in health and functional dyspepsia. Crossover study of gastric distensions with placebo and domperidone. Digestive Diseases and Sciences 36:52–8

29 Mearin F, Cucala M, Azpiroz F, Malagelada J-R 1991 The origin of symptoms on the brain-gut axis in functional dyspepsia. Gastroenterology 101:999–1006

30 Mayer EA, Gebhart GF 1994 Basic and clinical aspects of visceral hyperalgesia. Gastroenterology 107:271–93
31 Talley NJ 1994 A critique of therapeutic trials in *Helicobacter pylori*-positive functional dyspepsia. Gastroenterology 106:1174–84
32 Patchett S, Beattie S, Leen E, Keane C, O'Morain C 1991 Eradicating *Helicobacter pylori* and symptoms of non-ulcer dyspepsia. British Medical Journal 303:1238–40
33 McCarthy C, Patchett S, Collins RM, Beattie S, Keane C, O'Morain C 1995 Long-term prospective study of *Helicobacter pylori* in non-ulcer dyspepsia. Digestive Diseases and Sciences 40:114–19
34 Gorard DA, Farthing MJG 1994 Intestinal motor function in irritable bowel syndrome. Digestive Diseases and Sciences 12:72–84
35 Trotman IF, Misiewicz JJ 1988 Sigmoid motility in diverticular disease and the irritable bowel syndrome. Gut 29:218–22
36 Kellow JE, Gill RC, Wingate DL 1990 Prolonged ambulant recordings of small bowel motility demonstrate abnormalities in the irritable bowel syndrome. Gastroenterology 98:1208–18
37 Gorard DA, Libby GW, Farthing MJG 1994 Ambulatory small intestinal motility in 'diarrhea'-predominant irritable bowel syndrome. Gut 35:203–10
38 Prior A, Maxton DG, Whorwell PJ 1990 Anorectal manometry in irritable bowel syndrome: differences between diarrhea and constipation predominant patients. Gut 31:458–62
39 Whitehead WE, Holtkotter B, Enck P et al. 1990 Tolerance for rectosigmoid distension in irritable bowel syndrome. Gastroenterology 98:1187–92
40 Cook IJ, Van Eeden A, Collins SM 1987 Patients with irritable bowel syndrome have greater pain tolerance than normal subjects. Gastroenterology 93:727–33
41 Mayer EA, Raybould HE 1990 The role of visceral afferent mechanisms in functional bowel disorders. Gastroenterology 99:1688–1704
42 Whitehead WE, Crowell MD, Robinson JC, Heller BR, Schuster MM 1992 Effects of stressful life events on bowel symptoms: subjects with irritable bowel syndrome compared with subjects without bowel dysfunction. Gut 33:825–30
43 Siredy. Quoted by DeLangenhangen M. Muco-membranous colitis, JA Churchill, London, 1903
44 Da Costa JM 1871 Mucous enteritis. American Journal of Medical Sciences 62:321–35
45 White H 1905 A study of 60 cases of membranous colitis. Lancet ii:1129–35
46 Jordan SM, Keifer ED 1932 The irritable colon. Journal of the American Medical Association 95:592–5
47 Cohnheim 1909 Diseases of the digestive canal. JB Lippincott Co, Philadelphia and London
48 Bockus HL, Bank J, Wilkinson SA 1928 Neurogenic mucous colitis. American Medical Journal of Sciences 176:813–29
49 White BV, Jones CM 1940 Mucous colitis: a delineation of the syndrome with certain observations on its mechanism and on the role of emotional precipitating factors. American Journal of Internal Medicine 14:854–72
50 Feighner JP, Robins E, Guze SB 1972 Diagnostic criteria for use in psychiatric research. Archives of General Psychiatry 26:57–63
51 World Health Organisation 1978 Mental disorders: glossary and guide to their classification in accordance with the ninth revision of the International Classification of Diseases. Geneva
52 Spitzer RL, Williams JBW, Gibbon M et al. 1990 Structured Clinical Interview for DSM-III-R, Washington DC: American Psychiatric Association Press
53 American Psychiatric Association 1994 Diagnostic and Statistical Manual of Mental Disorders Fourth edition revised (DSM-IV). American Psychiatric Association, Washington DC 1994
54 McDonald AJ, Bouchier PAD 1980 Non-organic gastrointestinal illness: a medical and psychiatric study. British Journal of Psychiatry 136:276–83
55 Liss JL, Alpers D, Woodruff RA 1973 The irritable colon syndrome and psychiatric illness. Diseases of the Nervous System 70:151–7
56 Young SJ, Alpers DH, Norland CC, Woodruff RA 1976 Psychiatric illness and irritable bowel syndrome: practical implications for the primary physician. Gastroenterology 70:162–6
57 Haug TT, Svebak S, Wilhelmsen I, Berstad A, Ursin H 1994 Psychological factors and somatic symptoms in functional dyspepsia. A comparison with duodenal ulcer and healthy controls. Journal of Psychosomatic Research 38:281–91
58 Walker EA, Roy-Bryne PP, Katon WJ 1990 Irritable bowel syndrome and psychiatric illness. American Journal of Psychiatry 147:565–72
59 Lydiard RB, Fossey MD, Marsh W, Ballenger JC 1993 Prevalence of psychiatric disorders in patients with irritable bowel syndrome. Psychosomatics 34:229–34
60 Creed F, Guthrie E 1987 Psychological factors in the irritable bowel syndrome. Gut 28:1307–18
61 Hislop I 1971 Psychological significance of the irritable colon syndrome. Gut 12:452–7
62 Gomborone JE, Dewsnap PA, Libby GW, Farthing MJG 1993 Influence of psychiatric morbidity on self-appraisal of symptoms in irritable bowel syndrome. Gut 34 56:(Abstract)
63 Chaudhary N, Truelove S 1962 The irritable colon syndrome. A study of the clinical features predisposing causes and prognosis in 130 cases. Quarterly Journal of Medicine 31:307–23
64 Hill OW, Blendis L 1967 Physical and psychological evaluation of 'non-organic' abdominal pain. Gut 8:221–9
65 Sjodin I, Svedlund J 1985 Psychological aspects of non-ulcer dyspepsia: a psychosomatic view focusing on a comparison between the irritable bowel syndrome and peptic ulcer disease. Scandinavian Journal of Gastroenterology 20:51–8
66 Bass C 1986 Life events and gastrointestinal symptoms. Gut 27:123–6
67 Cannon W 1902 The movements of the intestines studied by means of Roentgenrays. American Journal of Physiology 6:251–77
68 Wolf S, Wolff H 1943 Human gastric function. Oxford University Press, New York
69 Abbott F, Mack M, Wolf S 1952. The relation of sustained contraction of the duodenum to nausea and

vomiting. Gastroenterology 20:238–48
70 Almy TP, Tulin M 1947 Alterations in colonic function in man under stress: experimental production of changes simulating the 'irritable colon.' Gastroenterology 8:616
71 Whorwell PJ, Houghton LA, Taylor EE, Maxton DG 1992 Physiological effects of emotion: assessment via hypnosis. Lancet 340:69–72
72 Waller S, Misiewicz J 1969 Prognosis of irritable bowel syndrome. Lancet ii:753–6
73 Brown G, Harris T 1978 Social origins of depression: the development of the Bedford College Life Events and Difficulties Schedule (LEDS). Tavistock, London
74 Craig T, Brown G 1984 Goal frustration and life events in the aetiology of painful gastrointestinal disorder. Journal of Psychosomatic Research 28:411–21
75 Creed F 1981 Life events and appendicectomy. Lancet i:1381–5
76 Creed F, Craig T, Farmer T 1988. Functional abdominal pain, psychiatric illness and life events. Gut 29:235–42
77 Dulmen AM, Fennis JF, Mokkink HG, Van Der Velden HG et al. 1995 Doctor-dependent changes in complaint-related cognitions and anxiety during medical consultations in functional abdominal complaints. Psychological Medicine 25:1011–1018
78 Gomborone JE, Dewsnap PA, Libby GW, Farthing MJG 1995 Abnormal illness attitudes in irritable bowel syndrome. Journal of Psychosomatic Research 39:227–30
79 Jones R, Lydeard S 1992 Irritable bowel syndrome in the general population. British Medical Journal 304:87–90
80 Heaton KW, O'Donnell LJD, Braddon FEM, Mountford RA, Hughs AO, Cripps PJ 1992 Irritable bowel syndrome in a British urban community: consulters and non-consulters. Gastroenterology 102:1962–7
81 Mechanic D 1962 The concept of illness behavior. Journal of Chronic Diseases 15:189–94
82 Heaton KW, Ghosh S, Braddon FEM 1991 How bad are the symptoms and bowel dysfunction of patients with the irritable bowel syndrome? A prospective controlled study with emphasis on stool form. Gut 32:73–9
83 Crockett RW 1952 Psychiatric findings in Crohn's disease. Lancet i:946–9
84 McMahon AW, Schmitt P, Patterson SF et al. 1973 Personality differences between inflammatory bowel disease patients and their healthy siblings. Psychosomatic Medicine 35:91–103
85 Spitzer RL, Endicott J 1975 Schedule for affective disorders and schizophrenia (SADS). 2nd e. New York
86 Eysenck HJ, Eysenck SB 1975 Manual for the Eysenck Personality Questionnaire. Education and Industrial Testing Service, San Diego
87 Zigmond AS, Snaith RP 1983 The Hospital Anxiety and Depression Scale. Acta Psychiatrica Scandinavica 67:361–70
88 Alexander F 1950 Psychosomatic medicine: its principles and application. WW Norton, New York
89 Murray CD 1930 Psychogenic factors in the aetiology of ulcerative colitis and bloody diarrhea. American Journal of Medicine and Sciences. 180:239–48
90 Feldman F, Cantor D, Soll S, Bachrach W 1990 Psychiatric study of a consecutive series of nineteen patients with regional ileitis disease. British Medical Journal 4:711–14
91 Jess P, von der Lieth L, Matzen P, Modsen P et al. 1989 The personality pattern of duodenal ulcer patients in relation to spontaneous ulcer healing and relapse. Journal of Internal Medicine 226:395
92 Goldberg D 1970 A psychiatric study of patients with diseases of the small intestine. Gut 11:459–65
93 Engel GL 1955 Studies of ulcerative colitis. III. The nature of the psychologic process. American Journal of Medicine 19:231
94 Drossman DA 1991 Psychosocial factors in the care of patients with gastrointestinal diseases. In: Yamada T (ed) Textbook of gastroenterology. JB Lippincott Philadelphia, pp 546–61
95 North CS, Alpers DH, Helzer JE et al. 1991 Do life events of depression exacerbate inflammatory bowel disease? Annals of Internal Medicine 114:381
96 Robertson DA, Ray J, Diamond I, Edwards JG 1989 Personality profile and affective states of patients with inflammatory bowel disease. Gut 30:623–6
97 Bauer B, Bergmann M 1981 Psychological factors in duodenal ulcers. Deutsche Zeitschrift fur Verdauungs und Stoffwechselkrankheiten. 41:288–94
98 Magni G, Rizzardo R, Di Mario F, Farini R, Aggio L, Naccarato R 1894 Personality and psychological factors in chronic duodenal ulcer. Their interactions with biological parameters. Schweizer Archiv fur Neurologie, 135:315–20
99 Sifneos PE 1988 Alexithymia and its relationship to hemispheric specialisation, affect and creativity. Psychiatric Clinics of North America 11:287–92
100 Marty P, Fain M, M'Ilzan Mde, David C 1968 The Dora Case and the psychosomatic viewpoint. Revue Francaise de Psychanalyse 32:679–714
101 Nakagawa T, Sugita M, Nakai Y, Ikemi Y 1979 Alexithymic feature in digestive diseases. Psychotherapy and Psychosomatics 32:191–203
102 Weinryb R, Rossel R 1986 Personality traits that can affect adaptation after colectomy. A study of 10 patients treated for ulcerative colitis either with proctocolectomy and ileostomy. Psychotherapy and Psychosomatics 45:57–65
103 Lyketsos CG, Lyketsos GC, Richardson SC, Beis, A 1987 Dysthymic states and depressive syndromes in physical conditions of presumably psychogenic origin. Acta Psychiatrica Scandinavica 76:529–34
104 Jonsson BH, Theorell 1991. Life events, abdominal pain and depression in peptic ulcer and depressive disorder. International Journal of Psychosomatics 38:27–32
105 Paulley JW 1959 Histologic and psychologic findings in idiopathic steatorrhoea. Proceedings of the World Congress in Gastroenterology 469–76
106 Sheffield BF, Carney MW 1976 Crohn's disease: a psychosomatic illness? British Journal of Psychiatry 128:446–50
107 Whybrow PC, Kane TJ, Lipton MA 1968 Regional ileitis and psychiatric disorder. Psychosomatic Medicine 30:209
108 Gazzard BG, Price HL, Libby GW, Dawson AM 1978

The social toll of Crohn's disease. British Medical Journal 2:1117–19

109 Ford CV, Golber GA, Castelnuovo-Tesesco P 1969 A psychiatric study of patients with regional enteritis. Journal of the American Medical Association 208:311–15

110 Helzer JE, Stillings WA, Chammas S, Norland CC, Alpers DH 1982 A controlled study of the association between ulcerative colitis and psychiatric diagnosis. Digestive Diseases and Sciences 27:513–18

111 Helzer JE, Chammas S, Norland CC, Stillings WA, Alpers DH 1984 A study of the association between Crohn's disease and psychiatric illness. Gastroenterology 86:324–30

112 Xiao S 1991 Psychologic correlates in peptic ulcer. Chinese Journal of Neurology and Psychiatry 24:282–5

113 Walker P, Luther J, Samloff IM, Feldman M 1988 Life events stress and psychosocial factors in men with peptic ulcer disease. II. Relationships with serum pepsinogen concentrations and behavioral risk factors. Gastroenterology 94:323–330

114 Sjodin I, Svedlund J, Dotevall G, Gillberg R 1985 Symptom profiles in chronic peptic ulcer disease. A detailed study of abdominal and mental symptoms. Scandinavian Journal of Gastroenterology 20:419–27

115 Beaumont W Experiments and Observations on the gastric juice and the physiology of digestion. FP Allen Plattsburg, New York

116 Jacobson E 1927. Spastic esophagus and mucous colitis. Archives of Internal Medicine 37:443

117 Young LD, Richter JE, Anderson KO, Bradley LA, Katz PO et al. 1987 The effects of psychological and enviromental stressors on peristaltic esophageal contractions in healthy volunteers. Psychophysiology 24:132

118 Lask B 1986 Psychological aspects of inflammatory bowel disease. Wiener Klinische Wochenschrift 98:544–7

119 Magni G, Di Mario F, Aggio L, Borgherini G 1986 Psychosomatic factors and peptic ulcer disease. Hepato-Gastroenterology 33:131–7

120 Garrett VD, Brantley PJ, Jones GN, McKnight GT 1991 The relation between stress and Crohn's disease. Journal of Behavioral Medicine 14:87–96

121 Piper DW, Tennant C 1993 Stress and personality in patients with chronic peptic ulcer. Journal of Clinical Gastroenterology 16:211–14

122 Nanda R, James R, Smith H, Dudley CRK, Jewell DP 1989 Food intolerance and the irritable bowel syndrome. Gut 30:1099–1104

123 Francis CY, Whorwell PJ 1994 Bran and irritable bowel syndrome: time for reappraisal. Lancet 344:39–40

124 Klein KB 1988 Controlled treatment trials in the irritable bowel syndrome: A critique. Gastroenterology 95:232–41

125 Poynard T, Naveau S, Mory B, Chaput JC 1994 Meta-analysis of smooth muscle relaxants in the treatment of irritable bowel syndrome. Alimentary Pharmacology and Therapeutics 449–510

126 Whorwell PJ, Prior A, Colgan SM 1987 Hypnotherapy in severe irritable bowel syndrome. Gut 28:423–5

127 Guthrie E, Creed F, Dawson D, Tomenson B 1991 A controlled trial of psychological treatment for the irritable bowel syndrome. Gastroenterology 100:450–7

128 Guthrie E, Creed F 1994 The difficult patient: treating the mind and the gut. European Journal of Gastroenterology and Hepatology 6:489–94

129 Gorard DA, Libby GW, Farthing MJG 1995 Effect of a tricyclic antidepressant on small intestinal motility in health and in diarrhea-predominant irritable bowel syndrome. Digestive Diseases and Sciences 40:86–95

130 Gorard DA, Libby GW, Farthing MJG 1994 5-Hydroxytryptamine and human small intestinal motility: effect of inhibiting 5-hydroxytryptamine uptake. Gut 34:496–500

131 Svedlund J, Sjodin I, Olloson JO et al. 1983 Controlled study of psychotherapy in irritable bowel syndrome. Lancet ii:589–91

132 Blanchard EB, Schwarz SP, Neff DF, Gerardi MA 1988 Prediction of outcome from the self-regulatory treatment of irritable bowel syndrome. Behavior Research and Therapy 26:187–90

133 Latimer PR 1978 Crohn's disease: a review of the psychological and social outcome. Psychological Medicine 8:649–56

134 Schwarz SP, Blanchard EB 1990 Inflammatory bowel disease: A review of the psychological assessment and treatment literature. Annals of Behavioral Medicine 12:95–105

135 Beck AT 1976 Cognitive therapy and emotional disorders. International Universities Press, New York

136 Whorwell PJ, Prior A, Faragher EB 1984 Controlled trial of hypnotherapy in the treatment of severe refractory irritable bowel syndrome. Lancet ii:1232–4

137 Harvey RF, Hinton RA, Gunary RM, Barry RE 1989 Individual and group hypnotherapy in treatment of refractory irritable bowel syndrome. Lancet I (8635):424–5

138 Prior A, Colgan SM, Whorwell PJ 1990 Changes in rectal sensitivity after hypnotherapy in patients with irritable bowel syndrome. Gut 31(8):896–8

139 Whorwell PJ 1991 Use of hypnotherapy in gastrointestinal disease. British Journal of Hospital Medicine 45(1):27–9

140 Milne B, Joachim G, Niedhardt J 1986 A stress management programme for inflammatory bowel disease patients. Journal of Advanced Nursing 11:561–7

141 Corney RH, Stanton R, Newell R, Clare A, Fairclough P 1991 Behavioral psychotherapy in the treatment of irritable bowel syndrome. Journal of Psychosomatic Research 35:461–9

142 Skinner JB, Erskine A, Pearce S, Rubenstein M, Taylor M, Foster C 1990 The evaluation of a cognitive behavioral treatment programme in outpatients with chronic pain. Journal of Psychosomatic Research 34:13–19

143 Smart HL, Mayberry JF, Atkinson M 1986 Alternative medicine consultations and remedies in patients with the irritable bowel syndrome. Gut 27(7):826–8

144 Zikmund V 1995 Problems with the limitations of medicine. Bratsisl Lek Listy 96(2):63–8

CHAPTER CONTENTS

8

Allergy

Alan Watkins

INTRODUCTION

Recent evidence suggests that the incidence and severity of allergic disease are increasing[1]. The prevalence of asthma has been estimated to be up to 10% in some populations,[2] which translates into 2–3 million people suffering asthmatic symptoms each year in the UK. Furthermore, despite the availability of highly efficacious drugs many asthmatics continue to suffer. For example, a survey of 7000 asthmatics reported that 40% are woken every night by their asthma, and 70% reported being woken at least once a week[3]. Similarly, 25% of all asthmatics reported feeling breathless on most days of the week and at least a quarter require at least one emergency hospital admission each year[4,5]. Sadly 2000 people still die each year from asthma, and this figure remains unchanged despite improved treatments and a greater understanding of the pathophysiology of the disease[6].

It has been estimated that asthma management alone currently imposes a financial burden on the NHS of about £400 million per annum, in addition to costing the Department of Social Security £60 million in sickness benefit and the nation £350 million in terms of lost productivity[7]. A large proportion of the NHS bill is due to pharmaceutical costs; with the total number of prescriptions for asthmatic drugs doubling during the 1980s, and prescriptions for inhaled corticosteroids increasing fourfold.

THE MIND AND ALLERGIES

Ever since Willis suggested, in 1679, that neural mechanisms may be important in the pathophysiology of allergic disease, the role of thoughts and feelings in the development of allergies has attracted scientific interest[8]. However, over the last 50 years the focus of scientific research has narrowed, and predominantly confined itself to investigating the changes seen in the airways at a cellular and subcellular level. The emotional, social and psychological aspects of allergic disease have received little serious scientific consideration. This molecular focus has resulted in significant advances in understanding of the pathophysiology of allergic disease. Thus, it is now widely believed that allergic reactions are inflammatory diseases, involving almost all the cells of the immune system.

However, recent scientific evidence has also shown that virtually all the immune cells involved in allergic inflammation are controlled in a complex and sophisticated manner by the central nervous system (CNS) through two neural mechanisms, namely the autonomic nervous system and neuroendocrine axis. Until very recently, the implications of this neuroimmunomodulation (NIM) for asthma and rhinitis have been largely overlooked[9]. This chapter will try to reintroduce the idea that the brain plays a pivotal role in regulating the inflammatory response that underlies much of the pathophysiology seen in allergic inflammation. In addition, it will review the evidence base for mind–body approaches in the treatment of allergic inflammation of the airways not only because there is a public desire for such approaches (see Ch. 2) but because such approaches may be effective, less expensive and may help reduce the financial burden to the nation.

AUTONOMIC DYSFUNCTION IN ALLERGY

It is widely recognized that the mucosal tissue in the airways is very richly innervated by the autonomic nervous system (ANS)[10]. However, assessment of the impact of autonomic innervation on allergic inflammation must not be restricted to the study of this sympathetic, parasympathetic, and non-adrenergic non-cholinergic (NANC) innervation of the airways, it must also include the innervation of the bone marrow and thymus, where immune cells develop[11,12], in addition to the autonomic innervation of regional lymph nodes, where respiratory antigens are presented[13].

Despite the complex innervation of all the tissues involved in mucosal immunity and the significant amount of data suggesting that the ANS regulates almost all the cells involved in allergic inflammation, all-embracing theories of autonomic imbalance have failed to explain the pathophysiology seen in the majority of asthmatics[14]. Theories of excessive cholinergic drive, β-adrenoreceptor hypofunction or α-adrenoreceptor hyperfunction have consistently foundered on contradictory data[15]. This failure is hardly surprising since β-receptor function and metabolism vary widely within each individual over time and vary according to asthma severity, with signal transduction failing during severe inflammation, and the presence of β-adrenergic receptors on diverse cellular populations in the airways[16]. Similarly, animal studies have failed to find consistent cholinergic changes[17,18].

Autonomic complexity

It is clear that a greater understanding of the complex nature of the interaction between the autonomic neural networks and the cells involved in airway inflammation, in the primary, secondary and tertiary lymphoid compartments will be required before the importance of autonomic innervation in allergic inflammation can be determined. Since it is now clear that a single population of nerves can release several neuropeptides, and therefore have either a bronchodilating or bronchoconstricting action, depending on the dynamic interplay of pro- and anti-inflammatory forces in the local milieu, studies doubting the importance of a particular neuropeptide, based on the inability to demonstrate significant immunohistochemical staining in asthmatic biopsies[19], may be overly simplistic.

The dynamic nature of the autonomic regulation of airway function is evidenced not only by the complexity of lymphoid tissue innervation, but also by the effects of the ANS on leucocyte migration and recruitment. Thus the sympathetic nervous system (SNS) may alter cellular recruitment to the airways either by modulating lymphocyte–endothelial interaction or by having a more direct effect on vascular tone[20]. The SNS effect on lymphocyte–endothelial interaction is probably indirect, altering the sensitivity of endothelial cells to cytokines which alter adhesion molecule expression rather than directly altering adhesion molecule expression itself[21]. In contrast, neuropeptides have been shown to directly alter β_2-integrin expression in vascular endothelium resulting in a rapid and sustained influx of neutrophils and eosinophils[22].

Functional studies

What is required in order to decipher the complex autonomic regulation of allergic inflammation are sophisticated in vivo studies in robust, functional animal models of allergic disease. For example, a recent study demonstrated that surgical denervation of the superior cervical ganglion reduced anaphylactic death by 68%, reduced neutrophil recruitment to the airways and dampened the normal rise in bronchoalveolar lavage fluid (BALF) immunoglobulin (Ig)-M, IgA and IgG levels in addition to reducing peritoneal histamine levels[23,24].

NEUROENDOCRINE REGULATION OF THE AIRWAYS

Allergic inflammation of the skin and airways is not only regulated in a complex manner by the ANS, but there is also a sophisticated modulation of immunity by neuroendocrine steroids and peptides[25,26]. Again assessment of the role of this neuroimmunomodulation should not be restricted to the effects of neuroendocrine molecules produced in the bronchial mucosa, but should incorporate the effects of these molecules on the primary, secondary and tertiary lymphoid organs, since neuropeptides and neurosteroids can have a profound effect on T cell differentiation, proliferation and function in the thymus or regional lymph nodes[27,28].

In addition, neuroendocrine steroids and peptides can modulate cholinergic transmission, mucus secretion, neurogenic microvascular leakage, T cell γ-IFN production, human cutaneous mast cells degranulation in vitro, T-lymphocyte–dependent antibody production and the expression of high affinity IL-2 receptors[29,30,31].

Thus autonomic and neuroendocrine 'mind–body' pathways have the capacity to profoundly alter local immunity. Furthermore, these pathways may act synergistically, since the hypothalamus receives a rich autonomic innervation and synthesizes catecholamines and hypothalamic hormone production can profoundly affect autonomic function[32,33].

STRESS AND ALLERGIC INFLAMMATION

This molecular evidence showing that the brain can modulate immunity at a cellular level provides a mechanistic explanation for how stress can disrupt airway function and contribute to the symptomatology of asthma and rhinitis[34]. Thus a number of recent animal studies demonstrated that the stress-induced inhibition of cell-mediated immunity and pulmonary infiltration were due to increased levels of circulating corticosteroids and catecholamines[35–38]. In fact there is evidence to suggest that stress may promote allergic inflammation by driving the immune system towards a Th2-dominated response and this effect may be mediated by corticosteroids[39–41].

In addition to this animal research there is substantial human evidence to suggest that the immunosuppression that can follow acute and chronic stress is mediated by the neuroendocrine response to that stress. However, very little of this in vitro research has focused on allergic disease per se. Direct investigation of the impact of psychological factors in asthma have utilized questionable psychological assessments and involved small numbers of patients[42–44]. Although one or two studies have demonstrated that high levels of stress increase the risk of contracting an upper respiratory tract infection[45].

DEPRESSION AND ALLERGIC INFLAMMATION

While there is substantial evidence demonstrating the immunosuppressive effects of negative emotional states on immunity[46,47], there are relatively little data on whether depression can increase the risk of developing allergic disease or exacerbate existing disease. Only a handful of studies have examined the effects of mood disorders on allergic disease. The studies that have been conducted employed a wide variety of psychological measurements, with the majority, but not all, reporting an increase in the association between depression or anxiety and asthma[48–54].

One study suggested that up to 25% of school-age children admitted for severe asthma were depressed, and 33% were coping poorly[55]. In addition, poor control of asthmatic symptoms has been associated with emotional or behavioral disturbance[56]. The importance of emotions in modifying asthma symptomatology was highlighted by the demonstration that tricyclic antidepressants improved symptomatology in 62% of all asthmatics, and 79% of asthmatic children[57,58]. Most of this research is correlational and does not clarify how emotional disruption exacerbates the physiological disruption that underlies allergic inflammation. One postulated mechanism of how mood can alter airway tone suggests that the increased cholinergic activity seen in depression precipitates the critical bronchospasm, sudden deterioration and subsequent death seen in some asthmatics[59]. Such a hypothesis has yet to be tested despite the widespread availability of simple technology capable of accurately measuring autonomic tone and the persistence of 2000 preventable deaths in the UK each year.

However, mood disorder may not only precipitate bronchospasm through autonomic dysregulation, there is good evidence to show that it also affects the neuroendocrine axis[60]. It is well established that many patients with a depressive illness have disturbed central glucocorticoid metabolism, with hypercortisolemia, increased levels of CRF in the cerebrospinal fluid, a blunted ACTH response to CRF or non-suppression of cortisol following administration of dexamethasone[61–65]. The hypothalamic disruption maybe interact, synergistically, with the autonomic dysfunction and exacerbate the immune disruption seen in allergic inflammation[64,65]. Thus mood may affect airway inflammation via both autonomic and neuroendocrine pathways.

PERSONALITY AND ALLERGIC INFLAMMATION

In addition to the strong circumstantial evidence suggesting that stress and mood disorder can significantly impact airway tone there is some evidence to suggest that various personality characteristics can identify asthmatics that are particularly 'at risk'. The majority of these studies were uncontrolled and descriptive and as a consequence a variety of descriptors, such as denial, repressed hostility, depression, emotional immaturity and a 'negative parental aura' have been associated with poor asthmatic control[66–68]. In the only case-controlled study to date 21 children who died from asthma following hospital discharge were matched for age, sex, race and severity of disease with 21 children who were alive at follow-up. Hospital records were evaluated for 57 physiological and psychological variables. A stepwise discriminate analysis revealed 14 variables which could distinguish the group of children that died from the control group. Ten of these differentiating characteristics reflected the psychological adaptation of the child or their family to the situation. The authors concluded that the psychological features that characterized the children who died were more than just a consequence of severe disease, and may be important in identifying children at high risk of dying[52].

MIND–BODY INTERVENTIONS IN ALLERGIC DISEASE

It is clear from the above discussion that there is a substantial amount of circumstantial evidence to suggest that the brain may play a vital role in regulating airway function and tone. But what is the evidence that mind–body inteventions can help in the management of allergic disease? There has been a significant volume of research into the efficacy of a wide variety of mind–body therapies. This evidence is reviewed below.

Hypnosis

Hypnosis has been used for many years to treat allergies and there are numerous anecdotal reports suggesting that it may be effective, particularly for skin disease[69]. More recently larger controlled studies have shown that hypnosis can reduce immediate and delayed-type hypersensitivity reactions to various cutaneous allergens[70–72]. However, not all authors have been able to demonstrate this effect even in highly hypnotizable subjects[73,74].

In a small study of chronic urticaria, more than 80% of patients either improved or showed a complete recovery as assessed by subjective and objective criteria[75]. In a more recent study in patients with chronic urticaria of up to 8 years' duration, hypnosis relieved the itching, but only in the hypnotizable group. At a follow-up appointment 90% of patients were either free of hives or had improved significantly[76]. Similarly, the severity of symptoms and reliance on medication were reduced by guided imagery in a small study of patients with atopic eczema[77].

It has been suggested that hypnosis simply promotes or inhibits cutaneous vasodilation rather than altering the inflammatory process[78]. There is no evidence to suggest that hypnosis can alter immune function in allergic disease; however hypnosis has been shown to alter immune parameters, such as natural killer cell activity and chemotaxis, in other clinical settings[79,80].

In contrast to a single anecdotal report on the use of hypnosis in allergic rhinitis[81], the efficacy of hypnosis in bronchial asthma has been widely studied. It has been suggested that over a third of all asthmatics may bronchoconstrict to suggestion or stress[82]. In contrast, bronchodilation is believed to be less susceptible to suggestion. Following a number of early uncontrolled reports suggesting a beneficial effect of hypnotic suggestion in asthma, a number of small scale controlled trials were conducted which demonstrated a reduction in morbidity and steroid usage in asthmatics following hypnotherapy[83,84].

More recently, a larger single center study confirmed the effectiveness of hypnosis in reducing the hospital admission rate, duration of stay, and need for systemic steroids in 16 subjects with inadequately controlled asthma[85]. However, no objective changes in airway function were demonstrated in this study, and it has been suggested that the observed subjective improvement may in fact be detrimental resulting in asthmatics underestimating the severity of their disease and thereby increase their risk of sudden death. In contrast to this single center study, the multicenter British Thoracic Society study was unable to confirm any subjective or objective benefit of hypnosis in 91 asthmatics[86].

A number of groups have investigated the effect of hypnosis on more specific, objective measures of airway function. These studies have reported improvements in airway caliber, response to hypercapnia, bronchial hyper-reactivity (BHR) as well as symptom scores and the use of bronchodilators[87–89]. However, some of these improvements only occurred in the highly susceptibile asthmatics.

Several groups have demonstrated that suggestion can promote bronchoconstriction or bronchodilation following saline inhalation[90–93]. It is interesting to note that the emotionally reactive subjects had the most reactive airways in response to hypnosis even though these individuals did feel that their asthma could be emotionally triggered. Hypnosis has also been shown to reduce exercise-induced bronchospasm[94].

A retrospective analysis of asthmatics treated with hypnotherapy indicated that more than

50% had a substantial objective improvement and 25% reported a significant subjective improvement[95]. Not suprisingly the more suggestible the subject the more likely they were to benefit. Hypnosis seems to be particularly effective in children: whether this is due to their greater suggestibility, or a result of a more reversible disease process is unclear[96,97]. Similarly, it is unclear whether hypnosis directly reduces airway inflammation or improves airway caliber by reducing emotional anxiety, which is a well recognized precipitant of acute bronchoconstriction. In addition, some benefit may be due to increasing patients' sense of control and involvement in their disease.

Acupuncture

The use of acupuncture in the treatment of cutaneous allergic reactions or rhinitis has received little attention. A small controlled study in rodents involving daily acupuncture for 3 days demonstrated a suppression of the delayed hypersensitivity reaction to trinitrochlorobenzene. The two reported trials of acupuncture in rhinitis produced contradictory results. The earlier trial studied 22 rhinitic subjects given six acupuncture treatments and reported a virtual eradication of symptoms in 50% of subjects, and a moderate reduction in symptoms in 34%. This subjective improvement was accompanied by a reduction in peripheral blood eosinophilia and nasal eosinophil recruitment in addition to reduced IgE levels[98]. In contrast, a later study concluded that any benefit produced was probably secondary to suggestion rather than acupuncture[99].

In contrast to the paucity of data on allergic rhinitis and dermatoses, acupuncture has been widely used in the treatment of asthma, and in some countries nearly a quarter of general practitioners believe it to be efficacious[100]. Some reviews have suggested that acupuncture is effective in acute asthma[101], with a few studies documenting an improvement in spirometric findings within 10 minutes of therapy[102]; however the effect is usually less than that seen following the use of a bronchodilator. Other authors have suggested that acupuncture has a greater effect on airway tone and therefore should be used as a preventative measure rather an acute treatment.

A recent review assessed the quality of 13 published trials on asthma treated with acupuncture. The authors highlighted a range of methodological weaknesses and reported that of the five methodologically weakest studies all reported beneficial effects on pulmonary function, drug requirements and symptoms. In contrast, only three of the best eight studies reported a beneficial effect. Therefore the authors concluded that claims that acupuncture was effective in the treatment of asthma were not based on well performed clinical trials[103]. Other reviewers have come to the same conclusion[104].

The three published studies not included in this review also produced contradictory results. A double-blind placebo-controlled crossover designed study involving 15 patients with stable asthma treated twice weekly for 5 weeks failed to find any subjective or objective improvement in asthma using acupuncture[105]. In contrast, a small trial involving nine patients with extrinsic asthma reported a significant reduction in pharmacotherapy following acupuncture[106].

A much larger series involving 192 patients from the Department of Acupuncture, Kaifeng city, China, reported a startling degree of success[107].

The majority of the above studies have only examined the short-term effects of a single or small number of acupuncture sessions and the results have been mixed. Only a handful of studies have examined the long-term effects of acupuncture treatment, its effects on airway hyper-reactivity or its effects on immune parameters and again the results have been mixed. For example, acupuncture had no effect on bronchial hyper-reactivity (BHR) provoked by histamine[108], but did protect against metacholine-induced BHR[109], although this effect was very short lived. Similarly acupuncture had no effect on IgE levels, spirometry or skin reactivity but did reduce 'leukocyte responsiveness'[110].

A small study did investigate the effects of a longer course of acupuncture, eight sessions, in chronic asthmatics. The evaluation was blind to treatment and employed a crossover design in which all 25 subjects received both true and sham acupuncture with a 3 or 4 week washout period between treatments. The study failed to show any significant benefit on daily symptom scores, medication usage, patients' subjective self-assessment or lung function[111].

A similar study investigated the effects of ten twice weekly sessions of acupuncture compared with ten sessions of sham acupuncture in 17 patients with chronic stable asthma. The results indicated a modest improvement in both subjective and objective measures of airway inflammation compared with sham treatment. In the true acupuncture group, peak flow increased by 22% in the morning and 7% in the evening, while daily medication decreased by 53%. This group remained significantly improved throughout the trial period of 11 weeks, although with decreasing benefits over time. While the authors acknowledged that the effects on lung function were modest, they suggested that the substantial reduction in medication intake may be valuable even in the absence of improvements in pulmonary function[112]. A reduction in pharmacotherapy with no alteration in pulmonary function has also been reported in a number of other studies involving patients with extrinsic asthma[110], and chronic obstructive airways disease.

There are a number of difficulties in interpreting these data. Firstly a wide variety of experimental paradigms, subject populations, and outcome measures were used. Secondly a variety of different acupuncture techniques were employed. Thus, the majority of studies utilized 'formula acupuncture', where needles are placed at the same points in all patients. This differs from 'classical Chinese acupuncture', which requires different acupuncture points depending on the unique characteristics of individual patients. In addition, classical Chinese acupuncture is normally used in conjunction with a wide range of herbal preparations. Finally the duration of acupuncture treatment is clearly an important factor and the duration of needle retention may also be vital in determining efficacy with 40 minutes being the optimum retention time[113].

Despite these problems, it seems that acupuncture may have a role to play in certain subgroups of patients such as drug-induced or allergic asthma and ineffective in other such as exercise-induced asthma[114]. Clearly, further large scale, well designed and well controlled studies assessing the long-term consequences of acupuncture are required before acupuncture can be recommended.

Homeopathy

Homeopathy is widely used by the general public for a variety of conditions including atopic dermatitis[115], and remarkable claims have been made for its efficacy in asthma[116]. However two recent large reviews of the role of homeopathy in clinical medicine concluded that except for the occasionally demonstrated benefit there was little scientific evidence to support the use of homeopathy in the majority of clinical settings[117,118].

Part of the difficulty is that there are a number of different homeopathic approaches to the management of allergy. Firstly, classical homeopathy aims to match the patient's symptoms to those produced by a particular herb or animal remedy, which is then given in a very dilute form. This approach is labor intensive and involves detailed history taking[119]. The second approach, termed complex homeopathy, uses a mixture of a herbs and homeopathic products. For example, a homeopathic remedy developed from the lungs of guinea pigs killed by anaphylactic shock has been shown to produce symptomatic improvements in asthmatics[120]. The third approach, which has been termed homeopathic immunotherapy (HIT), involves treating like with like. Thus HIT suggests that someone suffering from hay fever should be treated with a homeopathic dilution of the pollens to which they are allergic[121].

Only a handful of studies have been published on the use of homeopathy in rhinitis. For example, a study involving 164 patients with allergic rhinitis treated with 5 weeks of Galphimia D6 versus placebo failed to show any significant benefit, although a trend in favor of homeopathy was reported[122]. In contrast, a double-blind placebo-controlled study from Glasgow involving 144 patients with allergic rhinitis given HIT found a significant reduction in patient- and doctor-assessed symptom scores, which was associated with a 50% reduction in patients' antihistamine requirements[121]. In a more recent meta-analysis, combining the rhinitis data with data from two studies of HIT in asthma, the authors argued that the evidence to support HIT was unequivocal[123]. However, detractors have argued that the study only involved a small number of patients, and the major treatment effect was the patient's own perception of their asthma rather than objective measurements of lung function.

Therefore, although many homeopaths' clinical experience suggests that homeopathy may indeed help asthma, there is little clinical trial evidence to support such beliefs. This does not disprove the validity of homeopathy, but merely means that larger controlled studies are needed replicating Reilly's provocative data.

Yoga

While many asthmatics have been significantly helped by training in breathing techniques there has been little formal clinical research to assess their efficacy. There have been two controlled studies on the use of yoga techniques in asthma. The first involved 53 asthmatics trained over 2 weeks in an integrated set of yoga exercises, including breathing, physical postures and breath slowing techniques as well as training in meditation. Patients in the treatment and control groups were equally motivated to take up yoga at randomization and those randomized to the treatment arm were instructed to practice these techniques for 65 minutes every day. The control group consisted of 53 patients with asthma, matched for age, sex and severity who continued to take their usual drugs. Patients were followed for 6 weeks. Results demonstrated a significant reduction in the number of asthma attacks per week, the use of asthmatic medication and a significant improvement in peak expiratory flow rate (PEFR) in the yoga group compared with controls[124]. Recently these results were independently replicated[125].

This more recent randomized, double-blind, placebo-controlled, crossover trial assessed the effects of two pranayama yoga breathing exercise on airway reactivity, airway caliber, symptom scores and medication usage in patients with mild asthma. Following a 1 week run-in period the 18 patients with mild asthma practiced slow deep breathing for 15 minutes twice daily for 2 weeks. During this period, subjects were asked to breathe through a Pink City Lung Exerciser, a device which forces subjects to breathe slowly with a 1:2 inspiration: expiration ratio. This is equivalent to pranayama breathing methods. All patients entered improved while using the Lung Exerciser compared with a dummy placebo device, although the differences did not reach statistical significance. In contrast, there was a significant reduction in bronchial hyper-reactivity to histamine during pranayama breathing, but not with the placebo device. Taken together these studies suggest that asthmatics may be helped by training in breathing techniques. Whether such effects are brought about by increased endogenous glucocorticoid production folowing the practice of yoga[126], or changes in autonomic function[127], is unknown.

Chiropractic

Chiropractic is widely used in the UK for the treatment of arthritic and soft tissue disorders. However in some countries it is widely used in the treatment of asthma[128]. A 1980 survey reported that a substantial number of Danish children with chronic asthma were treated with chiropractic, and the vast majority of their parents considered the treatment beneficial[129]. Similarly an Australian survey conducted in 1985 reported that 45% of asthmatic families had consulted alternative therapists, most commonly chiropractors[130]. Despite this, there are very few controlled trials investigating the efficacy of chiropractic or osteopathy in allergic disease. A pilot study conducted over 20 years ago in patients with chronic obstructive pulmonary disease demonstrated non-significant increases in vital capacity, residual volume, total lung capacity and forced expiratory volume in the first second (FEV_1) in patients treated with spinal manipulation compared with controls[131]. Another poorly designed study reported improvements in pulmonary function and symptom scores, but the size of the control group precluded statistical analysis[132]. A more recent Australian study found only subjective improvements in symptoms with no improvements in lung function in asthmatics treated with chiropractic[133]. A recent review of the literature concluded that there was no evidence to support the role of chiropractic in allergic disease[134].

Herbal remedies

There has been a reasonable volume of research investigating a wide variety of herbal medicines in the treatment of allergic disease. For example, a recent study investigating the efficacy of a herbal tea in non-exudative steroid-resistant severe atopic eczema gave very promising results[135]. In a crossover study, with a 4 week washout period, 37 children aged 1–18 years drank a brew of herbal tea, or similarly tasting placebo, daily for 8 weeks. Erythema decreased by 51% on active treatment (vs. 6% on placebo), and 'cutaneous damage' decreased by 63% (vs. 6% on placebo). In addition, ability to sleep improved in 19 children during active treatment compared with only three on placebo. The herbal tea had no effect on asthmatic symptoms, serum IgE levels, eosinophil counts, or urinary cortisol excretion. Finally there was no short-term evidence of toxicity. In view of this very encouraging response the same remedy was prescribed to 40 adults with refractory widespread atopic dermatitis with equally dramatic results[136]. The authors suggested that the herbal preparation may have a combination of anti-inflammatory, antimicrobial, sedative and immunosuppressant effects. Intensive research is now under way to try and identify the active ingredients in this herbal brew.

A number of herbs commonly used in Ayurvedic medicine to treat asthma have been formally investigated. For example, Coleus forskholii, which has been shown to increase intracellular levels of cyclic AMP[137], has been shown to have a powerful bronchodilating effect, with fewer side effects than Fenoterol[138]. Similarly, Ginkgo biloba which contains several unique terpene molecules known to antagonize platelet activating factors (PAF) and hence limit bronchial hyper-reactivity, has been shown to improve pulmonary function, protect against exercise-induced asthma and decrease bronchial hyper-reactivity to nebulized house dust mite[139,140]. Finally, a number of animal and large controlled double-blind crossover studies in humans have suggested that Tylophora asthmatica is effective in the treatment of asthma, although these studies also reported that the asthmatics taking Tylophora frequently suffered minor side effects[141–144].

Recently, Saiboku-to, a herb widely used in traditional Chinese medicine for the treatment of bronchial asthma has attracted interest. It was reported to have a steroid sparing effect in 40 asthmatics who took the remedy regularly for between 6 and 24 months[145]. Furthermore, it was reported to act on β_2 adrenoreceptors and alter ACTH and cortisol levels while manifesting few side effects. A much smaller study involving nine patients taking Saiboku-to for over 1 year confirmed the steroid sparing effects[146]. The active ingredient in Saiboku-to may be the magnolol fraction.

Vitamin and mineral supplementation

The role of a variety of nutritional interventions have been investigated in allergic disease. For example, it has been suggested that sodium restriction or the ingestion of omega-3 fatty acids may be beneficial in reducing bronchial hyper-responsiveness[147,148]. In contrast, the role of vitamin C in allergic disease is debatable[149–152]. The treatment of acute asthma with intravenous magnesium has attracted interest with various authors arguing in favor or against its role[153,154].

Food allergy and intolerance

Environmental antigens whether they be aeroallergens or dietary allergens are widely implicated in the pathophysiology of allergic disease. House dust mite proteins are recognized as the major precipitant of allergic disease in the UK. Similarly there is good evidence that tartrazine, acetylsalicylic acid, biogenic amines and the preservative sodium metabisulfite which occur in yeast and cheeses, can provoke bronchoconstriction[155–158]. However, whether more commonly encountered food antigens can exacerbate allergic disease is controversial. Advocates argue strongly that food allergy is a very important cause of asthma, and is often overlooked[159]. The problem may arise in discriminating between allergy, which is mediated by specific antibodies detectable in the serum, and intolerance, whose mechanism is unclear. Individuals with food intolerance frequently have a negative skin prick test (SPT) and radioallergen absorbent test (RAST)[160]. Their negative immunological results and the fact that they often present with multiple symptoms and multiple claimed intolerances frequently leads to these patients' suffering being dismissed by clinical immunologists. While some of these individuals may actually have underlying psychological or even psychiatric disorders, clinical experience suggests that many are genuinely troubled by their diet.

The most common food sensitivity in asthmatic patients is milk closely followed by egg, and wheat. Wheat intolerance is more frequent in older patients than in young asthmatics[159]. There are four studies, all employing slightly different methodology, which suggest that food intolerance might contribute to asthmatic symptomatology[158,160–162].

Guidelines have been published for the diagnosis of food intolerance and the development of avoidance diets[163]. The use of double-blind placebo-controlled food challenge in the diagnosis of food intolerance is questionable and therefore the most useful approach is simply to institute a dietary avoidance regime and monitor for any empirical improvement. Such an approach must be instituted carefully under very controlled conditions for it is very easy to drift into a severely limiting diet which is unpalatable and may promote vitamin and mineral deficiency. Clearly a great deal more research is required before the importance of nutritional antigens in allergic disease is clarified, and therefore such an approach should only be advocated when there is a very robust clinical history and avoidance can show clearcut improvement in objective disease parameters or symptoms.

CONCLUSION

There is a substantial evidence to suggest that the brain plays a vital role in the development and manifestation of allergic disease and should not be dismissed as an occasional trigger in a small minority of patients. Attention to the mind–body interface may change autonomic tone and the neuroendocrine milieu in which the allergic disease manifests. In addition, there is sufficient evidence to suggest that mind–body therapies may have something to offer patients with allergies. Clearly further research conducted in skeptical centers of excellence is required. However, in patients whose symptoms are inadequately controlled or who have limited therapeutic options, such approaches may be considered not as an alternative to conventional treatment, but as complementary treatments in the fight against what is an increasing clinical problem.

REFERENCES

1 Burney PGJ, Chin S, Rona RJ 1990 Has the prevalence of asthma increased in children? Evidence from the national study of health and growth 1973–86. British Medical Journal 300:1306–10

2 Levy L, Bell 1984 General practice audit of asthma in childhood. British Medical Journal 289:1115–8

3 Turner-Warwick M 1989 Nocturnal asthma: A study in general practice. Journal of the Royal College of General Practice 39:239–43

4 Gellert AR, Gellert SL, Iliffe SR 1990 Prevalence and management of asthma in a London inner city general practice. British Journal of General Practice 40:197–201

5 Anderson HR, Bailey PA, Cooper JS et al. 1983 Morbidity and school absence caused by asthma and wheezy illness. Archives of the Diseases of Childhood 58:777–84

6 Berrill WT 1993 Is the death rate from asthma exaggerated? Evidence from West Cumbria. British Medical Journal 306:193–4

7 Glaxo Pharmaceuticals 1990 The occurrence and cost of asthma

8 Willis T 1679 Pharmaceutice Rationalis, Vol 2. Dring, Harper Leigh, London

9 Busse WW, Kielcot-Glaser JK, Coe C et al. 1995 Stress and asthma: NHBLI Workshop Report. American Journal of Critical Care Medicine Jan:248–252

10 Barnes PJ 1986 State of the art. Neural control of human airways in health and disease. American Review of Respiratory Disease 134:1289–1314

11 Calvo W 1968 Innervation of the bone marrow in laboratory animals. American Journal of Anatomy 123:315

12 Williams JW, Peterson RG, Shea PA et al. 1980 Sympathetic innervation of mouse thymus and spleen: evidence for a functional link between nervous and immune systems. Brain Research Bulletin 6:83

13 Felton DL, Felten SY, Bellinger DL et al. 1987 Noradrenergic sympathetic neural interactions with the immune system: Structure and function. Immunological Review 100:225–60

14 Watkins AD 1997 Neuropharmacology. In: Kay AB (ed) Allergies and allergic disease. Blackwell Press (in press)

15 Casale TB 1987 Neuromechanisms of asthma. Annals of Allergy 59:391–8

16 Bai TR, Mak JCW, Barnes PJ 1992 A comparison of beta adrenergic receptors and in vitro relaxant responses to isoproterenol in asthmatic airway smooth muscle. American Journal of Respiratory Cell and Molecular Biology 6:647–51

17 Sorkness R, Clough JJ, Castleman WL et al. 1994 Virus induced airway obstruction and parasympathetic hyperresponsiveness in adult rats. American Journal of Critical Care Medicine 150(1):28–34

18 Elwood W, Sakamoto T, Barnes PJ et al. 1993 Allergen induced airway hyper-responsiveness in Brown Norway rat: role of parasympathetic mechanisms. Journal of Applied Physiology 75(1):279–84

19 Howarth PH, Djukanovik R, Reddington T et al. 1995 Neuropeptide containing nerves in endobronchial biopsies from asthmatic and nonasthmatic subjects. American Journal of Respiratory Cell and Molecular Biology 13:288–296

20 Ottaway CA, Husband AJ 1994 The influence of neuroendocrine pathways on lymphocyte migration. Immunology Today 15(11):511–17

21 Bourdoulous S, Durieu-Trautmann O, Strosberg AD 1993 Catecholamines stimulate MHC class I, class II, and invarient chain gene expression in brain endothelium through different mechanisms. Journal of Immunology 150:1486–95

22 Smith CH, Barker JNWN, Morris RW et al. 1993 Neuropeptides induce rapid expression of endothelial cell adhesion molecules and elicit granulocytic infiltration in human skin. Journal of Immunology 151:3274–82

23 Ramaswamy K, Mathison R, Carter L et al. 1990 Marked anti-inflammatory effects of decentralisation of the superior cervical ganglia. Journal of Experimental Medicine 172:1819–30

24 Mathison R, Carter L, Mowatt C et al. 1994 Temporal analysis of the anti-inflammatory effects of decentralisation of the rat superior ganglia. American Journal of Physiology 266:R1537–43

25 Blalock JE 1994 The immune system: Our sixth sense. Immunologist 2:8–15

26 Reichlin S 1993 Neuroendocrine-immune interactions. New England Journal of Medicine Oct 21:1246–53

27 Moreno J, Vincente A, Heijnen I 1994 Prolactin and early T cell development in embryonic chicken. Immunology Today 15(11):524–6

28 Dardenne M, Savino W 1994 Control of thymus physiology by peptidic hormones and neuropeptides. Immunology Today 15(11):518–23

29 Brown SL, Van Epps DE 1986 Opioid peptides modulate production of interferon-gamma by human mononuclear cells. Cell Immunology 103:19–28

30 Casale JB, Bowman S, Kaliner M 1984 Induction of human cutaneous mast cell degranulation by opiates and endogenous opioid peptides: Evidence for opiate and non opiate receptor participation. Journal of Allergy and Clinical Immunology 73:775–81

31 Johnson HM, Smith EM, Torres BA et al. 1982 Regulation of the in vitro antibody response neuroendocrine hormones. Proceedings of the National Academy of Sciences of the USA 79:4171–4

32 O'Flynn K, O'Keane V, Lucey JV 1991 Effect of fluoxetine on noradrenergic mediated growth hormone release: a double blind, placebo controlled study. Biological Psychiatry 30(40):377–82

33 Terao A, Oikawa M, Saito M. 1993 Cytokine induced changes in hypothalmic norepinephrine turnover: involvement of corticotrophin-releasing hormone and prostaglandins. Brain Research 622:257–61

34 Coe CL 1993 Psychosocial factors and immunity in nonhuman primates: a review. Psychosomatic Medicine 55:298–308

35 Sheridan JF, Feng N, Bonneau RH 1991 Restraint stress differentially affects anti-viral cellular and humoral immune responses in mice. Journal of Neuroimmunology 31:245–55

36 Hemann G, Beck FM, Tovar CA et al. 1994 Stress-

induced changes attributable to the sympathetic nervous system during experimental influenza viral infection in DBA/2 inbred mouse strain. Journal of Immunology 53(2):173–80
37 Dobbs CM, Vasquez M, Glaser R et al. 1993 Mechanisms of stress-induced modulation of viral pathogenesis and immunity. Journal of Neuroimmunology 48(2):151–60
38 Kusnecov AV, Grota LJ, Schmidt SG 1993 Decreased herpes simplex viral immunity and enhanced pathogenesis following stressor administration in mice. Journal of Immunology 38:129–38
39 Rook GAW, Hernandez-Pando R, Lightman SL 1994 Hormones, peripherally activated prohormones and regulation of the Th1/Th2 balance. Immunology Today 15(7):301–3
40 Karp JD, Cohen N, Moynihan JA 1994 Quantitative differences in interleukin-2 and interleukin-4 production by antigen-stimulated splenocytes from individually and group-housed mice. Life Science 55(10):789–95
41 Moynihan JA, Karp JD, Cohen N et al. 1994 Alterations in IL-4 and antibody production following pheromone exposure: role for glucocorticoids. Journal of Neuroimmunology 54:51–8
42 Wistuba F 1986 Significance of allergy in asthma from a behavioral medicine viewpoint. Psychotherapy and Psychosomatics 45(4):186–94
43 Hollaender J, Florin I 1983 Expressed airway conductance in children with bronchial asthma. Journal of Psychosomatic Research 27(4):307–11
44 Michel FB 1994 Psychology of the allergic patient. Allergy 49 (18 Suppl):28–30
45 Cohen S, Tyrell DA, Smith AP 1991 Psychological stress and the susceptibility to the common cold. New England Journal of Medicine 325:606–12
46 Stein M, Miller AH, Trestman RL 1991 Depression and the immune system. In: Ader R, Cohen N (eds)Psychoneuroimmunology, 2nd edn. Academic Press, San Diego, pp 897–931
47 Denney DR, Stephenson LA, Penick EC et al. 1988 Lymphocyte subclasses and depression. Journal of Abnormal Psychology 97:499–502
48 Yellowless PM, Haynes S, Potts N 1988 Psychiatric morbidity in patients with life-threatening asthma: initial report of a controlled study. Medical Journal of Australia 149:246–9
49 Badoux A, Levy DA 1994 Psychological symptoms in asthma and chronic urticaria. Annals of Allergy 72:229–33
50 Lyketsos CG, Lyketsos GC, Richardson SC et al. Dysthymic states and depression syndrome in physical conditions of presumably psychological origin. Acta Psychiatrica Scandinavica 76:529–34
51 Lyketsos GC, Karabetsos A, Jordanoglou J et al. 1984 Personality characteristics and dysthymic states in bronchial asthma. Psychotherapy and Psychosomatics 41:177–85
52 Strunk RC, Mrazak DA, Fuhrmann GS et al. 1985 Physiologic and psychological characteristics associated with deaths due to asthma in childhood. A case-controlled study. JAMA 254(9):1193–8
53 Rubin NJ 1993 Severe asthma and depression. Archives of Family Medicine 2(4):433–40
54 Janson C Bjornsson E, Hetta J et al. 1994 Anxiety and depression in relation to respiratory symptoms and asthma. American Journal of Asthma and Critical Care Medicine 149(4):930–4
55 Klinnert M, Miller B, LaBrecque J et al. 1985 Psychological and social problems in severely asthmatic children. Paper presented at the 32nd Annual Meeting of the American Academy of Child Psychiatry 1:37–8
56 Norrish M, Tooley M, Godfrey S 1977 Clinical and psychological study of asthmatic children attending a hospital clinic. Archives of Diseases of Childhood 52:912–17
57 Meares R, Mills J, Horvath T 1971 Amitryptaline and asthma. Medical Journal of Australia 2:25–28
58 Sugihara H, Ishihara K, Noguchi H 1965 Clinical experience with amitryptaline (trytanol) in the treatment of bronchial asthma. Annals of Allergy 23:422–9
59 Miller BD 1987 Depression and asthma: a potentially lethal mixture. Journal of Allergy and Clinical Immunology 80(3):481–6
60 Charlton BG, Ferrier IN 1989 Hypothalamo-pituitary-adrenal axis abnormalities in depression: a review and a model. Psychosomatic Medicine 19:331–6
61 Gold PW, Chrousos G, Kellner C 1984 Psychiatric implications of basic and clinical studies with corticotrophin releasing factor. American Journal of Psychiatry 141:619–27
62 Gold PW, Goodwin FK, Chrousos GP 1988 Clinical and biochemical manifestations of depression. Relation to neurobiology of stress. New England Journal of Medicine 319:413–20
63 Sacha EJ 1982 Endocrine abnormalities in depression. In: Paykel ES (ed) Handbook of affective disorders. Guildford, New York, pp 191–201
64 Kronful A, House JD 1984 Depression cortisol and immune function. Lancet 1:1026–7
65 Dorian B, Garfinkel P 1987 Stress, immunity and illness — a review. Psychological Medicine 17:393–407
66 Dirks J, Kinsman R 1982 Death in asthma: a psychosomatic autopsy. Journal of Asthma 19:177–87
67 Santiago S, Klaustermeyer W 1980 Mortality in status asthmatics: a nine year experience in a respiratory intensive care unit. Journal of Asthma Research 17:75–9
68 Pinkerton P 1972 Depression v. denial in childhood asthma: equivalent fatal hazards. In: Depressive states in childhood and adolescence. Almquist and Wiskell, Stockholm, pp 187–92
69 Fry L, Mason AA, Pearson RSB 1964 Effect of hypnosis on allergic skin responses in asthma and hay fever. British Medical Journal 1:1145–8
70 Zachariae R, Bjerring P 1993 Increase and decrease of delayed cutaneous reactions obtained by hypnotic suggestions during sensitization. Allergy 48:6–11
71 Zachariae, Bjerring P, Arendt-Nielsen L 1989 Modulation of type I immediate and type IV delayed immunoreactivity using direct suggestion and guided imagery during hypnosis. Allergy 44:537–42
72 Zacharaie R, Bjerring P 1990 The effect of hypnotically induced analgesia on flare reaction of cutaneous histamine prick test. Archives of Dermatological Research 54:539–43

73 Jensen P 1990 Alternative therapy for atopic dermatitis and psoriasis: patient reported motivation, information and effect. Acta Dermato-Venereologica 70(5):425–8

74 Locke SE, Ransil BJ, Covino NA 1987 Failure of hypnotic suggestion to alter immune response to delayed-type hypersensitivity antigens. Annals of the New York Academy of Sciences 496:745–9

75 Kaneko Z, Takaishi N 1963 Psychosomatic studies on chronic urticaria. Folia Psychiatrica et Neurologica Japonica 17:16–24

76 Shertzer CL, Lookingbill DP 1987 Effects of relaxation therapy and hypnotizability in chronic urticaria. Archives of Dermatology 123:913–6

77 Horne DJ, White AE, Varigos GA 1989 A preliminary study of psychological therapy in the management of atopic eczema. British Journal of Medical Psychology 62:241–8

78 Barber TX 1984 Changing 'unchangeable' bodily processes by (hypnotic) suggestions: a new look at hypnosis, cognitions, imaging, and the mind-body problem. In: Sheikh AE (ed) Imagination and healing. Baywood, New York, pp 69–127

79 Zachariae R, Kristensen JS, Hokland P et al. 1990 The effect of psychological intervention in the form of relaxation and guided imagery on cellular immune function in healthy subjects — an overview. Psychotherapy and Psychosomatics 54:32–9

80 Zachariae R, Bjerring P 1991 Monocyte chemotactic activity in sera after hypnotically induced emotional states. Scandinavian Journal of Immunology 34:71–9

81 Mason A, Black S 1958 Allergic skin responses abolished under treatment of asthma and hayfever by hypnosis. Lancet 1:877–80

82 Isenberg SA, Lehrer PM, Hochran S 1992 The effects of suggestion and emotional arousal on pulmonary function in asthma: a review and a hypothesis regarding vagal mediation. Psychosomatic Medicine 54:192–216

83 Macer-Loughnan GP, Macdonald N, Mason AA et al. 1962 Controlled trial of hypnosis in the symptomatic treatment of asthma. British Medical Journal 2:371–6

84 Morrison JB 1976 Report on 33 asthmatic patients whose treatment was modified by hypnotherapy. Proceedings of the British Society of Medical Dental Hypnosis 2:9–23

85 Morrison JB 1988 Chronic asthma and improvement with relaxation induced by hypnotherapy. Journal of the Royal Society of Medicine 81:701–4

86 Committee of the British Tuberculous Association 1968 Hypnosis in asthma: a controlled trial. British Medical Journal 4:71–6

87 Neild JE, Cameron IR 1985 Bronchoconstriction in response to suggestion: its prevention by an inhaled anticholinergic agent. British Medical Journal 290:674

88 Sato P, Sargur M, Schoene RB 1986 Hypnosis effect on carbon dioxide chemosensitivity. Chest 89:828–31

89 Ewer TC, Stewart DE 1986 Improvement in bronchial hyper-responsiveness in patients with moderate asthma after treatment with a hypnotic technique: a randomised controlled trial. British Medical Journal 292:1129–32

90 Isenberg SA, Lehrer PM, Hochron S 1992 The effects of suggestion on airways of asthmatic subjects breathing room air as a suggested bronchconstrictor and inhaled bronchodilator. Journal of Psychosomatic Research 36:769–76

91 Janson-Bjerklie S, Boushey HA, Carrieri VK et al. 1986 Emotionally triggered asthma as a predictor of airway response to suggestion. Research in Nursing and Health 9:163–70

92 Horton DJ, Suda WL, Kinsman RA et al. 1978 Bronchoconstrictive suggestion in asthma: a role for airways hyper-reactivity and emotions. American Review of Respiratory Disease 117:1029–38

93 Butler C, Steptoe A 1986 Placebo responses: an experimental study of psychophysiological processes in asthmatic volunteers. British Journal of Clinical Psychology 25:173–83

94 Ben-Zvi Z, Spohn WA, Young SH et al. 1982 Hypnosis for exercise-induced asthma. American Review of Respiratory Disease 125:392–5

95 Collison DR 1975 Which asthmatic patients should be treated by hypnotherapy? Medical Journal of Australia 1:776–81

96 Diamond HH 1959 Hypnosis in children: complete cure in forty cases of asthma. American Journal of Hypnosis 1:124–9

97 Aronoff GM, Aronoff S, Peck LW 1975 Hypnotherapy in the treatment of bronchial asthma. Annals of Allergy 34(6):356–62

98 Lau BH, Wong DS, Slater JM 1975 Effect of acupuncture on allergic rhinitis: clinical and laboratory evaluations. American Journal of Chinese Medicine 3:263–70

99 Czubalski K, Zawisza E, Borzcecki M et al. 1977 Acupuncture and phonostimulation in pollenosis and vasomotor rhinitis in the light of psychosomatic investigations. Acta Otolaryngology (Stockholm) 84:446–9

100 Knipschild P, Kleijnen J, Reit ter G 1990 Belief in the efficacy of alternative medicine among general practitioners in the Netherlands. Social Science and Medicine 31:625–6

101 Virsik K, Kritufek D, Bangha O et al. 1980 The effect of acupuncture on bronchial asthma. Progress in Respiratory Research 14:271–5

102 Tandon MK, Soh PFT 1989 Comparison of real and placebo acupunture in histamine induced asthma: a double blind crossover study. Chest 96:102–5

103 Kleijnen J, Reit ter G, Knipschild P 1991 Acupuncture and asthma: a review of controlled trials. Thorax 46:799–802

104 Aldridge D, Pietroni PC 1987 Clinical assessment of acupuncture in asthma therapy: a discussion paper 80:222–4

105 Tandon MK, Soh PF, Wood AT 1991 Acupuncture for bronchial asthma? A double blind crossover study. Medical Journal of Australia 154(6):409–12

106 Sternfield M, Fink A, Bentwich Z et al. 1989 The role of acupuncture in asthma: changes in airway dynamics and LTC4 induced LA1. American Journal of Chinese Medicine 17:129–34

107 Zang 1990 Immediate antiasthmatic effect of acupuncture in 192 cases of bronchial asthma. Journal of Traditional Chinese Medicine 10:89–93

108 Tandon MK, Soh PFT 1989 Comparison of real and placebo acupuncture in histamine induced asthma: a double blind crossover study Chest 96:102–5

109 Tashkin DP, Bresler DE, Kroenig RJ et al. 1977 Comparison of real and simulated acupuncture and

isoproterenol in methacholine-induced asthma. Annals of Allergy 39:379–87

110 Sternfield M, Fink A, Bentwich Z 1989 The role of acupuncture in asthma: changes in airway dynamics and LTC4 induced LA1. American Journal of Chinese Medicine 17:129–34

111 Tashkin DP, Kroenig RJ, Bresler DE 1885 A controlled trial of real and simulated acupuncture in the management of chronic asthma. Journal of Allergy and Clinical Immunology 76:855–64

112 Christensen PA, Laursen LC, Taudorf E 1984 Acupuncture and bronchial asthma. Allergy 39:379–85

113 Zang J 1990 Immediate antiasthmatic effect of acupuncture in 192 cases of bronchial asthma. Journal of Traditional Chinese Medicine 10:89–93

114 Morton AR, Fazio SM, Miller 1993 Efficacy of laser-acupuncture in the prevention of exercise induced asthma. Annals of Allergy 70(4) 295–8

115 Jensen P 1990 Alternative therapy for atopic dermatitis and psoriasis: patient reported motivation, information and effect. Acta Dermato-Venereologica 70(5):425–8

116 Vincenzo F 1987 A clinical case: asthma and Staphysagria and homeo-mesotherapy. Homeopathology International 1(2):13,22

117 Hill C, Doyon F 1990 Review of randomised trials in homoeopathy. Revue de Epidemiologie et de Sante Publique 38:138–47

118 Kleijnen J, Knipschild P Riet ter G 1991 Clinical trials of homoeopathy. British Medical Journal 302:316–22

119 Boyd H 1981 Introduction to homoeopathic medicine. Beaconsfield, UK

120 Boucinhas JC, Boucinhas ID de M 1990 Prophylaxie des crises d'asthma bronchique chex l'enfant par l'usage de Pouman histamine 5CH. Homeopathie Francaise 78:35–9

121 Reilly DT, Taylor MA 1986 Is homoeopathy a placebo response? Controlled trial of homoeopathic potency with pollen in hay fever as a model. Lancet 2:881–6

122 Wiesenauer M, Gaus W 1985 Double-blind trial comparing the effectiveness of the homeopathic preparation Galphimia potentiation D6, Galphimia dilution 10(-6) and placebo on pollinosis. Arzneimittelforschung 35:1745–7

123 Reilly D Taylor M, Beattie G et al. 1994 Is evidence for homoeopathy reproducible? Lancet 334:1610–6

124 Nagarathna R, Nagendra HR 1985 Yoga for bronchial asthma: a controlled study. British Medical Journal 291:172–4

125 Singh V, Wisniewski A, Britton J et al. 1990 Effect of yoga breathing exercises (pranayama) on airway reactivity in subjects with asthma. Lancet 335:1381–3

126 Udupa KN, Singh RH 1972 The scientific basis of yoga. JAMA 220:1365

127 Benson H, Lehmann JW, Malhotra MS et al. 1982 Body temperature changes during the practices of gTum-mo yoga. Nature 295:234–6

128 Jamison JR, Leskovec K, Lepore S et al. 1986 Asthma in chiropractic clinic: a pilot study. Journal of Australian Chiropractic Association 16:137–43

129 Amtsraadsforeningen 1980 Statistik over kiropraktisk behandling — den specielle undersoegelse, Sygesikringens Forhandlingudvalg, Copenhagen, Denmark

130 Donnelly WJ, Spykerboer JE, Thong YH 1985 Are patients who use alternative medicine dissatisfied with orthodox medicine? Medical Journal of Australia 142:439–41

131 Miller WD 1975 Treatment of visceral disorders by manipulative therapy. In: Goldstein M (ed). The research status of spinal manipulative therapy. NINCDS Monograph, US Department of Health, Education and Welfare, Bethesda, pp 295–301

132 Hviid C 1978 A comparison of the effect of chiropractice treatment on respiratory function in patients with respiratory distress symptoms and patients without. Bulletin of the European Chiropractic Union 26:17–34

133 Jamison JR, Leskovek K, Lepore S 1986 Asthma in chiropractic clinic: a pilot study. Journal of the Australian Chiropractic Association 16:137–43

134 Renaud CI, Pichette D 1990 Chiropractice management of bronchial asthma: a literature review. American Chiropractic Association 27:25–6

135 Sheehan MP, Atherton DJ 1992 A controlled trial of traditional Chinese medicinal plants in widespread non-exudative eczema. British Journal of Dermatology 126–84

136 Shehan MP, Rustin MHA, Atherton DJ et al. 1992 Efficacy of traditional Chinese herbal therapy in adult atopic dermatitis. Lancet 340:13–17

137 Kaik G, Witte PU 1986 Protective effect of forskolin in acetylcholine provocation in healthy probands. Comparison of 2 doses with fenoterol and placebo. Weiner Medizinische Wochenschrift 136(23–24):637–41

138 Bauer K 1993 Pharmacodynamic effects of inhaled dry powder formulations of fenoterol and colforsin in asthma. Clinical Pharmacological Therapy 53(1):76–83

139 Wilkens JH 1990 Effects of PAF-antagonist (BN 52063) on bronchoconstriction and platelet activation during exercise induced asthma. British Journal of Clinical Pharmacology 29(1):85–91

140 Guinot P 1987 Effect of BN 52063, a specific PAF-acether antagonist, on bronchial provocation test to allergens in asthmatic patients. A preliminary study. Prostaglandins 34(5):723–31

141 Gupta S 1979 Tylophora indica in bronchial asthma — a double blind study. Indian Journal of Medical Research 69:981–9

142 Shivpuri DN, Singhal SC, Parkash D 1972 Treatment of asthma with an alcoholic extract of Tylophera indica: a crossover, double blind study. Annals of Allergy 30:402–12

143 Shivpuri DN, Singhal SC, Parkash D 1969 A crossover double blind study on Tylophora indica in the treatment of asthma and allergic rhinitis. Journal of Allergy 43(3):145–50

144 Thiruvengadam KV 1978 Tylophera indica in bronchial asthma (a controlled comparison with a standard anti-asthmatic drug). Journal of the Indian Medical Association 71(7):171–6

145 Nakajima S, Tohda Y, Ohkawa K et al. 1993 Effect of Saiboku-to (TJ-96) on bronchial asthma. Annals of the New York Academy of Sciences 685:549–60

146 Homma M, Kitaro O, Kobayashi H et al. 1993 Impact of free magnolol excretions in asthmatic patients who responded well to Saiboku-tu, a Chineses herbal medicine. Journal of Pharmaceutical Pharmacology 45:844–6

147 Burney 1989 The effect of changing dietary sodium on

the bronchial response to histamine. Thorax 44(1):36–41
148 Burney PG 1986 Response to inhaled histamine and 24 hour sodium excretion. British Medical Journal 292:1483–6
149 Schwartz J, Weiss ST 1990 Dietary factors and their relation to respiratory symptoms. The Second National Health and Nutrition Examination Survey. American Journal of Epidemiology 132(1):67–76
150 Malo JL 1986 Lack of acute effects of ascorbic acid on spirometry and airway responsiveness to histamine in subjects with asthma. Journal of Allergy and Clinical Immunology 78(6):11532–58
151 Mohsenin V 1987 Effect of vitamin C on NO_2-induced airway hyper-responsiveness in normal subjects. American Review of Respiratory Disease 136:1408–11
152 Bucca C 1990 Effect of vitamin C on histamine bronchial responsiveness of patients with allergic rhinitis. Annals of Allergy 65:311–14
153 Chyrek-Borowska S, Obrzut D, Hofman J 1978 the relation between magnesium, blood histamine level and eosinophilia in the acute stage of the allergic reaction in humans. Archives of Immunological Therapy and Experimentation (Warsz) 26(1–6):709–12
154 Allen M 1992 Serum magnesium levels in asthmatic patients during acute exacerbations of asthma. American Journal of Emergency Medicine 10(1):1–3
155 Baker GJ, Collett P, Allern DH 1981 Bronchospasm induced by metabisulphite-containing food and drugs. Medical Journal of Australia ii:614–16
156 Lockley SD 1977 Hypersensitivity to tartrazine and other dyes and additives present in foods and pharmaceutical products. Annals of Allergy 38:206–210
157 Monoret-Vautrin DA 1987 Food intolerance masquerading as food allergy. In: Brostoff J, Challacombe SJ (eds) Food allergy and intolerance. Balliere Tindall, London, pp 836–49
158 Stenius BSM, Lemola M 1976 Hypersensitivity to acetylsalicylic acid and tartrazine in patients with asthma. Clinical Allergy 6:119–29
159 Wraith DG Asthma. In: Brostoff J, Challacombe SJ (eds) Food allergy and intolerance. Balliere Tindall, London, pp 486–97
160 Wraith DG, Merrett J, Roth A et al. 1979 Recognition of food allergic patients and their allergens by the RAST technique and clinical investigation. Clinical Allergy 9:25–36
161 Stevenson DD, Simon RA 1981 Sensitivity to ingested metabisulphites in asthmatic subjects. Journal of Allergy and Clinical Immunology 68:26–32
162 Wraith DG, Young GVW, Lee TH 1979 The management of food allergy with diet and Nalcrom. In: Pepys J, Edwards AM (eds) The mast cell: its role in health and disease. Pitman, Tunbridge Wells, pp 443–6
163 Radcliffe M 1987 A diagnostic use of dietary regimes. In: Brostoff J, Challacombe SJ (eds) Food allergy and intolerance. Balliere Tindall, London, pp 806–23

CHAPTER CONTENTS

9

Non-specific ill health: a mind–body approach to functional somatic symptoms

Michael Sharpe
Simon Wessely

INTRODUCTION

In this chapter we review the conceptual issues encountered in the discussion of so-called functional somatic symptoms, and briefly review the main theoretical standpoints from which these symptoms have been viewed. We conclude that in order to successfully comprehend and manage this group of conditions it is necessary to adopt an integrated mind–body perspective which transcends the traditional dualistic approach. Such a perspective is described and the associated approach to management outlined. Finally we describe the application of this approach using the chronic fatigue syndrome as an example.

What are functional somatic symptoms?

While the terms 'illness' and 'disease' are often used interchangeably, it is useful to differentiate between them[1]. *Illness* may be defined in terms of the patient's experience of there being 'something wrong', whereas *disease* implies the presence of objectively identifiable biological abnormalities in the structure and/or function of the bodily organs and systems. A person who feels ill and cannot perform their daily tasks is clearly not well. Yet in many such cases the doctor cannot find evidence of organic bodily disease. What is wrong with them? If the person's symptoms are predominantly psychological they may be diagnosed as having a psychiatric, or 'mental' illness. When their complaints are somatic, however, the diagnosis is often problematic[2]. What should we call these complaints? Are they 'real physical illnesses' or are they 'all in the mind'? Are they 'psychiatric' or 'medical'? How should they be treated? These are the questions we will attempt to answer in this chapter.

TERMS AND DEFINITIONS

Having identified the clinical problem, it is necessary to briefly review the names that have been used to refer to it. Dualistic assumptions about the nature of the problem are apparent in the literal meaning of many of the terms.

Terms implying psychological cause

Originally referring to the action of emotional influences on physical symptoms *psychosomatic* now covers all associations between psychological variables and physical symptoms[3]. Indeed it could be argued that its usage has become so wide as to be meaningless. *Somatization* is a related term[4] that clearly implies the conversion of psychological distress into somatic symptoms. There are various definitions, one of the most widely quoted being: 'an idiom of distress in which patients with psychosocial and emotional problems articulate their distress primarily through physical symptomatology'[5]. However the concept of somatization remains inherently dualistic[6] and the associated implication that the somatic symptoms it refers to are really 'mental' has failed to convince physicians and patients alike[7]. In their efforts to be atheoretical, the authors of DSM-III (American Psychiatric Association, 1987)[8] introduced the related term *somatoform*. The term is essentially mentalist and retains strong associations with somatization and simple psychogenesis. It is also rather ugly.

Interestingly, many terms that originally implied a physical cause for symptoms are now used to imply a psychogenic origin. *Hysteria* is one of the oldest terms and has a long and varied history[9]. Its original and literal meaning refers to the physical disease caused by the migration of the uterus around the body[10]. Because of its misconceived and misogynist origins it is now generally avoided, but continues as conversion disorder and dissociative disorder in the classifications (American Psychiatric Association, 1994)[11]. *Hypochondriasis* is another ancient term. Its original and literal meaning referred to the hypochondrium but it now has the connotation of a mental illness. *Neurasthenia* originally implied weak nerves. The term was popular at the turn of the century and was originally believed to have an organic basis. It is now used as a psychiatric diagnosis for unexplained fatigue and implies that this is a mental condition[12].

Terms implying physical causation

Just as the older medical terms have come to imply a psychological cause newer medical terms such as myalgic encephalomyelitis, irritable bowel syndrome, and fibromyalgia imply a physical causation[13].

Non-dualistic terms

More recently introduced terms have attempted to escape from the dualistic trap, but with only limited success. These include *medically unexplained physical symptoms*[14], and *unexplained physical symptoms*[15]. These terms beg the question 'unexplained by what?' To say they are *medically unexplained* introduces an implicit distinction between physical medicine and psychiatric medicine, and assumes that physicians cannot make psychiatric diagnoses. The most explicit term '*medical symptoms not explained by organic disease*', employed for the purpose of a joint venture between the British Royal Colleges of Physicians and Psychiatrists[16] is a more precise, almost operational definition, but still begs important theoretical questions about the definition of organic disease. It is also cumbersome to the point of impracticality.

We therefore return to our original term of *'functional somatic symptoms'*[17]. Functional implies that there is an abnormality in the physical functioning of the body, but this is not of a type or degree that can be detected in terms of gross structural changes and does not exclude a psychological component. Although dualistic thinking has tended to distort the original meaning of this term so that it implies psychogenesis[18], we prefer to retain its original meaning[19].

None of the terms in current use are entirely satisfactory. All may be used to dismiss patients' complaints, all are to a greater or lesser extent predicated on a mind–body division, and most are regarded by patients as pejorative. We have decided wherever possible to employ the term *functional somatic symptoms.* This has been defined by Kellner as 'somatic symptoms not caused by disease detectable by physical examination or routine laboratory investigations, although specific physiologic changes can be detected in some of these symptoms by special techniques'[20]. Functional has the advantage of neither evoking a hypothetical organic process, nor indicating that the origin of the patient's symptoms lies entirely in 'the mind'. Rather it implies that there is a real abnormality in the way the organism is functioning, and as such sets the stage for a more open minded approach.

DO FUNCTIONAL SOMATIC SYMPTOMS MATTER?

Prevalence

Symptoms are common in the general population. The lifetime prevalence of a number of somatic symptoms as elicited in a US population survey is listed in Box 9.1. The main point to note is that one-third of all the symptoms reported were *unexplained* by disease[21].

Box 9.1 Lifetime prevalence of functional somatic symptoms[21]

• Joint pains	37%
• Back pain	32%
• Headache	25%
• Fatigue	25%
• Chest pain	25%
• Arm and leg pain	24%
• Abdominal pain	24%
• Dizziness	23%

Disability and distress

Functional somatic symptoms are also of clinical importance. They tend to persist[22] and are associated with considerable distress and disability. For example, chronic pain and fatigue syndromes are associated with depression, distress and disability[23,24]. In some cases disability can be severe[25].

Use of medical resources

As many as one in five new consultations in primary care are for somatic symptoms for which no specific cause can be found[26]. Whilst many of these complaints are transient, a sizeable proportion are persistent[27]. Furthermore, many patients with functional complaints remain dissatisfied despite the considerable cost of investigating their complaints[22,28]. Functional somatic complaints are also among the commonest reasons for hospital out-patient referral from primary care and are especially frequent in certain specialist clinics. Particularly common are abdominal and bowel symptoms in gastroenterology clinics and chest pain and palpitations in cardiac out-patients. One-third of all patients seen in neurology, cardiology and gastroenterological clinics in Manchester received a final diagnosis of a 'functional' disorder. For most of these patients, the physician's role began and ended with the exclusion of organic disease — hardly any received treatment[29].

The proportion of hospital in-patients with predominantly functional complaints would appear to be lower than that in out-patients. Nonetheless they consume a considerable amount of medical resources. Fink used Danish case registers to document the medical and surgical treatment resources used by the relatively small number of patients who, during an 8 year period, were admitted at least ten times to general hospitals for physical symptoms for which no organic case was found. They had consumed 3% of the budget for admissions to non-psychiatric departments[30].

Ineffectiveness of current medical care

Contrary to what many physicians appear to believe, long-term follow-up studies suggest that many patients who present to out-patient clinics with worry about physical problems are not reassured by negative physical investigations[31]. Any reassurance achieved tends only to be short term[32]. The ineffectiveness of conventional care in these patients is presumably because negative investigations, and hence physicians, tell patients what is *not* wrong with them, rather than what is. So what is wrong with patients suffering from functional complaints?

WHAT IS THE CAUSE OF FUNCTIONAL SOMATIC SYMPTOMS?

All in the mind?

The patient who suffers somatic symptoms for which the doctor can find no demonstrable organic disease is often told that the illness is all in his or her mind[33]. This is the traditional psychiatric perspective. Thus if medical investigations are negative, the problem is not 'physical', and if it is not physical, it must be 'mental'. This mentalist approach conceives of functional somatic symptoms as psychiatric disorders produced by mental mechanisms. The mentalist view has been conceptualized in several ways. The simplest is malingering. The patients do not really have the symptoms. They are simply lying about them to achieve something[34].

A more sophisticated version of this view is to invoke unconscious mental processes. Psychodynamic theory refers to the conflict between different psychic processes, both conscious and unconscious. From the psychodynamic standpoint, functional somatic symptoms are produced by the unconscious mind to serve a purpose. Thus the symptoms might serve to allow the expression of feelings or needs that would be otherwise unacceptable (e.g. the expression of dependency needs), or alternatively to defend the person against a threat to his/her psychic equilibrium (e.g. protecting self-esteem by avoiding blame for perceived failure). This process has been called *primary gain*. The symptoms may also facilitate a desired change in the patient's external world, for example the avoidance of responsibility at work, or even financial advantage. This latter process had been called *secondary gain*[35].

A more recent approach arises from the idea that the symptoms are a consequence of *distorted information processing*. The essence of this approach is that fears and beliefs about minor symptoms (which may have an emotional origin) leads to them becoming a focus of attention and effectively being amplified[36,37]. The patient's distorted interpretation of the symptom may serve to perpetuate the original symptoms. An example would be misinterpretation of functional pain as indicating disease, leading to coping by avoidance of activity, increasing depression and disability, and further preoccupation with the pain[38].

Finally, the social learning approach focuses on the interpersonal causes. Thus patients' 'illness behavior'[39] is learned from others, or from previous experience of disease. The behavior functions as a social communication by which the person attempts to gain legitimacy for the 'sick role'[40]. Validation of the sick role usually requires that it is legitimized by a doctor.

In summary, there are various ways of conceptualizing these symptoms as existing 'above the neck'. These include lying, unconscious conflicts, distorted bodily perception and social learning. But are these descriptions adequate?

All in the body?

An alternative approach to regarding such medically unexplained symptoms as 'all in the mind' is to regard them as 'all in the body'.

They may be assumed to be a manifestation of a hitherto unidentified organic disease or a manifestation of disturbed physiology. This is the traditional and largely prevalent biomedical perspective. In this way many functional somatic complaints are attributed to infection with a virus[41]. Other hypothetical disease processes have been proposed to explain and indeed define specific functional syndromes — these include myalgic encephalomyelitis (ME) as an explanation for chronic fatigue[10], and repetitive strain injury (RSI) for painful hands[42]. The evidence for these hypothetical disease processes is weak.

Yet other explanations may focus exclusively on measurable physiological processes. These commonly involve activity in the autonomic nervous system, and skeletal muscle tension[43]. Examples include increased motility and contractions in the gut of patients with the irritable bowel syndrome[44], hyperventilation in patients reporting non-cardiac chest pain[45] and muscle tension in chronic back pain[46]. There is some empirical support for these explanations, but generally they do not lead to effective treatments.

Mind versus body

Thus functional somatic symptoms are typically viewed from one of two distinct and polar perspectives; one is mentalist or psychiatric, the other physicalist or biomedical. The pervasive, if not always explicit assumption, that mind and body are separate (mind–body dualism) leads to illness being regarded as *either* 'physical' *or* 'mental' in nature[2]. This dichotomization is further complicated by moralistic prejudices which assume that illnesses classified as mental imply a degree of personal weakness or inferiority on the part of the sufferer[47].

MEDICAL OR PSYCHIATRIC?

The dualistic conceptualization of illness is reflected in the way we classify functional somatic symptoms. On the one hand the *medical* approach to medically unexplained illness assumes that the condition is due to a bodily disease, the cause of which will eventually be found. The diagnoses used by exponents of this approach include fibromyalgia, irritable bowel syndrome, repetitive strain injury and myalgic encephalomyelitis. On the other hand the *psychiatric* approach tends to regard these conditions as mental disorders (such as depression or anxiety) which by some perversity, or process of somatization, present as somatic disorders. All seems in order until we find that when these systems are applied simultaneously many patients with 'medical' functional somatic syndromes also meet criteria for 'psychiatric' diagnosis[48]. Are they medical or psychiatric patients?

AN INTEGRATED MEDICAL-PSYCHIATRIC APPROACH

Causation

We suggest that the mental or psychiatric approach to functional somatic symptoms fails to adequately explain the mechanism by which functional somatic symptoms are produced and is unacceptable to many patients. The physical approach of hypothesizing occult disease models has often led up blind alleys such as chronic brucellosis, or the search for a retrovirus to account for chronic fatigue syndrome, and does not lead to effective treatments. We therefore propose an integrated psychophysiological approach to the clinical care of patients suffering from functional somatic symptoms.

Classification

The very fact that there are two overlapping diagnostic systems in existence reflects the traditional and profoundly unhelpful split between the intellectual traditions of psychiatry and that of other medical specialities. Although potentially confusing to the clinician who wishes to obtain the best of both psychiatric and medical knowledge for his patient, it may be less of a problem in practice than it initially appears to be. We advocate the use of precise operational diagnoses based on an adequate assessment of *both* the physical *and* mental state. The absence of identifiable disease should not deter the clinician from the use of clinically valid, reliable and etiologically neutral terminology with which to describe commonalities in patients' illnesses. However, we would discourage the use of diagnoses that do not have explicit criteria for their use, that include unproven assumptions about etiology or imply hypothetical ideas concerning pathology. We suggest that until the medical and psychiatric diagnostic systems are successfully combined the clinician should consider the use of descriptive diagnoses from both systems. For example if the patient meets criteria for both chronic fatigue syndrome and depression both diagnoses may be made as, in the current state of knowledge, the combination of diagnoses conveys more information than either alone.

We consider that management begins with the patient's first contact with the medical services and includes the process of history taking, examination and investigation, the giving of an explanation and advice to the patient, and if appropriate, the prescription of medication, or psychotherapy. Throughout this process the doctor–patient relationship is of crucial importance.

Assessment

Wherever the patient is seen, adequate assessment is the *sine qua non* of management. The specific aims of assessment are:

1. To clarify the nature of the patient's complaints
2. To understand what the patient wants
3. To elicit the patient's fears and beliefs about their illness
4. To exclude organic disease
5. To identify emotional disorder and distress
6. To identify relevant psychological and social stressors.

Formulation

Diagnosis alone is inadequate to determine the treatment of the patient with functional somatic symptoms. Rather, each patient should be assessed individually and a simple formulation produced. A useful formulation should consider multiple etiological factors. These can be conveniently divided into biological, psychological and social realms. It should also distinguish between those factors that may have predisposed the person to develop the illness, those that precipitated it and those that are acting to perpetuate it. Treatment must focus on the perpetuating factors. The formulation may be represented as a grid (see Table 9.1 for an example).

Table 9.1 General approach to formulation

	Predisposing factors	Precipitating factors	Perpetuating factors
Biological	Genetics Temperament	Trauma Infection	Pathophysiological processes
Psychological and behavioral	Habitual modes of thinking Experience of illness	Stress	Belief in disease Fear of disease Avoidance of activity
Social	Quality of relationships Chronic difficulties	Conflict Employment stress Relationship problems	Reinforcement of sick role Ongoing stress

General aspects of treatment

There are a number of general aspects of treatment that must be implemented before more specific measures are considered. These are:

1. Make the patient feel understood
2. Establish a positive collaborative relationship
3. Correct misconceptions about disease and give a positive explanation of symptoms
4. Avoid unnecessary investigation and treatment
5. Negotiate a formulation and treatment plan with the patient.

A satisfactory doctor–patient relationship is essential for treatment success. It is particularly important in the case of patients with functional somatic symptoms who are likely to have experienced disbelief or even dismissal of their symptoms by other doctors[33,49]. Not infrequently an impasse develops in the doctor–patient relationship as a consequence of a mismatch between the patient's expectations and what the doctor is able to provide[50]. We have found that this situation is best managed by shifting the emphasis of the doctor–patient relationship from the traditional pattern, in which the doctor provides all the answers, to a collaborative exploration of the problem and its treatment. This type of therapeutic relationship is central to the practice of cognitive behavior therapy (see below) and has been termed called 'collaborative empiricism'[51].

Patients want an explanation of the origin of their symptoms. Before attempting to do this the doctor should elicit the patient's own theory. This may be close to the doctor's own medical understanding, but may on occasion be idiosyncratic and even bizarre[52]. The first step in the explanation is to try to correct the patient's erroneous beliefs. This often requires sensitivity if the patient is not to feel misunderstood or even humiliated. The second step is to provide as clear and unambiguous a statement as possible about the absence of a sinister disease. The final step is to educate the patient about the actual cause of their symptoms. This explanation should be in positive terms and, if possible, should start from the patient's own theory and be consistent with their own experience.

Box 9.2 Specific treatment measures

- Behavioral and lifestyle change
  - Lifestyle advice
  - Graded increases in activity
  - Relaxation
- Pharmacological
  - Antidepressant drug therapy
  - Other drugs
- Specific psychological interventions
  - Dynamic psychotherapy
  - Cognitive behavior therapy
  - Group therapy
  - Family therapy
- Occupational and social interventions
  - Liaise with employer
  - Occupational counseling
  - Problem solving for social problems

Whenever possible, explanation should be in terms of an integrated physiological and psychological understanding[43]. In some cases (irritable bowel syndrome, pelvic pain and atypical chest pain) plausible and specific physiological mechanisms of symptom production, for which there is reasonable evidence may be incorporated, whereas in other cases the physiological mechanism must be more speculative.

Another important aspect of the management of the patient with functional somatic symptoms is the limiting of further medical opinions, examinations and investigations unless these are likely to offer new and useful information[53]. In addition to these general aspects of treatment there are a number of specific interventions that may be useful. These are best chosen on the basis of the individual formulation. They are listed in Box 9.2.

Behavioral and lifestyle change

There is considerable evidence for the benefits of simple behavioral and lifestyle changes in the management of functional somatic symptoms. The main targets for such changes are (a) stress and lifestyle; and (b) activity and physical fitness. Many symptoms have their origin in anxiety and tension[54,55]. Therefore helping the patient to be aware of tension, to identify sources of 'stress', and to manage these effectively are important therapeutic techniques. Clinical experience suggests that many patients with functional complaints suffer stress because of maladaptive coping strategies. These include excessively high standards, lack of assertiveness, and avoidance of interpersonal conflict. Some may be helped by simple advice about these issues, others will benefit from more specific instruction in relaxation and breathing control, often combined as anxiety management programs[56], whilst yet others may require more specialized psychotherapeutic interventions (see below).

Increased activity and improving physical fitness are of benefit in patients with fatigue and musculoskeletal pain, and are a component of many treatment programs[57]. Activity programs should start at a reasonable level and progress slowly. Initial increases in activity can aggravate symptoms and consequently lead to poor compliance. The patient may therefore need encouragement and help to attribute any increase in symptoms to the physiological effects of activity, rather than to worsening of disease.

Drug therapy

A large number of pharmacological agents have been advocated for the treatment of various functional symptoms[58]. Most are symptomatic remedies, few are of proven efficacy and some may even be harmful. The prescribing of pharmacological agents may also have psychological effects. On the one hand the patient may benefit from a placebo effect[59]; on the other a prescription may serve to reinforce the patient's conviction that they have disease, and to undermine any verbal reassurance given to the contrary[60]. In particular, the use of analgesics may actually perpetuate rather than relieve chronic pain[61]; opiates present their own special problems of addiction. Polypharmacy risks dangerous drug interactions and, in general, should be avoided.

Probably the most useful currently available agents for patients with functional complaints are the so-called 'antidepressant' drugs. The rationale for their use is fully discussed elsewhere[62]. Their applicability extends beyond the treatment of depressive syndromes and includes anxiety and panic, poor sleep, and pain. There is particularly good evidence of their efficacy in the treatment of fibromyalgia[63], chest pain[64] and irritable bowel syndrome[65]. There is also some evidence to support their use in other functional syndromes such as chronic fatigue[66]. The relative usefulness of the newer agents such as the SSRI antidepressants and the reversible MAO inhibitors remains to be established, but they may be found to have specific advantages for particular symptoms. One of the principal problems in using antidepressant drugs is compliance with treatment. This may be maximized by fully discussing the reason for prescribing the drug, its possible side effects and likely benefits, with the patient, and by careful follow-up.

Complementary and alternative therapies

Various terms have been used to describe non-orthodox approaches. *Complementary medicine* implies they work alongside orthodox medicine whilst *alternative therapies* indicates a rival form of therapy. A British Medical Association Working Party (1993)[67] preferred the term *non-conventional therapies* which it defined as 'those forms of treatment which are not widely used by orthodox health care professionals, and skills of which are not taught as part of the undergraduate curriculum of orthodox medicine and medical health care courses'. These non-conventional therapies are very diverse, ranging from those that are at least partially accepted by orthodox practitioners (such as chiropractic and osteopathy) to alternative procedures (such as radionics) which are rejected by virtually all doctors. Non-conventional medical therapies — especially osteopathy, acupuncture and homeopathy — attract patients with functional somatic symptoms. The principal reason is that these patients have understandably become dissatisfied with orthodox medicine.

They are unlikely to have been provided with a credible or comprehensible explanation for their somatic complaints. In contrast, alternative therapists often provide positive explanations which appeal to many patients, and are closely in tune to contemporary ideas of illness and the environment.

There have been far too few adequate evaluations of alternative and complementary treatments to come to any clear conclusions about efficacy, partly because many alternative practitioners reject the concept of a randomized controlled trial (British Medical Association, 1993)[67].

Non-conventional therapy may offer the patient an acceptable answer to symptoms which are of short duration and not of serious medical significance. There are a number of reasons for this. Firstly, some, such as the manipulation therapies for back pain, appear to be effective. Secondly, the placebo benefits can be considerable, especially in patients with functional symptoms. Thirdly, a number of complementary treatments involve relaxation and simple psychotherapy which may be of considerable benefit to this patient group. The dangers of non-conventional approaches are that more appropriate and effective orthodox treatments will be delayed or missed entirely, and the patients may pay large sums of money that can be ill-afforded for unsuccessful therapies.

In summary the manifest failure of the dualistic approach to functional somatic complaints is an important factor driving many patients into the arms of non-conventional therapists. By listening, taking time and adopting an integrated approach to the patient's illness such therapists may enjoy a degree of success. The main problems are that such approaches may deter patients from obtaining more effective conventional care and encourage the further elaboration of already unhelpful illness beliefs. Ideally conventional medicine would embrace an integrated approach rendering much non-conventional care redundant. However the resulting demand would undoubtedly swamp services[68]. The approach we would advocate is to be tolerant of non-conventional therapies provided that they are not interfering with a potentially effective management plan in a patient with significant disability or distress.

Specific psychological therapies

The initial assessment and explanation given to the patient is a *general* psychological treatment of great importance and potential efficacy. It is a skill that should be possessed by all doctors. A variety of *specific* psychotherapies have been employed in the management of patients with functional somatic symptoms. The most commonly practiced are cognitive behavioral and brief dynamic psychotherapies. Ingredients common to both these types of psychotherapy include helping the patient to make sense of their symptoms, to shift their focus of concern from somatic symptoms to relevant psychological and social issues, and to actively deal with relationship and lifestyle problems. There are also differences between them; cognitive behavioral therapies focus more on practical methods of managing symptoms in the present, and dynamic therapies on their historical origins and on relationships, including that of the patient with the therapist[69].

There is currently considerable evidence for the efficacy of cognitive behavioral therapies in the treatment of functional syndromes. Although there has been less systematic evaluation of the efficacy of dynamic psychotherapy in such patients it has been shown to be useful in patients with 'treatment resistant' irritable bowel syndrome[70]. In practice these relatively sophisticated therapies will only be necessary for a minority of patients.

Although usually administered on a one-to-one basis, psychotherapy may also be given in a group setting[71,72] thereby saving skilled therapist time. Therapeutic groups can be difficult to conduct however and the need for careful preparation of each session may mean that less time is saved than might be anticipated.

Family interventions

It is important not to neglect the patient's family and other relationships. These may be relevant to their illness in a variety of ways. First, they may be a major cause of stress. Second, the patient's family may hold strong beliefs about the nature of the patient's illness. Third the behavior of others may shape the patient's adoption of the sick role[73,74]. Where the assessment indicates that they are relevant, these interpersonal factors must be addressed. Perhaps the simplest measure is to arrange a joint interview with patient and spouse or partner in order to explain the nature of the patient's illness and the intended treatment[75]. More formal family therapy has also been advocated for the treatment of functional complaints[76], although it has not been systematically evaluated for this purpose. The family is of particular importance in the management of children and adolescents[77].

The management of occupational and social factors

The workplace may be a source of both psychological and physical stress, and changes in working practice may be important in the management of musculoskeletal pain[78]. Problems with return to work because of dissatisfaction with employment, and reluctance on the part of the employer to permit a gradual return to full duties are major potential obstacles to rehabilitation. Negotiation with occupational physicians or the patient's employers can therefore be important in achieving a return to work[79].

Social factors appear to shape functional illnesses, and may also give rise to 'fashions' in the form such illnesses take[80]. Compensation payments and state benefits can influence the course of functional illness and can be difficult for the individual doctor to influence[81,82].

PRACTICAL TREATMENT IMPLICATIONS

Faced with a patient whose symptoms are functional, how should management be planned and organized? The available evidence suggests that there is, in fact, little specificity in the relationship between a given symptom or syndrome and a given treatment. This means that the pharmacological, psychological and social interventions outlined above may be useful across the range of functional syndromes. The choice of intervention should therefore be more greatly influenced by the formulation of the patient's illness, and by practical considerations than by the specific symptom presented.

Plan of approach

We recommend a stepped care approach to treatment. This means starting with the most simple treatments and only employing more complex and expensive therapies for those who do not respond to simpler measures.

After assessment all patients should be given education and advice, and where possible the patient's spouse or partner should also be interviewed. Care should be taken to avoid iatrogenic harm by not making presumptive diagnoses of disease, ordering excessive investigation or prescribing inappropriate treatment.

If there is evidence of depression, or if there is evidence that the syndrome may respond to an antidepressant, then a trial of an appropriate drug should be considered. The practitioner who feels able to give a brief psychological therapy may use this as an alternative to, or in combination with drug treatment.

If these measures prove to be ineffective, referral for specialist treatment and assessment may be considered. Review by a specialist physician or surgeon may be useful in reassuring both the patient, and the referring doctor, that the problem is not one of occult organic disease, and in facilitating referral for psychological assessment and treatment. Alternatively the doctor may choose to refer the patient for psychological treatment directly. The choice of specific therapy will be dependent both on the availability and on the patient's preference. In most cases we would favor a cognitive behavioral approach, but for patients treated outside research studies it may be more effective to adopt an eclectic approach[83]. This can almost always be administered on an out-patient basis, but in patients who are severely disabled in-patient treatment may be required.

Treatment combinations

Treatment should be kept simple, and targeted at the factors that the assessment indicates are perpetuating the illness. In practice, as with all chronic illness, multiple factors may be important. Combined treatments may include a biological intervention (e.g. an antidepressant), a psychological intervention (e.g. re-attribution of symptoms from disease to functional syndrome), and an interpersonal component (e.g. education of the spouse or partner how to respond to patient's complaints).

Which patients should be treated?

Clearly not every patient who presents with a functional symptom requires specific treatment. The decision to treat must be based on the degree of distress, disability and the duration of the symptoms. Patients who were well-adjusted before becoming ill are more likely to respond to reassurance and other brief treatments. Aims should be less ambitious for those patients who have exhibited lifelong difficulty in social and occupational adjustment.

IMPLICATIONS FOR MEDICAL SERVICES

Ideal care would be based on skilled management by primary care physicians who would assess and treat the majority of patients. Those patients who could not be effectively managed in primary care would be further assessed in the out-patient clinic of the appropriate speciality, their fears discussed, and education given about how to cope with their symptoms. Patients with persistent or severe problems would be seen in specialist clinics run jointly by physicians and specialist psychiatrists or psychologists. These clinics would have ongoing treatment programs for patients with severe functional complaints, probably incorporating some form of cognitive behavioral program[84]. A small in-patient rehabilitation unit would also be available. Clearly most services currently fall far short of this ideal[85].

CHRONIC FATIGUE SYNDROME

Chronic fatigue syndrome (CFS) is a topical and important example of a functional somatic syndrome. In this case the issues of mind versus body have been writ large. Here the meaning and moral status of the illness regarded as psychological are important in shaping the behavior of those with the illness[86,87].

One of the most important areas of progress has been the near universal adoption of uniform case definitions for CFS. The most recent case definition for chronic fatigue syndrome is based on an international consensus of researchers including both psychiatrists and physicians. It represents a clear 'stepping back' from the idea of identifying a new disease, toward an explicit acceptance that it represents nothing more than a working definition of a clinical problem, pending further understanding. This new simpler definition has reduced the number of symptoms required and requires the exclusion of only a small number of specified psychiatric syndromes[88].

Clinical example

A typical patient will be found in the infectious disease department of the hospital. Her principal complaint is of fatigue, poor concentration, and muscle pain. These symptoms are exacerbated by physical and mental exertion, and have led to a substantial reduction in daily activities. The history is of an acute onset of symptoms after a 'viral illness'. Appropriate enquiry often reveals symptoms suggestive of depression or anxiety, but without prominent mood change. The patient believes the illness to be 'medical' rather than 'psychiatric'. When the patient admits to distress, she explains it as a result of the illness rather than its cause. How is her illness best approached? Following the general principles we have described, it is important that a combined medical and psychiatric assessment is performed in every case.

Excluding organic disease

A few of those patients who present with severe

chronic fatigue will be found to have occult organic disease. How frequently organic disease is found will depend on how thorough an assessment the patient has already received. Even if disease is not evident at assessment, it is wise to remain vigilant to this possibility and to reinvestigate if new clinical signs appear. The conditions to be considered include hypothyroidism, anemia, Addison's disease and sleep disorder. In most cases of chronic fatigue simple assessment is adequate. Studies suggests that if a careful history and physical examination do not suggest a specific disease, routine laboratory investigations are likely to add little and should therefore not be routinely performed[89,90]. Although changes have been noted in various other parameters, such as antinuclear factor, immune complexes, immunoglobulin subsets and so on, these are encountered only in a minority, and are rarely substantial. Their significance is for researchers rather than clinicians[91]. Studies of pediatric populations suggest a similar picture — only one alternative diagnosis was uncovered when 55 children with chronic fatigue were fully evaluated in one center[92].

Identifying psychiatric syndromes

All patients should have a psychiatric history taken and their mental state examined. It is worth identifying a number of psychiatric syndromes, because they may guide treatment. The assessment should seek evidence of major depression, anxiety and panic disorder, and also evaluate any suicidal intent. The psychiatric assessment should be systematic as hidden distress is common and casual estimates of the patient's degree of distress may be misleading. Assessing certain symptoms, such as anhedonia (loss of pleasure, characteristic of depression) and avoidance (characteristic of phobic disorder) can be particularly difficult in the setting of profound exhaustion.

Additional patient characteristics

An adequate individual patient assessment must identify all the important obstacles to recovery. It often needs to go beyond diagnosis and to include a systematic individualized description of each case. The aspects to be considered in the systematic description include the individual's beliefs about their illness, their coping behavior, emotional state, and physiological condition as well as interpersonal and occupational problems and the family's understanding of the illness.

The patients' illness beliefs are best elicited by asking them to describe how they understand the cause of their illness, and then probing the answer with questions such as 'what made you think that?' Such enquiries may reveal important misconceptions. A related question is how they cope with their symptoms. Here the assessor is particularly seeking evidence of avoidance of symptom associated activities, unproductive attempts to function normally, or fluctuation between these states. Enquiries into the patient's emotional state will give clues to anxious, depressed or frustrated reactions to the illness and other life difficulties. The patient's physiological state may be directly assessed in a variety of ways although indirect clinical estimation of physiological processes is more common. For example, the capacity for exercise may be assessed by formal exercise testing, or the degree of physiological deconditioning may be estimated from the duration of inactivity. Finally it is almost always useful to interview other family members to obtain both an account of the patient's premorbid personality, as well as the family's beliefs about the illness and its management.

Diagnosis and formulation

The choice of diagnosis should be pragmatic[2]. There is little point in giving a diagnosis of CFS if the patient's symptoms are clearly those of depression or anxiety, and they are accepting of this diagnosis. In other cases a diagnosis of CFS may be the most appropriate: it offers the patient a coherent label for their symptoms and will therefore lessen the risk that they will embark on a fruitless search for a 'better' explanation. The label CFS also avoids the misleading connotations of 'pseudo-disease' labels such as chronic Epstein–Barr virus infection or myalgic encephalomyelitis. Without such a label it is almost impossible to organize dealings with family, friends and work. Patients prefer it — and will vote with their feet until they find a doctor who will validate their illness experience.

We believe that a positive diagnosis of CFS has a place in clinical practice, providing that it is used in a constructive fashion. Above all it is most important that neither the physician nor the patient stops at this diagnosis, but goes on to identify any obstruction to recovery in each case. A diagnosis of CFS, like that of fibromyalgia or irritable bowel syndrome, can be of use in clinical practice as a structure for patient understanding and a model for treatment. What should have no place is affirming a label of CFS, and following this with something along the lines of 'there is no treatment' or 'you will just have to wait until it goes away'.

Individual case description

A multidimensional description provides a comprehensive picture of the factors that may be relevant to the patient's illness and is an important supplement to diagnosis[93,94]. Its use can be illustrated by returning to the case example.

Approach to clinical example

Assessment of the patient described at the beginning of this review revealed that she believed that her symptoms were caused by an ongoing virus infection and that she should beware of exacerbating her symptoms. She consequently avoided activity and had been profoundly inactive for over a year, often lying in bed and sleeping for long periods. She was therefore likely to be physiologically deconditioned. She was frustrated with her inability to do things and sometimes felt low in mood about her predicament. Her job had been very stressful, but since becoming ill she had been unable to work. She had now lost her job and was cared for by her mother who also believed she had permanent disability. Her doctor said that the best thing was rest. The formulation is shown in Table 9.2.

Table 9.2 General approach to formulation

	Perpetuating factors
Biological	Effect of profound inactivity Effect of chronic emotional arousal Other?
Psychological and behavioral	Belief in viral infection Fear of making disease worse Avoidance of activity/problems
Social	No job Reinforcement of sick role by mother and doctor

HOW TO TREAT CHRONIC FATIGUE SYNDROME

The management of patients with CFS should be based on both the diagnostic and individualized formulation of the problem. It can be divided into general and specific treatments. The five basic steps essential to the care of patients with CFS are a prerequisite to any more specialized form of treatment.

1. Acknowledge the reality of the patient's symptoms and the distress and disability associated with them.
2. Provide appropriate education about the nature of the syndrome to both the patient and their family, while avoiding unproductive arguments.
3. Treat identifiable depression and anxiety disorder.
4. Gently encourage a return to normal functioning by overcoming avoidance and regaining the capacity for physical activity.
5. Help the patient to overcome occupational and interpersonal obstacles while maintaining their self-esteem.

Pharmacological treatments

Many pharmacological treatments have been suggested for patients with CFS. To date, none are of proven efficacy and several are potentially harmful[58]. However as described above, patients who are clearly depressed should be offered treatment with so-called antidepressant drugs. There is some evidence to support the use of these drugs even in the absence of definite depressive disorder[66]. Although clinical experience suggests that the SSRI antidepressants may be better tolerated, a recent randomized trial of fluoxetine did not find it to be beneficial[95]. The clinical similarities of CFS to 'atypical' depression may suggest a role for monoamine oxidase inhibitors, but so far there have been no trials of this agent. However, patients are often reluctant to take antidepressants and careful explanation and follow-up are required. Other pharmacological agents should only be used with care and preferably only as part of randomized controlled trials.

Complementary and alternative therapies

No-one can doubt the popularity of alternative approaches to unexplained symptoms in general, and chronic fatigue in particular. As already noted, narrowly defined medical approaches are not particularly effective in the management of chronic fatigue. The popularity of alternative approaches may therefore stem from the recent observation that the general public perceives orthodox medicine as particularly ineffective in the area of chronic fatigue[96]. That leaves the prosaic consideration of efficacy. As yet no complementary approach to the problem of chronic fatigue has been proven to be effective, largely because of the absence of systematic studies[97]. The results of those that have been studied have not been encouraging[98,99,100]. We believe that the effects of complementary therapies are hard to distinguish from those due to the charisma of the practitioner, and that the additional efficacy of the intervention, even if proven, will be small. Therefore we cannot, at present, recommend such approaches for chronic fatigue.

Exercise therapy

This should be considered for patients who are physically inactive. In both fibromyalgia and CFS a modest amount of evidence suggests that *graded* increases in physical activity are helpful in improving function and relieving symptoms[101,102]. However, the simplistic application of exercise regimens, particularly if given without explanation and follow-up, is unlikely to be helpful, and may be harmful by damaging the patient's confidence.

Psychotherapy

Psychosocial difficulties may be targeted using psychotherapy. Reluctance to consider the role of psychological factors in CFS and related syndromes makes the application of psychotherapy potentially difficult, but not impossible. While family therapy[103] and brief psychodynamic therapy[104] may have a place in the management of selected patients, and family approaches are particularly relevant when dealing with children, cognitive behavioral approaches have been the most systematically researched. This form of therapy is especially suited to the task of helping patients to achieve a more helpful view of the illness, and to adopt more effective coping strategies. Several forms of cognitive behavior therapy have been evaluated in patients specifically diagnosed as having CFS. Encouraging results from an initial study[105] were unfortunately not replicated in a further trial[106]. However two recent randomized trials of a form of cognitive behavior therapy especially designed for patients with CFS both achieved a considerable reduction in disability and fatigue, compared with conservative medical care[107], or an equivalent number of relaxation sessions[108]. This form of cognitive behavior therapy placed particular emphasis on helping patients to reappraise their illness beliefs, as well as on increasing activity and solving social problems, and consisted of between 12 and 16 weekly individual treatment sessions. We may conclude that cognitive behavior therapy offers a potentially useful approach to the rehabilitation of patients with CFS. However, it also has the limitation of requiring skilled therapists, and will not help all patients.

CONCLUSIONS

In this chapter we have outlined the concept of functional somatic symptoms and syndromes, and drawn attention to their prevalence and public health importance. We have also discussed models for understanding these conditions, and, in keeping with the philosophy underlying this book, have emphasized the need to develop multifactorial models of illness, to supersede ideas still prevalent of disease as either physical or psychiatric. We hope that we have convinced the reader that functional somatic symptoms and syndromes cannot be adequately understood either as simple expressions of physical pathology, or in terms of a traditional psychiatric framework. Instead, we suggest that this can only be achieved by introducing a biopsychosocial framework, and the idea that what starts (precipitates) an illness needs to be distinguished from what perpetuates it. Finally, we have chosen the example of chronic fatigue syndrome to illustrate the application of these principles in clinical practice.

REFERENCES

1 Susser M 1990 Disease, illness, sickness: impairment, disability and handicap. Psychological Medicine 20:471–3
2 Mayou R, Sharpe M 1995 Diagnosis, illness and disease. Quarterly Journal of Medicine 88:827–31
3 Lipowski ZJ 1984 What does the word 'psychosomatic' really mean? A historical and semantic inquiry. Psychosomatic Medicine 46:153–71
4 Murphy MR 1989 Somatisation: embodying the problem. British Medical Journal 298:1331–2
5 Katon WJ 1984 Depression: relationship to somatization and chronic medical illness. Journal of Clinical Psychiatry 45:4–12
6 Mumford D 1992 Does 'somatization' explain anything? Psychiatry in Practice Spring: 11–14
7 Mace CJ, Trimble MR 1991 Hysteria, functional or psychogenic? A survey of British neurologist's preferences. Journal of the Royal Society of Medicine 84:471–5
8 American Psychiatric Association 1987 Diagnostic and Statistical Manual of Mental Disorders, Third edition. American Psychiatric Association, Washington, DC
9 Mersky H 1986 The importance of hysteria. British Journal of Psychiatry 149:23–8
10 Richmond C 1989 Myalgic encephalomyelitis, Princess Aurora, and the wandering womb. British Medical Journal 298:1295–6
11 American Psychiatric Association 1994 Diagnostic and Statistical Manual of Mental Disorders, Fourth edition. American Psychiatric Association, Washington, DC
12 Wessely S 1991 History of postviral fatigue syndrome. British Medical Bulletin 47:919–41
13 Kellner R 1991 Psychosomatic syndromes and somatic symptoms. American Psychiatric Press, Washington, DC
14 Mayou RA 1991 Medically unexplained physical symptoms. British Medical Journal 303:534–5
15 Escobar JI, Canino G 1989 Unexplained physical complaints. Psychopathology and epidemiological correlates. British Journal of Psychiatry 154:24–7
16 Creed F, Mayou R, Hopkins A 1992 Medical symptoms not explained by organic disease. The Royal College of Psychiatrists and the Royal College of Physicians of London, London
17 Stearns AW 1946 A History of the development of the concept of functional nervous disease during the past twenty-five hundred years. American Journal of Psychiatry 103:289–308
18 Lipkin M 1969 Functional or organic? A pointless question. Annals of Internal Medicine 5:1013–17
19 Trimble MR 1982 Functional diseases. British Medical Journal 285:1768–70
20 Kellner R 1985 Functional somatic symptoms and hypochondriasis. Archives of General Psychiatry 42:821–33
21 Kroenke K, Price RK 1993 Symptoms in the community. Prevalence, classification, and psychiatric comorbidity. Archives of Internal Medicine 153:2474–80
22 Kroenke K, Mangelsdorff D 1989 Common symptoms in ambulatory care: incidence, evaluation, therapy and outcome. American Journal of Medicine 86:262–6
23 Dworkin SF, Von Korff M, LeResche L 1990 Multiple pains and psychiatric disturbance. An epidemiologic investigation. Archives of General Psychiatry 47:239–44
24 Wessely S, Powell R 1989 Fatigue syndromes: a comparison of chronic 'postviral' fatigue with neuromuscular and affective disorder. Journal of Neurology, Neurosurgery and Psychiatry 52:940–8
25 Smith GR, Jr., Monson RA, Ray DC 1986 Patients with multiple unexplained symptoms. Their characteristics, functional health, and health care utilization. Archives of Internal Medicine 146:69–72
26 Bridges KW, Goldberg DP 1985 Somatic presentation

of DSM III psychiatric disorders in primary care. Journal of Psychosomatic Research 29:563–9
27 Kroenke K, Spitzer RL, Williams JB, Linzer M, Hahn SR, deGruy FV, 3rd, Brody D 1994 Physical symptoms in primary care. Predictors of psychiatric disorders and functional impairment. Archives of Family Medicine 3:774–9
28 Kroenke K, Arrington ME, Manglesdorff D 1990 The prevalence of symptoms in medical outpatients and the adequacy of therapy. Archives of Internal Medicine 150:1685–9
29 Hamilton J, Campos R, Creed F 1996 Anxiety, depression and the management of medically unexplained symptoms in medical clinics. Journal of the Royal Society of Medicine 30:18–21
30 Fink P 1992 Surgery and medical treatment in persistent somatizing patients. Journal of Psychosomatic Research 36:439–47
31 Channer KS, James MA, Papouchado M, Rees JR 1987 Failure of a negative exercise test to reassure patients with chest pain. Quarterly Journal of Medicine 63:315–22
32 Sox HC, Jr., Margulies I, Sox CH 1981 Psychologically mediated effects of diagnostic tests. Annals of Internal Medicine 95:680–5
33 Ware NC 1992 Suffering and the social construction of illness: the delegitimation of illness experience in chronic fatigue syndrome. Medical Anthropology Quarterly 6:347–61
34 Miller E 1988 Defining hysterical symptoms. Psychological Medicine 18:275–7
35 M'Uzan M, de 1974 Psychodynamic mechanisms in psychosomatic symptom formation. Psychotherapy and Psychosomatics 23:103–10
36 Barsky AJ 1992 Amplification, somatization, and the somatoform disorders. Psychosomatics 33:28–34
37 Salkovskis PM 1989 Cognitive behavior therapy for psychiatric problems Hawton K, Salkovskis PM, Kirk J, Clark DM (eds) Oxford Medical Publications, Oxford, pp 235–276
38 Philips HC 1987 Avoidance behavior and its role in sustaining chronic pain. Behavior Research and Therapy 25:273–9
39 Mechanic D 1962 The concept of illness behavior. Journal of Chronic Diseases 15:189–94
40 Parsons T 1951 The social system. Free Press of Glencoe, New York.
41 Cope H, David A, Mann A 1994 'Maybe it's a virus?' beliefs about viruses, symptom attributional style and psychological health. Journal of Psychosomatic Research 38:89–98
42 Hall W, Morrow L 1988 'Repetition strain injury': an Australian epidemic of upperlimb pain. Social Science in Medicine 27:645–9
43 Sharpe M, Bass C 1992 Pathophysiological mechanisms in somatization. International Reviews in Psychiatry 4:81–97
44 Camilleri M, Ford MJ 1994 Functional gastrointestinal disease and the autonomic nervous system: a way ahead? Gastroenterology 106:1114–8
45 Chambers J, Bass C 1990 Chest pain with normal coronary anatomy: a review of natural history and possible etiologic factors. Progress in Cardiovascular Disease 33:161–84
46 Flor H, Turk DC, Birbaumer N 1985 Assessment of stress-related psychophysiological reactions in chronic back pain patients. Journal of Consulting and Clinical Psychology 53:354–64
47 Kirmayer LJ 1988 Biomedicine Examined Lock M, Gordon D (eds) Kluwer, Dordrecht, pp 57–92
48 Simon GE, VonKorff M 1991 Somatization and psychiatric disorder in the NIMH Epidemiologic Catchment Area study. American Journal of Psychiatry 148:1494–500
49 Reid J, Ewan C, Lowy E 1991 Pilgrimage of pain: the illness experiences of women with repetition strain injury and the search for credibility. Social Science in Medicine 32:601–12
50 Sharpe M, Mayou R, Seagroatt V, Surawy C, Warwick H, Bulstrode C, Dawber R, Lane D 1994 Why do doctors find some patients difficult to help? Quarterly Journal of Medicine 87:187–93
51 Beck AT Rush AJ Shaw BF, Emery G 1979 Cognitive therapy of depression. Guilford Press, New York
52 Wright AL, Morgan WJ 1990 On the creation of 'problem' patients. Social Science in Medicine 30:951–9
53 Todd JW 1984 Investigations. Lancet ii:1146–7
54 Sainsbury P, Gibson JG 1954 Symptoms of anxiety and tension and the accompanying physiological changes in muscular system. Journal of Neurology, Neurosurgery and Psychiatry 17:216–24
55 Tyrer P 1976 Institute of Psychiatry Maudsley Monograph 23: The role of bodily feelings in anxiety. Oxford University Press, Oxford
56 Sorby NG, Reavley W, Huber JW 1991 Self help programme for anxiety in general practice: controlled trial of an anxiety management booklet. British Journal of General Practice 41:417–20
57 Scordo KA 1991 Effects of aerobic exercise training on symptomatic women with mitral valve prolapse. American Journal of Cardiology 67:863–8
58 Gantz NM, Holmes GP 1989 Treatment of patients with chronic fatigue syndrome. Drugs 38:855–62
59 Shepherd M 1993 The placebo: from specificity to the non-specific and back. Psychological Medicine 23:569–78
60 Elks ML 1994 On the genesis of somatization disorder: the role of the medical profession. Medical Hypotheses 43:151–4
61 Pither CE 1989 Treatment of persistent pain. British Medical Journal 299:1239–40
62 Katon W, Sullivan M 1995 Treatment of Functional Somatic Symptoms. Mayou R, Bass C, Sharpe M. (eds) Oxford University Press, Oxford
63 Goldenberg DL 1989 Treatment of fibromyalgia syndrome. Rheumatic Diseases Clinics of North America 15:61–71
64 Cannon RO, Quyyumi AA, Mincemoyer R, Stine AM, Gracely RH, Smith WB 1994 Imipramine in patients with chest pain despite normal coronary angiograms. New England Journal of Medicine 330:1411–17
65 Greenbaum DS, Mayle JE, Vanegeren LE, Jerome JA, Mayor JW, Greenbaum RB, Matson RW, Stein GE, Dean HA, Halvorsen NA et al. 1987 Effects of

desipramine on irritable bowel syndrome compared with atropine and placebo. Digestive Disease and Science 32:257–66
66 Lynch S, Seth R, Montgomery S 1991 Antidepressant therapy in the chronic fatigue syndrome. British Journal of General Practice 41:339–42
67 British Medical Association 1993 Complementary Medicine. New approaches to good practice. Oxford University Press, Oxford
68 Eisenberg DM, Kessler RC, Foster C, Norlock FE, Calkins DR, Delbanco TL 1993 Unconventional medicine in the United States — prevalence, costs and pattern of use. New England Journal of Medicine 328:246–52
69 Altshuler KZ, Rush AJ 1984 Psychoanalytic and cognitive therapies: a comparison of theory and tactics. American Journal of Psychotherapy 38:4–17
70 Guthrie E, Creed F, Dawson D, Tomenson B 1991 A controlled trial of psychological treatment for the irritable bowel syndrome. Gastroenterology 100:450–7
71 Stern R, Fernandez M 1991 Group cognitive and behavioural treatment for hypochondriasis. British Medical Journal 303:1229–31
72 Melson SJ, Rynearson EK 1986 Intensive group therapy for functional illness. Psychiatric Annals 16:687–92
73 Benjamin S, Mawer J, Lennon S 1992 The knowledge and beliefs of family care givers about chronic pain patients. Journal of Psychosomatic Research 36:211–17
74 Turk DC, Flor H, Rudy TE 1987 Pain and families. I. Etiology, maintenance, and psychosocial impact. Pain 30:3–27
75 Flor H, Turk DC, Rudy TE 1987 Pain and families. II. Assessment and treatment. Pain 30:29–45
76 Griffith JL, Griffith ME, Slovik LS 1989 Mind-body patterns of symptom generation. Family Process 28:137–52
77 Rikard-Bell CJ, Waters BGH 1992 Psychosocial management of chronic fatigue syndrome in adolescence. Australian and New Zealand Journal of Psychiatry 26:64–72
78 Brooks P 1993 Repetitive strain injury: does not exist as a separate medical condition. British Medical Journal 307:1298
79 Peel M 1988 Rehabilitation in postviral syndrome. Journal of Social and Occupational Medicine 38:44–5
80 Shorter E 1995 Sucker-punched again! Physicians meet the disease-of-the-month syndrome. Journal of Psychosomatic Research 39:115–18
81 Lucire Y 1988 Social iatrogenesis of the Australian disease 'RSI'. Community Health Studies 12:146–50
82 Binder LM, Rohling ML 1996 Money matters: a meta-analytic review of the effects of financial incentives on recovery after closed-head injury. American Journal of Psychiatry 153:7–10
83 Murphy M 1993 Psychological treatment in disease and illness Hodes M, Moorey S (eds) Gaskell, London, pp 65–87
84 Speckens AEM, Van Hemert AM, Spinjoven P, Hawton KE, Bolk JH, Rooijmans GM 1995 Cognitive behavioral therapy for medically unexplained physical symptoms: a randomized clinical trial. British Medical Journal 311:1328–32
85 Royal Colleges of Physicians and Psychiatrists 1995 Joint Working Party Report: The psychological care of medical patients; recognition of need and service provision. Royal College of Physicians and Royal College of Psychiatrists, London
86 Wessely S 1994 Chronic fatigue syndrome. In: Straus, S E (ed) Marcel Dekker Inc., New York, pp 3–44
87 Sharpe M 1996 Chronic fatigue syndrome. Psychiatric Clinics of North America 19:549–73
88 Fukuda K, Straus SE, Hickie I, Sharpe M, Dobbins JG, Komaroff AL 1994 Chronic fatigue syndrome: a comprehensive approach to its definition and management. Annals of Internal Medicine 121:953–9
89 Swanink CM, Vercoulen JH, Bleijenberg G, Fennis JF, Galama JM, Van der Meer JW 1995 Chronic fatigue syndrome: a clinical and laboratory study with a well matched control group. Journal of Internal Medicine 237:499–506
90 Valdini AF, Steinhardt S, Feldman E 1989 Usefulness of a standard battery of laboratory tests in investigating chronic fatigue in adults. Family Practice 6:286–91
91 Bates DW, Buchwald DS, Lee J, Kith P, Doolittle T, Rutherford C, Churchill WH, Schur PH, Wener M, Wybenga D et al. 1995 Clinical laboratory test findings in patients with chronic fatigue syndrome. Archives of Internal Medicine 155:97–103
92 Feder HM, Jr., Dworkin PH, Orkin C 1994 Outcome of 48 pediatric patients with chronic fatigue. A clinical experience. Archives of Family Medicine 3:1049–55
93 Turk DC, Flor H 1989 Primary fibromyalgia is greater than tender points: toward a multiaxial taxonomy. Journal of Rheumatology Supplement 19:80–6
94 Vercoulen JH, Swanink CM, Fennis JF, Galama JM, Van der Meer JW, Bleijenberg G 1994 Dimensional assessment of chronic fatigue syndrome. Journal of Psychosomatic Research 38:383–92
95 Vercoulen JH, Swanink CM, Zitman FG, Vreden S, Hoofs M, Fennis JF, Galama JM, Van der Meer JW, Bleijenberg G 1996 Randomized, double-blind, placebo-controlled study of fluoxetine in chronic fatigue syndrome. Lancet 347:858–61
96 Vincent C, Furnham A 1994 The perceived efficacy of complementary and orthodox medicine: preliminary findings and the development of a questionnaire. Complementary Therapies in Medicine 2:128–34
97 Dowson D 1993 The treatment of chronic fatigue syndrome by complementary medicine. Complementary Therapies in Medicine 1:9–13
98 Kaslow J, Rucker L, Onishi R 1989 Liver extract-folic acid-cyanocobalamin vs placebo for chronic fatigue syndrome. Archives of Internal Medicine 149:2501–3
99 Morris D, Stare F 1993. Unproven diet therapies in the treatment of chronic fatigue syndrome. Archives of Family Medicine 2:181–6
100 Martin R, Ogston S, Evans J 1994 Effects of vitamin and mineral supplementation on symptoms associated with chronic fatigue syndrome with Coxsackie B antibodies. Journal of Nutritional Medicine 4:11–23
101 McCain GA, Bell DA, Mai FM, Holliday PD 1988 A controlled study of the effects of a supervised cardiovascular fitness training programme on the mainfestations of primary fibromyalgia. Arthritis and Rheumatism 31:1135–41

102 Burckhardt CS, Mannerkorpi K, Hedenberg L, Bjelle A 1994 A randomized, controlled clinical trial of education and physical training for women with fibromyalgia. Journal of Rheumatology 21:714–20

103 Graham H 1990 Family interventions in general practice: a case of chronic fatigue. Journal of Family Therapy 13:225–30

104 Taerk G, Gnam W 1994 A psychodynamic view of the chronic fatigue syndrome: the role of object relations in etiology and treatment. General Hospital Psychiatry 16:319–25

105 Butler S, Chalter T, Ron M, Wessely S 1991 Cognitive Behavior therapy in chronic fatigue syndrome. Journal of Neurology, Neurosurgery and Psychiatry 54:153–8

106 Lloyd AR, Hickie I, Brockman A, Hickie C, Wilson A, Dwyer J, Wakefield D 1993 Immunologic and psychologic therapy for patients with chronic fatigue syndrome: a double-blind, placebo-controlled trial. American Journal of Medicine 94:197–203

107 Sharpe M, Hawton K, Simkin S, Surawy C, Hackmann A, Klimes I, Peto T, Warrell D, Seagroatt V 1996 Cognitive behavior therapy for chronic fatigue syndrome: a randomized controlled trial. British Medical Journal 312:22–6

108 Deale A, Chalder T, Everitt B, Marks I, Wessely S 1997 Cognitive behavior therapy for chronic fatigue syndrome: a randomized controlled trial. American Journal of Psychiatry 154:408–414

CHAPTER CONTENTS

10

Psychological health: helping people in stress and distress

Simon Easton

INTRODUCTION

Stress and distress appear to be part and parcel of human experience, and at times almost all of us are subject to intense periods of stress or distress. Occasionally, stress is positively sought out, but more frequently it is seen as highly undesirable. Many people are unclear what they should do about stress and think it is just something they simply have to put up with. Distress, on the other hand, is usually seen as undesirable, and it normally provokes attempts to stop or reduce the distressing experience.

Stress has commanded much attention because it is commonly seen as a prime cause of distress. As a result, better management of stress seems attractive because it deals with the cause rather than the effect.

Stress can lead to significant, but avoidable, costs for the individual, employers and the wider society in which they live. It has been suggested that more than 40% of absenteeism at work can be attributed to stress[1], and the costs of stress to society are huge when reduced productivity, health care costs and other indirect consequences of an individual's experience of stress are taken into account.

Prolonged stress is now recognized even at governmental level as playing a major part in the onset of mental and physical health problems[2]. Stress has been shown to play a key role in the onset and maintenance of an ever-increasing list of health problems such as depression, hypertension, and ischemic heart disease[3,4,5].

Stress might be expected to affect an individual's well-being in various ways. The 'fight or flight' response to stress, involving hormonal and chemical defense mechanisms may adversely affect an individual's well-being if those defense mechanisms are frequently triggered, or if they are activated over a longer period[6,7].

Alternatively, stress may lead to behaviors which can adversely affect an individual's health, as, for example, when an individual turns to drinking alcohol excessively, or as appetite and eating habits change. Psychological approaches often focus on both preventing the fight and flight response, and on behavioral or situational change.

Stress management training, one-to-one counseling and educational programs on stress reduction have all been shown, in various settings, to give rise to a range of benefits which frequently include affective and physiological changes, as well as practical changes, such as reduction in absenteeism from work[8].

The psychological interventions used in stress management are based on the psychotherapies which have been shown to be generally effective when used with individuals in clinical settings with moderate and severe psychological difficulties[9]. Thus the talking therapies may play a part in preventing stress and its consequences, as well as helping people to manage physical illness and to adapt their behavior to foster recovery of health.

Stress can strike at the heart of an individual's quality of life, both directly and indirectly. It can trigger ill health and it can delay or thwart recovery from ill health. The psychological coping strategies of an individual, and their experience of stress and distress are at the center of a comprehensive understanding of an individual's mental and psychological health. Therefore, it is argued that not only is stress management likely to be cost-effective, but the effects of stress reduction on the quality of life may be dramatic. It could be argued that psychological health warrants as much, if not more, attention in primary care than physical health.

DEFINITIONS AND PERCEPTIONS

Despite a wealth of research on the theoretical effects of stress on a wide variety of diseases, and some agreement on the importance of stress in some specific diseases, the incorporation of stress management into health care in everyday practice is some way off. This is partly due to a problem with the word 'stress', itself. Unfortunately, stress is used both to describe the stimulus and the response — both the cause and the reaction. In addition, confusion springs from the idea that stress can be good ('eustress') or bad. Even greater confusion springs from the wider use of the word to include physical stress experienced by an individual.

Sutherland and Cooper (1990)[10] accurately reflect the broad agreement in the psychological literature when they state that 'the contemporary approach to understanding stress embraces an interactive viewpoint (i.e. stress is in the eye of the beholder)'. They add, however: 'it is necessary to be aware of potential stressors in the environment'. Cohen et al. (1991)[11] underlined this point when they showed that reaction to a common cold virus was associated both with an individual's perception of stress and their experience of stressors in the environment. Thus stress is not only the product of our perceptions; it can also be produced by environmental stressors which may be too small to consciously impinge on our perceptions.

A number of factors, such as cognitive appraisal, experience and physical resources have been proposed as central to our understanding of stress[12,13,14]. In practical terms, this means that individuals might try to manage stress by avoiding unnecessary stressors and/or by changing their perception of those stressors which are unavoidable. Alternatively, they might seek to improve their resistance to the stressors they encounter.

Lazarus' model of stress draws attention to the importance of both an individual's appraisal of an event, and their appraisal of their coping abilities and resources. When an individual perceives that the threat is high and their ability to cope is low, then they tend to experience stress[13].

Some individuals may find certain stressors more difficult to manage. For example, 'schizophrenia' as described by Zubin and Spring (1977)[15] may be understood in terms of a lowered resistance to stressors in genetically vulnerable individuals. Problems with the reliability and validity of the diagnosis of 'schizophrenia'[16] have led to confusion in attempts to develop this theme. However, recent research, which emphasizes the role of coping mechanisms, has led to a 'dynamic vulnerability formulation' of mental illness[17]. Such a model suggests that many people labeled 'schizophrenic', and others, might benefit from stress management training. It also suggests that an attempt to reduce the level of stressors in an individual's environment would be valuable. Such approaches have proven effective in work with whole families[18,19].

PSYCHIATRIC CONTINUUM

This emphasis on the role of stress in the etiology of distress and mental ill health tends to reduce the emphasis on formal psychiatric diagnoses, moving away from a 'them and us' approach to a more dynamic approach which addresses the commonality of experience. An emphasis on the continuum of experience between happiness, mild unhappiness, depression and misery, for example, encourages a recognition of each individual's resources and capabilities which will be needed for change, without ignoring the role played by other physical or social factors. Bentall (1992)[20] has underlined many of the problems associated with diagnoses in mental health in a (tongue in cheek) proposal to classify happiness as a psychiatric disorder.

A focus on understanding an individual's unique set of circumstances is of ultimate importance in helping them tackle distress. Generalizations inherent in psychiatric diagnosis seem to hinder, rather than help an understanding of stress and distress[21]. Time spent on distinguishing between anxiety or depression might be better spent trying to understand the individual's circumstances and developing ideas about interventions based on a formulation specific to the individual. This approach promotes a consideration of all factors, rather than a preoccupation with any one factor in isolation. In addition, it attempts to identify causes as well as effects. Thus the concepts of stress and distress and their role in the etiology of mental ill health are central to any understanding of an individual's psychological well-being.

Overall, stress remains a complex area for theory and research. A focus on an individual's perception of stress and their perception of their ability to meet the demands made upon them would appear to be beneficial in helping them reduce, avoid, or more effectively manage stressors.

TALKING THERAPIES IN STRESS AND DISTRESS

Individuals in distress will often seek an opportunity to talk to someone else about their situation. The help offered can be informal, for instance when a general practioner offers advice or gives someone the opportunity to 'offload' their problems; or it can be more formally offered as counseling. When more formal help is likely to be of use, the question arises as to the most appropriate form that talking therapy should take. Is talking therapy a highly skilled task or simply a straightforward process of listening and guidance? Does training confer special skills in the talking therapies?

Issues of competence, qualifications, expertise and professionalism in the talking therapies are only very slowly being tackled. The very titles of counselor, psychotherapist and psychologist, among others, offer little consistent guidance as to the skills, qualifications and legitimacy of those offering help to individuals in distress. Even the widely used title of counsellor does not clearly indicate the nature of the service to be expected. Counseling can refer to many things, including listening and sympathy, lengthy psychoanalysis, and interventions drawing upon healing and religious beliefs.

Attempts to define the essence of counseling, as distinct from structured psychological therapies, have been difficult. However, such attempts to identify the most appropriate level of expertise required by those seeking help do warrant the effort if people are to receive the help they need.

Typically, counseling is seen as a process aimed at strengthening, rather than changing, an individual's defenses and their ability to cope with stressful situations. Counseling tends to draw upon general listening skills and helps people to help themselves. Psychological therapy not only draws upon counseling processes, but also offers individuals the opportunity to develop and, if necessary, change, strategies and defenses. Thus, counseling and psychological therapy might usefully be seen as points on a continuum of expertise. Such a distinction between the role of counsellors and psychological therapists may help both referrers and individuals in distress to identify the most appropriate level of expertise needed.

THE ESSENCE OF THE THERAPEUTIC RELATIONSHIP

A good psychotherapeutic relationship depends, to a large extent, on the therapist, and it does appear that the therapist's well-being is likely to enhance outcome[22]. However, a therapist's well-being is not necessarily enhanced by personally undergoing therapy[23]. A therapist needs to be comfortable enough to be able to focus their attention on the needs of the client. It may, however, be helpful to remember that feeling comfortable and at ease with oneself does not necessarily require psychotherapy.

While it has been argued that the essence of counseling is to provide a good human relationship[24], some confusion has arisen as to when formal counseling is or isn't taking place. Counseling is used to refer to everything from disciplining to the information-giving that might accompany the prescription of drugs. The British Association for Counselling has suggested that counseling occurs 'when a counselor offers or agrees in an explicit way to offer someone the opportunity to explore, discover and clarify ways of living in a more resourceful and satisfying way'[25]. This endeavor to define counseling is not merely an attempt to undermine the value of advice, information-giving and other ways of helping: rather, it is an attempt to highlight the idea that counseling has a distinct identity. Counseling differs from other forms of helping in its central focus on the counselor's establishing an empathic, accepting, collaborative and genuine relationship with the counselee[26].

Rogers (1957)[24] suggested that warmth, acceptance of the client, accurate empathy and openness were essential, and perhaps entirely sufficient in helping people in distress. Counseling is presented as being about establishing a good human relationship, which might, in itself, be enough to help someone feel better emotionally.

The observation that widely differing forms of psychotherapy appear to have largely similar success rates, and all tend to be more successful (on average) than no intervention[27], has supported this view that the relationship, rather than the psychotherapeutic technique, might be of central importance. The widely differing theories and philosophies behind different approaches to counseling and psychological therapy may play little part in establishing the relationship. Major reviews on the role of different psychotherapeutic strategies have disagreed on whether all therapies are equivalent[28] or whether specific techniques, such as cognitive therapy or behavior therapy might be more successful at helping people tackle specific difficulties[29,30]. It is not clear whether the difficulties associated with research in this area have obscured real differences in effectiveness of the various approaches, or whether the specific psychotherapeutic approach used is irrelevant so long as it does not disrupt the essential relationship.

It may be that counseling and psychological therapy simply offer something straightforward, such as friendship[31], or direct feedback[32,33]. At this stage, however, 'it is possible that all the models are equally unsound scientifically, but they energize therapists and provide useful fictions to activate the patients to lead somewhat more satisfying lives'[34]. Counselors need some theory (or myth) to guide them in their dealings with clients, which makes them look and feel competent[33]. Alternatively it might be that all the various therapies are trying to say the same thing, struggling towards some kind of 'truth'; they merely differ in the way they are trying to express that 'truth'.

The common factors in psychotherapy are often defined, regardless of the school of training or theory, in such a way that the emphasis is more on the process than on the technical detail of interventions. Thus, Frank (1985)[35] has suggested that psychotherapeutic intervention is no more than an elaboration or adaptation of healing processes that have been used since human beings first noticed the distress of those around them and tried to help. He emphasizes the setting in which therapy tends to be offered. Within western culture, today, psychotherapists would typically have credentials as a healer and they would be expected to behave in certain ways that imply some underlying theory. Some form of ritualistic behaviour would be typical and, in theory at least, the interaction between therapist and client would be targeted entirely on the needs of the client.

In other cultures, however, it may be that such a socially accepted process and the implicit aim of fostering increased autonomy for the individual might be seen as rather strange — indeed, it has been suggested that many Hindus would see the fostering of some dependency on others (rather than fostering independency and autonomy) as an essential part of any endeavor to help people in distress[36].

It may therefore be that the 'truth' for one cultural group might be quite different from that which would be appropriate for another. Psychotherapeutic interventions and counseling might, therefore, need to be tailored to address factors such as ethnic background culture of clients[37].

WHICH TALKING THERAPY?

Acceptance of the apparent equivalence of therapies has been questioned by many[28,38]. Some have seen the failure of research to guide practice as proof that counseling is an art. Others have interpreted the confusion in the research findings as allowing them to do what they feel is right, hoping that any future research will vindicate their choice of approach in counseling. Alternatively, some theorists have endeavored to use the research on the process of therapy to draw together what they see as the effective elements of different therapies in a cookbook approach, matching the intervention to the symptom[39,40].

Others, however, have suggested that the available evidence is strong enough to indicate that certain therapeutic approaches might be more effective for different groups of problems. Rosenhan and Selligman (1989)[41], for example, summarized what they saw as the broad consensus in suggesting that the more simple fears and anxieties could be most successfully treated with behavioral approaches, and that depression could be most effectively tackled with cognitive therapy.

Straightforward counseling (i.e. listening and helping someone clarify their concerns) may be most useful for mild problems, and in a range of situations, such as helping people manage grief, make decisions, or make choices. There are a few specific approaches which may be helpful for some problems (e.g. Masters and Johnsons' interventions for sexual problems (1970))[42], but a competent therapeutic approach may well serve as a basis for helping individuals in distress understand and tackle their problems, whatever they may be.

While counseling skills might be used in brief consultations, counseling and psychological interventions, the establishment of a good therapeutic relationship needed for counseling and therapy, usually involves rather more time. If empathy, warmth, and acceptance are to be present, and perceived as genuine, then a relationship must be established effectively in such a way as to promote and foster these qualities. Other aspects of counseling which have been described as characteristic, such as confession, atonement and encouragement[35], would usually be offered within the context of an established relationship. Unfortunately, attempts to rigorously explore such constructs in the counseling setting have been woefully unsuccessful[43].

In the absence of clear guidance from the research literature to date, it would still appear sensible to develop therapeutic approaches based on sound theory and empiricism. Even though some of the more bizarre therapies cannot be shown to be less effective, and have been criticized as being no more relevant than medieval theology[44], a balance has to be struck between considered conservatism in approach and open-mindedness towards new ideas.

Nevertheless, as the consensus does suggest that psychotherapy is better than nothing, it seems fair to say that appropriate referral for counseling or psychological therapy would generally be worthwhile. Beyond that, the suggestion that cognitive therapies might be useful for people feeling depressed, and behavioral therapies might be most useful for people experiencing fear and anxiety could be of use, but such therapeutic approaches can only be successful if the relationship between helper and client is sound.

WHICH THERAPIST?

Recognized accreditation or registration, along with personal recommendation and information on the counselor's approach may offer the best basis for selection for referral. Sex, age, race, and class of the therapist seem to have little relevance to effectiveness, but it may be sensible to think twice about referral to therapists who hold extremist views, or who exhibit behavior significantly removed from the cultural norm[23].

Many of the ideas developed for established professions which help shape appropriate behaviour might serve as guidelines for counselors and psychological therapists. Bell (1989)[45] has suggested that quality assurance and values training for therapists, along with collaborative relationships in therapy can play an important part in protecting clients from inappropriate influence by therapists. In the UK, confusion about the qualifications needed has led to accreditation of counselors by the British Association for Counselling, which is the major body representing counselors in the UK. Similarly, the British Psychological Society has established a charter to which recognized clinical psychologists are appointed. A counselor accredited by the British Association of Counselling or a chartered clinical psychologist should therefore be bound by a code of conduct and they would have been judged competent to practice. However, the scarcity of these qualifications and the availability of other well qualified individuals continues to lead to confusion.

An initial session with a therapist or counselor should always be seen as assessment of that particular helper's apparent experience and competence. If the client does not feel comfortable or reasonably confident that the helper can assist them, then it may be better to try another helper rather than persist. A good helper would make it clear that a client's choice is acceptable, whatever the outcome.

The choice of therapist may also depend simply on likes and dislikes. Someone's strong dislike or disinterest in counseling and psychological therapy would usually suggest that they are unable or unlikely to benefit[46]. The idea that you can take a horse to water but you can't make him drink holds true for counseling and psychological therapy.

SOME PITFALLS OF THERAPY

Intelligence

Burnard (1992)[47] has suggested that counseling can clarify problem issues and facilitate problem-solving, as well as fostering understanding and insight more effectively for people who can articulate their problems and who feel able to self-disclose. However, the evidence that counseling can only help those with a certain level of intelligence who are able to articulate their problems is weak. It must not be assumed that individuals with an average or below average intelligence could not benefit from counseling and psychological therapies. A frequently expressed fear among some therapists is that clients might indulge in 'intellectualization', thereby avoiding confronting their problems. A focus on helping clients help themselves, rather than an emphasis on the actions of the therapist may well overcome such dangers. Talking therapies should be available to all if they are thought worthwhile; people with special needs would be likely to want help just as much as anyone else.

Friendship — help or hindrance?

Frank (1995)[35] suggested that counseling and psychological therapy are aimed directly or indirectly at combating demoralization. Rogers'

(1957)[24] suggestion that a counselor should offer non-possessive warmth, genuineness and empathy has been taken by many counselors to imply that some specific 'counseling skills' are crucial to effective counseling. However, some have criticized this focus on techniques saying that it is misplaced[48]. As mentioned earlier, it may be that what Rogers was describing were the qualities of a good friend, not just a counselor or therapist.

While genuineness and empathy may be adequately provided by a general practitioner as part of the process of consultation, by a counselor with someone who is confused or anxious, or by somebody drawing upon more complex psychological therapy approaches, Dryden (1984)[49] has suggested that these basic factors may not be sufficient to deal with more complex difficulties.

Parry (1989)[50] described three levels of 'psychological skill', where level 1 involved basic or intuitive skills and techniques of helping. A friend might combine these level 1 skills with level 2 skills such as the use of specific psychological strategies or interventions. Where these more basic or intuitive skills prove insufficient, then a more intensive therapeutic endeavor might be necessary, drawing upon more complex psychological theories and approaches. Parry suggested that almost all health care workers use skills from levels 1 and 2, and additional training and education might take professionals through to level 3 skills; a level of help and expertise most friends would not be in a position to offer.

However, the Rogerian qualities in a relationship can serve to foster a sense of social support and counter feelings of helplessness and social isolation. There are indications that perceived social support and a sense of control alone can buffer or lessen the effects of stress[51,52].

Inducing helplessness

Giving advice and information or taking action on someone's behalf may all be valuable in some circumstances for some people, sometimes. Although education and direct action can play an important part in psychological therapies, they are typically seen as distinct from traditional counseling. If the therapy becomes focused on the action taken by the therapist on behalf of the client, problems may arise, since this may only serve to reinforce the client's feelings of helplessness. Similarly, very directive behavior by the therapist can foster ideas of dependency and undermine a client's motivation to help themselves. An active therapist can also lead a client to believe that the therapist sees the client as unable to help themselves; as someone who is helpless.

Inappropriate behavior by a therapist

While it is difficult to identify all possible forms of inappropriate intervention because any dogmatic statement inevitably gives rise to potential exceptions, Wolberg (1967)[53] has identified a list of therapist behaviours which are unlikely to be helpful in counseling. Wolberg suggests that moralistic judgements, exclamations of surprise and overconcern might best be avoided, as would discussions of political or religious issues. Arguing, ridiculing and belittling a patient or client may seem obviously unhelpful, but such aggressive styles of 'helping' appear to easily creep into the repertoire of many 'helpers'. Wolberg's suggestion that therapists and counselors should avoid probing of traumatic material begins to tread on the toes of therapists who would see it as essential to explore, at length, an individual's childhood experiences whatever the current problem.

Given the varying definitions of mental health, any overly rigid adherence to the mainstream or more traditional forms of psychological therapy may be questionable, especially given suggestions that different therapies may merely be different pathways to mental health[28]. When criticisms of the defensive conservatism of psychotherapy as a profession are taken into account, then the use of non-traditional forms of psychotherapy might more usefully seen as a valuable resource, especially when approaches supported by empirical research appear to have failed, or when traditional therapies are unacceptable to individuals in distress.

GROUP THERAPY

Counseling and psychological therapy need to be offered with an awareness of the social context for the individual in distress. In some circumstances, working with couples can be useful. At other times, spouses and other family members can be effectively enlisted to foster and support change. The stress management and family approaches used with people labeled 'schizophrenic' are a good example of the way in which interventions can be targeted at an individual's wider environment. Most therapists, however, continue to work with individuals rather than couples, possibly due to the sheer additional complexity of helping two people (rather than one) to make sense of their thoughts and feelings. Individual counseling often appears essential, in any case, as a precursor to working with a couple.

Group therapy can be based on as wide a range of theories and approaches as individual counseling. Where the efficacy of group versus individual treatment has been studied, no clear picture emerges and views differ widely on who might best benefit from the different forms of intervention[54].

Where group therapy or couples counseling are available, they may be useful for individuals experiencing relationship difficulties and for those who would find individual counseling to be too intimate and threatening. While groups offer the potential attraction of cost-effectiveness, difficulties frequently arise when aims and objectives of those in any therapeutic group differ widely or when members of a group collude in an endeavor to reduce the threat of change. Group therapy offers an individual the opportunity to draw upon the resources of a group of other people, rather than with just one therapist, but groups can also give rise to powerful forces which cannot easily be controlled by the therapist, and which may be harmful[55].

In practice, the decision to direct an individual towards group or couples therapy may be determined more by the availability of such therapies or by the desire of an individual for that sort of approach than by any clear or absolute rules governing such a decision.

EFFECTIVE COUNSELING

Whether in group settings or in one-to-one work, effective counseling focuses on listening rather than advising, the aim being to help the individual make sense of their experience rather than to offer interpretations, judgements and views which reflect the opinion and beliefs of the counselor. The balance must be struck between an overly non-directive approach, which leaves a confused individual, already feeling lost in his or her distress, even more unhappy than before, and a directive approach, in which advice prematurely provided is simply ignored. Lengthy silences at one extreme, and 'all you've got to do is ...' at the other are rarely helpful, but surprisingly prevalent, nevertheless. The effective counseling process is often conceived as involving three phases[56], although not all of these may be necessary:

Phase 1: Empathic listening

An initial phase of exploration offers an individual warmth, empathy and acceptance as the counselor simply listens and reflects or summarizes what he or she is told. In some situations, it has been suggested that simple ventilation of anxieties, sadness and other feelings may be useful[57], and therefore this phase of exploration may be sufficient for some people in distress.

The apparently simple goal of providing warmth and empathy, as well as listening, in this first and essential phase of a counseling relationship is not as easy for everyone as it might at first seem. Bell (1989)[45] has suggested that counseling and psychological therapy can actually work against an individual acquiring a sense of competency, independence and personal power. The offer of care can be manipulative, and a therapist might induce dependency in a client to serve the therapist's need to be needed. It has been suggested that an endeavor to help others may be adversely affected by confused motives on the part of the helper, along with unhelpful styles of helping[53,58,59].

The likelihood that the position of power held by the therapist will actually harm the client is generally exaggerated by clients and some therapists. Abuse of the relationship does occasionally occur, however, and the regulation of counselors and therapists has an important part to play in reducing the risks, as is the case in most other professions.

Phase 2: Defining the problem

A second phase, focusing on understanding, offers the opportunity for someone to clarify and elaborate their experience before exploring alternative perspectives and frameworks. Simply seeing a situation in another way, or a little more objectively, can be valuable for someone in distress — an attempt to help people who 'can't see the wood for the trees'.

These first two stages in interventions may, again, be sufficient in themselves for some people. Simply helping individuals stop and take stock of their situations can allow them to use their problem-solving skills and change circumstances in which they experience distress. These two stages can help an individual recover self-confidence, which may then allow them to carry on coping or take steps to resolve a difficulty.

Phase 3: Problem-solving

Where something else seems necessary, a further stage of problem-solving can be useful. This third stage can often be complex and involved, but it can also be brief. Brief problem-solving interventions can be highly effective in depression or attempted suicide[60].

Brief problem-solving typically involves defining a problem clearly, before exploring and evaluating potential solutions with a view to active implementation of a strategy. The effectiveness of a solution then needs to be evaluated and the process repeated if necessary.

PROBLEM-SOLVING IN PRIMARY CARE

Gath and Mynors-Wallis (1992)[61] studied the provision of problem-solving in primary care, and concluded that problem-solving should be seen as a practical and effective approach to helping difficult emotional disorders in the primary care setting (Box 10.1).

Box 10.1 A problem–solving approach, having established an alliance based on trust, respect, and acceptance

1. Clarification and definition of problem(s)
2. Identification of achievable goals
3. Generation of alternative solutions
4. Choice of preferred solution
5. Detailing of steps to achieve solution
6. Implementation of strategy and evaluation.

Two major advantages of a problem-solving strategy are that it emphasizes a collaborative approach, and it encourages individuals to take responsibility for their action and choices. Such brief and straightforward counseling or problem-solving have been shown to be as effective as anxiolytic medication[62]. Gath and Mynors-Wallis (1992)[61], however, suggest that approximately one-third of patients in general practice do not respond to such simple measures. When individuals experience persistent problems then a more structured psychological approach may be necessary.

The efficacy of the talking therapies is often subjected to a more rigorous appraisal than many psychopharmacological interventions, and a highly critical approach suggesting these therapies are 'second best' is not borne out by the research. Many of the psychological therapies have been shown to be more effective than placebo, and the major approaches, such as cognitive therapy, have repeatedly been shown to be equal to, or more effective than, pharmacotherapeutic interventions[9]. The finding that vastly different psychotherapies appear equally effective, however, leads to difficulty in trying to make an informed choice about therapy for any one individual in distress.

Given the efficacy of psychological interventions, and the general distrust of medications for psychological problems, the choice of therapy might sensibly, therefore, place much greater weight on client preferences, although consideration of cost should not be forgotten. Increasingly, an emphasis on cost-effectiveness has fostered interest in brief approaches in psychological intervention, particularly as the longer term psychodynamic and psychoanalytic approaches have consistently failed to show any significant superiority over shorter term interventions. This relative failure springs largely from the additional costs associated with greater duration of therapy, and the difficulty in showing benefits proposed for psychoanalytic or psychodynamic approaches.

Brief psychotherapy appears to be most effective with individuals experiencing job-related stress, anxiety problems, mild depression and grief reactions as well as other less severe problems[27].

WHEN COUNSELING IS NOT ENOUGH — COGNITIVE THERAPY?

In *The Skilled Helper*, Gerrard Egan[56] presented a method of counseling which he described as based on a problem management model, drawing upon cognitive behavioral approaches. The cognitive emphasis in counseling and psychological therapy has developed rapidly following the failure of scientific research to support psychoanalytic approaches, in addition to the dissatisfaction with behavior therapy, which was perceived as trying to explain human experience too simplistically[63,64].

It has been suggested that revisions of other therapies leads to convergence towards cognitive therapy of the kind described by Beck (1976)[65]. Cognitive therapy typically provides the practical framework for challenging thinking styles and interpretations[66]. It has been argued that revisions of psychoanalytic therapy have merely produced alternative presentations of cognitive therapy or that psychoanalytic therapy could be usefully simplified along the lines of the cognitive therapy framework[67].

Interventions using cognitive therapy in practice might be more accurately described as cognitive behavior therapy[68], because endeavors to help people solve problems often place great emphasis on directly changing behavior and environments.

Awareness of the relevance of reward and reinforcement[69], and the success of behavioral treatment for fears and anxiety[70], has led to a desire to draw upon the benefits and strengths of behavior therapy, and incorporate them into interventions focused on challenging interpretations, beliefs and assumptions. The validity of discussing a client's thinking and the attractiveness of linking therapeutic process to the philosophy of Cicero, Emperor Marcus Aurelius and the Stoics has, nevertheless, been balanced by reservations and criticisms[71].

The Stoics were among the first to put forward the ideas which underlie the cognitive approach, in suggesting that distress might be seen as the product of thinking. They suggested that thinking and logic, however, should be seen as potentially flawed and open to change, and that distress might be avoided if thinking changes. Whilst linking a down-to-earth practical focus on a psychological intervention to broader philosophical questions might offer the client an opportunity to explore their own assumptions, such a development is not essential.

Socratic questioning has been used in cognitive psychotherapy, where client and therapist identify hypotheses and beliefs which lead to an individual's distress, with a view to challenging and questioning underlying assumptions. The aim is to assist individuals in identifying rationales, whether they be 'right' or 'wrong', which avoid the experience of distress. If such an approach reduces distress, the question of whether the rationale or belief is 'true' or not is less important.

Cognitive-behavior therapists place great emphasis on establishing the core conditions associated with Rogerian therapy, as the foundation on which to use other ideas to help individuals reduce their experience of stress or distress.

Cognitive therapy has become widely recognized as a treatment of choice for people experiencing depression[72], and it has been effectively used to tackle a range of difficulties including eating problems, fears and anxieties, and habit problems. It has also proven effective in helping people experiencing delusions or hallucinations[67].

Evaluation of cognitive therapy has shown it to be at least as effective as antidepressants for mild and moderate depression[73]. Where depression is severe, then some form of medication may be necessary before someone can make use of cognitive therapy to tackle the cause of their unhappiness. The supposition that cognitive therapy tackles the causes rather than the symptoms of depression has led to the scrutiny of rates of recurrence of depression following cognitive therapy. If someone's thinking styles and beliefs are central to the etiological course of the depression, then cognitive therapy should lead to lower relapse rates than antidepressant medication, for most people. While absolute claims would be premature, research indicates that cognitive therapy alone is rarely, if ever, less effective than 'antidepressant' medication alone in outcome studies, and it often leads to much lower relapse rates[74].

So-called 'endogenous' depression responds to both cognitive therapy and 'antidepressant' medication[75]. Cognitive therapy and medication in combination are often more effective than either component alone[76].

THE ESSENCE OF COGNITIVE THERAPY

The essence of a cognitive behavioral approach lies in helping an individual understand their thinking, feelings and behaviour. Often, this will mean helping an individual explore the reasons why they continue to do things which they find unhelpful or undesirable. This approach would emphasize the need to be specific when describing problems, detailing the causes and consequences of thoughts, emotional reactions and behaviours. Often, an individual would be encouraged to keep a diary of their relevant behaviour, thinking and underlying assumptions, with a view to their identifying and testing personal theories. This process promotes client commitment and involvement in the process, and makes it clear that psychological therapy is not a passive experience.

Careful consideration of an individual's personal beliefs or theories can often lead to a need for information on how to counter unhelpful or inaccurate assumptions and beliefs. An educational component, where individuals are given information about the mechanisms of the stress reaction or the grief process, is seen as central to helping people manage stress[77].

The cognitive model underlying cognitive behavioral therapy aims to help an individual recognize and challenge their perceptions and interpretations. It attempts to encourage an individual understanding of stress and distress, rather than rely on generalizations which can be meaningless for any one person. This cognitive behavioral approach emphasizes that an individual's situation can be interpreted in various ways, and it highlights the benefits of changing those interpretations. The underlying theory suggests that emotions such as anxiety and depression are produced not by the situation, but by the individual's interpretation of a situation; that interpretation can be fallible, and there may be various alternative interpretations. Those various interpretations may lead to wholly different emotional reactions.

The cognitive approach is not merely 'positive thinking', which may be ineffective over the longer term. False optimism, on the part of a therapist, has no place in effective intervention. But, as mentioned previously, the most helpful way of thinking may not necessarily have to be the 'right' or morally/socially/ethically acceptable way of thinking. It has been suggested that people who are happy most of the time may actually be overly optimistic, but it would be thought arrogant and foolish to try to 'correct' their thinking[78].

Changes in thinking need to be genuine if they are to free an individual from distress. An individual's endeavor to think positively may simply mean that they try to deceive themselves or trick themselves, and such self-deception would be unlikely to be sustainable. Cognitive therapy needs to be carefully explained and presented to ensure that individuals do not simply blame themselves for unhelpful thinking. Individuals may need to be helped to understand the process of their distress before they are in a position to help themselves.

The instillation of hope in the relationship between therapist and client should be based upon a realistic assessment that psychological intervention will help, rather than an inappropriate promise of success.

Box 10.2 The cognitive model

Situations Thoughts Events	>	Interpretation (based on experience)	>	Emotional reaction

Cognitive behavioral therapy aims to help individuals become aware of their styles of thinking and interpreting situations with a view to helping them challenge and change unhelpful assumptions and beliefs. It suggests that emotions are best seen as the product of thinking and interpretations, which need therefore to be changed if an individual is to avoid distress (Box 10.2).

In practice, cognitive behavioral therapy uses specific examples to help individuals identify what might be an unhelpful style of thinking. For example, polarization or dichotomous thinking, where people see things as either black or white, may be inflexible and hinder the development of new strategies. It may be beneficial to countenance shades of grey, and avoid jumping to conclusions. An awareness of unhelpful thinking can, sometimes, be sufficient, in itself.

Unhelpful thinking styles include:

- All or nothing thinking; e.g. 'I need to get it absolutely right or else it is (I am) a failure.'
- Catastrophizing; e.g. assuming that the worst possible outcome is bound to happen.
- Ignoring the positive; e.g. 'OK, so I've got promoted to a job I wanted, with the best staff — but they've stopped my free supply of pencils!'

Where an awareness of unhelpful styles of thinking is not sufficient, then the individual's thinking style can be explored further. Patterns of thinking can be identified, as the underlying assumptions and beliefs are discovered, and directly challenged or tackled.

Challenging assumptions in people experiencing depression, for example, focuses on issues such as pessimism, low self-esteem or feelings of failure. When using this approach for anxiety or fears, assumptions about risks or the undesirability of outcomes can be identified and challenged. Where anger is a problem, then it may be useful to assist an individual in the exploration of their beliefs about what they may see as 'the rules' which, when broken, promote mild annoyance or outbursts of anger.

MANAGING STRESS AND DISTRESS

A comprehensive approach to helping someone in stress or distress might, therefore, simply start with the provision of a safe, accepting and empathic relationship. Within the framework of this relationship an individual could be encouraged to describe and express their difficulties, if necessary, using a problem-solving approach. Some structure to the consultation might be desirable, since recitation of difficulties can be pointless, and distressing. The therapist can provide relevant education and information, while helping the individual to identify the causes and possible explanations of their difficulties.

Simple straightforward reassurance can, at times, be very valuable — 'No, you are not the only one/going mad/beyond all help...!'

A detailed description of an individual's difficulties in specific situations, or a diary of difficult situations can help to identify changes in their behavior or environment that might be useful. In addition, helping an individual to identify and challenge unhelpful styles of thinking which promote feelings of anxiety, depression, anger, or guilt can be beneficial.

Identification of new cognitive strategies and behavioral approaches may help in situations of stress and distress. These must be consolidated through regular practice until the new behavioral and cognitive habits become established in place of the old. Once established, strategies must be devised to maintain the new habits and monitor their effectiveness.

EDUCATION AND INFORMATION

Since much of the information individuals require on stress and many of the skills, such as stress management, assertiveness, and relaxation, are relevant to a very large proportion of individuals in distress, educational materials and group approaches can be highly cost-effective. Approximately 40% of what is said during a medical consultation may be immediately forgotten. Since memory has been associated with compliance[79], attention to helping clients remember the key points in a consultation may be particularly important in the talking therapies, given the potential breadth of discussion.

Ley and Spelman (1967)[79] emphasized the benefits of providing written educational materials where relevant. It might well be good practice in counseling and the talking therapies to summarize, in written form, ideas and suggestions made during the counseling session. A few lines at the end of an appointment can play an important part in promoting further thought and action outside the session. As cognitive behavioral therapy sees rehearsal of new behavioral and thinking habits to be central to the process of change, if the client fails to remember what was agreed that they should endeavor to do, then progress may be thwarted.

GROUP PROGRAMS

In some circumstances, it may be both cost-effective and desirable for individuals to tackle their problems in a group setting. A group approach to stress, for example, counters social isolation and encourages the development of social support which has frequently been shown to be important in the maintenance of mental health[80]. An extensive study on the provision of stress management programs, based on a cognitive approach in New Zealand by Raeburn et al. (1993)[81], showed significant reductions in anxiety and increases in happiness. In this study, ten 90-minute sessions covered time management and relaxation skills, family approaches, assertiveness, general health issues and the development of individual stress management plans.

While multi-component stress management programs in the workplace have shown significant reductions in anxiety, depression and hostility, they often appear to be no more effective than other single focus approaches, such as relaxation training or education/social support groups[82]. Even if some statistically significant benefit can be shown, offering everyone stress management training may be less cost-effective than an approach which targets individuals who are actually at risk of experiencing stress, or who report distress. It should never be forgotten, however, that it may be much more appropriate, or cost-effective, to alter the environment which leads to individuals experiencing distress; stepping out of the lion's cage may be far more sensible than trying to see lions as less threatening!

STRESS MANAGEMENT PROGRAMS

Stress management approaches typically focus on three stages; awareness, understanding and change. Only when someone is aware of their difficulties can they understand the causes and processes underlying their problems. Change or intervention is more likely to be useful if a situation is adequately understood — effort wasted on irrelevant action can further sap resources needed to take the necessary steps.

An effective intervention, and successful stress management will be primarily defined from the individual's perspective. Absolute resolution of problems may be an ideal goal, but more effective coping in an unchanged situation may be just as valid. Personal styles of coping, such as avoidance or denial, can be highly effective, and striving for total resolution may be inappropriate and unobtainable. The aim is to help people in distress identify and implement the most effective coping strategies for them[83].

The contents of stress management programs vary widely when it comes to teaching specific skills. However, relaxation training is usually given in one form or another, along with assertiveness training, anger or time management, and encouragement to develop good sleeping, eating and exercise habits. The individual components may not be that important, since the attention to the problem, finding out that other people have similar problems, and encouragement may be the active ingredients.

Most of these ideas are unlikely to do any harm, but poor matching of intervention to individual needs can lead to frustration. For example, teaching relaxation to someone who is anxious without tackling the cause of that anxiety is a common mistake. Being told the answer is to relax while some threat is perceived to exist can be very unhelpful — if you think you are in the lion's den, relaxation is unlikely to be much use.

The fact that common ingredients and 'doing something' feature in most psychological interventions may go some way to explaining why so many apparently contradictory psychological therapies appear to be useful in helping people tackle stress and reduce distress. If blaming your parents helps relieve distress it may be a useful short-term strategy.

It is better to be pragmatic than dogmatic, and better to have an active, critical appraisal of interventions, with a realistic approach to the adoption of coping strategies. However, haphazard intervention may not be entirely useless. Lazarus (1993)[83] has cautioned against arbitrary, unsystematic eclecticism in which incompatible theories and techniques are combined in a well meant, but unhelpful intervention. If several schools of thought are combined in an attempt to help, the helper must carefully consider the costs and benefits of leaving the apparent security of adherence to a particular approach based on some attempts at coherent theory, however imperfect that theory may be.

CONCLUSION

Whatever the theories of research may say, the acid test of any attempt to help someone in distress will be whether or not they feel better and less distressed. Stress management 'works' if someone feels better for it and more able to manage the stress they were experiencing. The most important factor in a helper's efforts will probably be the establishment of a therapeutic alliance, and problem-solving may be better based on an understanding of each individual's specific situation, rather than on any psychiatric diagnosis or psychological generalization.

Advice, information-giving, and direct intervention may be helpful for some distressed individuals. Where something more is needed, then counseling based on listening and helping the individual to gain a greater understanding of their experiences may be more appropriate. This can be done on the basis of a clear agreement with someone (e.g. a physician) who also offers help in other ways. Alternatively, it may require referral on to helpers, be they trained or not, who have made clear the principles which will guide (and restrict) their actions in offering counseling.

Specific problem-solving techniques may guide a counselor's work with a client, and stress management can bring together education, problem-solving techniques and the management of other social and physical factors. The link between a counselor and a referring physician may need to be very closely maintained in some circumstances if therapeutic benefit is to be sustained. Competent counselors and psychological therapists can offer a relevant service at this level.

Where problems are more complex, or where various attempts at amelioration have already failed, then referral to a psychological therapist offers the opportunity to move beyond counseling and stress management to a more in-depth exploration of the factors underlying an individual's distress. Recognized qualifications or accreditation, personal recommendation, and some recognition of the need to make interventions as brief as possible, while still effective, can guide referrers.

The theoretical orientation of a therapy may be less relevant than the client's existing beliefs and preferences regarding interventions in determining outcome. The referrer should be guided by this fact when encouraging an individual to establish a powerful alliance with a counselor or therapist. This may mean helping an individual to establish a good friendship with a therapist or counselor who knows how to avoid acting unhelpfully. While 'unhelpful' interventions can be identified to some degree, the specifics of what is 'helpful' in an intervention seem rather more difficult to define at this time.

REFERENCES

1 Health and Safety Executive 1988 Mental health at work. HMSO, London
2 Department of Health 1994 ABC of mental health in the workplace. HMSO, London
3 Krantz DS, Raisen SE 1988 Environmental stress, reactivity and ischaemic heart disease. British Journal of Medical Psychology 61:3–16
4 Brown GW, Harris TD, 1978 Social origins of depression: study of psychiatric disorder in women. Free Press, New York
5 Fredrickson M, Matthews KA 1990 Cardiovascular responses to behavioral stress and hypertension: a meta-analytic review. Annals of Behavioral Medicine 12:30–39
6 Cannon WB 1935 Stresses and strain of homeostasis. American Journal of Medical Science 189(1):1–14
7 Melhuish A 1978 Executive health. Business Books, London
8 Murpy LR 1988 Workplace interventions for stress reduction and prevention. In Cooper CL, Payne R (eds) Causes, coping and consequences of stress at work. Wiley, London
9 Lambert MJ, Bergin AE 1994 The effectiveness of psychotherapy. In: Bergin AE, Garfield SL 1994 Handbook of psychotherapy and behaviour change, 4th edn. Wiley, Chichester
10 Sutherland VJ, Cooper CL 1990 Understanding stress. Chapman and Halls, London
11 Cohen S, Tyrell J, Smith AP 1991 Psychological stress and susceptibility to the common cold. New England Journal of Medicine 325:606–12
12 Selye H 1974 Stress without distress. JB Lippincott, Philadelphia
13 Lazarus RS 1968 Emotions and adaptation: Conceptual and empirical relations. In: Arnold W (ed) Nebraska Symposium on motivation. University of Nebraska Press, Lincoln
14 Cox T 1985 Stress. MacMillan, London
15 Zubin J, Spring B 1977 Vulnerability — a new view of schizophrenia. Journal of Abnormal Psychology 86:103–26
16 Bentall RP, Jackson HF, Pilgrim D 1988 Abandoning the concept of schizophrenia: some implications of validity arguments for psychological research into psychotic phenomena. British Journal of Clinical Psychology 27:303–24
17 Nicholson IR, Neufeld RWJ 1992 A dynamic vulnerability perspective on stress and schizophrenia. American Journal of Orthopsychiatry 62(1):117–30
18 Lam D 1991 Psychosocial family intervention in schizophrenia: a review of empirical studies. Psychological Medicine 21:423–41
19 Gilhooly M, Whittick J 1989 Expressed emotion in caregivers of the dementing elderly. British Journal of Medical Psychology 62:265–72
20 Bentall RP 1992 A proposal to classify happiness as a psychiatric disorder. Journal of Medical Ethics 18:94–8
21 Temerlin MK 1970 Diagnostic bias in community mental health. Community Mental Health Journal. 6:110–17
22 Beutler LE, Crago M, Arizmendi TG, 1986 Therapist variables in psychotherapy process and outcome. In: Garfield SL, Bergin AE (eds) Handbook of psychotherapy and behaviour change, 3rd edn. Wiley, New York
23 Bergin AE, Garfield SL 1994 Handbook of psychotherapy and behaviour change, 4th edn. Wiley, Chichester
24 Rogers CR 1957 The necessary and sufficient conditions of therapeutic personality change. Journal of Consulting Psychology 21:95–103
25 British Association for Counselling 1993 Code of Ethics and Practice for Counselors
26 Orlinsky DE, Grawe K, Parks BK 1994 Process and outcome in psychotherapy. In: Bergin AE, Garfield SL (eds) Handbook of psychotherapy and behaviour change, 4th edn. Wiley, Chichester
27 Smith ML, Glass GV, Miller TI 1980 The benefits of psychotherapy. The Johns Hopkins University Press, Baltimore
28 Stiles WB, Shapiro DA, Elliott R 1986 Are all psychotherapies equivalent? American Psychologist 41:165–80
29 Beck AT, Rush AJ, Shaw BF, Emery G 1979 Cognitive therapy for depression. Guilford, New York
30 Marks IM 1969 Fears and phobias. Heinemann, London
31 Schofield W 1964 Psychotherapy and the purchase of friendship. Prentice Hall
32 Goldfried MR 1980 Toward a delineation of therapeutic change principles. American Psychologist 35:991–999
33 Frank JD 1973 Persuasion and healing. Schocken Books, New York
34 Stavynski A, Greenberg D 1992 The psychological management of depression. Acta Psychiatrica Scandinavia 85:407–14
35 Frank JD 1985 Therapeutic components shared by all therapies. In: Mahoney MJ and Freeman A (eds) Cognition and psychotherapy. Plenum, Oxford
36 Neki JS 1973 Guru-Chela relationship: the possibility of a therapeutic paradigm. American Journal of Orthopsychiatry 32:755–66
37 Sue S, Zane N, Young K 1994 Research on psychotherapy with culturally diverse populations. In: Bergin AE, Garfield SL Handbook of psychotherapy and behaviour change, 4th edn. Wiley, Chichester
38 Rachman SJ, Wilson GT 1980 The effects of psychological therapy, 2nd edn. Pergamon Press, New York
39 Lazarus AA 1973 Multimodal behaviour therapy: treating the BASIC ID. Journal of Nervous and Mental Disease 156:25–31
40 Lazarus AA 1989 The practice of multimodal therapy. Johns Hopkins University Press, Baltimore
41 Rosenhan DL, Seligman MEP 1989 Abnormal psychology, 2nd edn. Norton, New York
42 Masters WH, Johnson VE 1970 Human sexual inadequacy. Little-Brown, Boston
43 Barkham M 1988 Empathy in counseling and psychotherapy. Counseling Psychology Quarterly 1(4):407–428
44 Howarth I 1989 Psychotherapy: who benefits? The Psychologist April:150–52
45 Bell L 1989 Is psychotherapy more empowering to the therapist than the client? Clinical Psychology Forum 23:12–14

46 Matthews AM, Johnston DW, Shaw PM, Gelder MG 1974 Process variables and the prediction of outcome in behaviour therapy. British Journal of Psychiatry 125:256–64
47 Burnard P 1992 What is counseling? Gale Centre Publications, Essex
48 Bozarth JD 1984 Beyond reflection: Emergent modes of empathy. In: Levant R, Shelin J (eds) Client centered therapy and the person-centered approach. Praeger, New York
49 Dryden W 1984 Individual therapy in Britain. Harper and Rowe, London
50 Parry G 1989 Care for the future. The Psychologist, Oct: 436–438
51 Steptoe A, Appels A 1989 Stress, personal control and health. Wiley, Chichester
52 Cohen S, Wills TA 1985 Stress, social support and the buffering hypothesis. Psychological Bulletin 98:310–57
53 Wolberg LR 1967 The technique of psychotherapy, 2nd edn. Grune and Stratton, New York
54 Vandervoort DJ, Fuhriman A 1991 The efficacy of group therapy for depression: a review of the literature. Small Group Research 22:320–38
55 Lieberman M, Yalom I, Miles M 1973 Encounter groups: first facts. Basic Books, New York
56 Egan G 1990 The skilled helper: A systematic approach to effective helping, 4th edn. Brooks/Cole, Pacific Grove, California
57 Silver R, Wortman C 1980 Coping with undersirable life events. In: Garber J, Seligman MP (eds) Human helplessness. New York, Academic Press
58 Malan D 1979 Individual psychotherapy and the science of psychodynamics. Butterworths, London
59 Meares RA, Hobson RF 1977 The persecutory therapist. British Journal of Medical Psychology 50:349–59
60 Salkovskis PM, Atha C, Storer D 1990 Cognitive behavioral problem solving in the treatment of patients who repeatedly attempt suicide. British Journal of Psychiatry 157:871–6
61 Gath D, Mynors-Wallis L 1992 Emotional problems in general practice: are psychological treatments better than drugs? In: Hawton K, Cowen P (eds) Practical problems in clinical psychiatry. Oxford University Press, Oxford
62 Catalan J, Gath DJ, Edmonds G, Ennis J 1984 The effects of non-prescribing of anxiolytics in general practice. British Journal of Psychiatry 144:593–602
63 Farkas GM 1980 An ontological analysis of behavior therapy. American Psychologist 35:364–74
64 Peterfreund E 1983 The process of psychoanalytic therapy. Lawrence Erlbaum Associates, Hillsdale
65 Beck AT 1976 Cognitive therapy and the emotional disorders. International Universities Press, New York
66 Bernier D 1989 Stress management: A review. Canada's Mental Health September: 15–19
67 Perris C 1988 The foundations of cognitive psychotherapy and its standing in relation to other psychotherapies. In: Perris C, Blackburn IM, Perris H (eds) Cognitive psychotherapy. New York, Springer-Verlag
68 Wilson GT 1984 Behavior therapy. In: Corsini RJ (ed) Current psychotherapies. FE Peacock, Itasca
69 Skinner BF 1938 The behavior of organisms: An experimental analysis. Appleton-Century Crofts, New York
70 Wolpe J, Lazarus A 1966 Behavior therapy techniques. Pergamon Press, New York
71 Gurnani PD, Wang M 1990 Some reservations concerning the current cognitive emphasis in therapy. Counseling Psychology Quarterly 3(1):21–41
72 Dobson KS 1989 A meta-analysis of the efficacy of cognitive therapy for depression. Journal of Consulting and Clinical Psychology 57(3):414–19
73 Wilson PH 1989 Cognitive-behavior therapy for depression: empirical findings and methodological issues in the evaluation of outcome. Behavior Change 6(2):85–95
74 Blackburn I 1995 The relationship between drug and psychotherapy effects. In: Aveline M, Shapiro DA (eds) Research foundations for psychotherapy practice. Wiley, London
75 Whisman MA 1993 Mediators and moderators of change in cognitive therapy of depression. Psychological Bulletin 114(2):248–65
76 Evans MD, Hollon SD, DeRubeis RJ, Piasecki JM, Grove WM, Garvey MJ, Tuason VB 1992 Differential relapse following cognitive therapy and pharmacotherapy for depression. Archives of General Psychiatry 33:802–808
77 Romano JL 1988 Stress management counseling: from crisis to prevention. Counseling Psychology Quarterly 1(2 & 3):211–19
78 Taylor SE, Brown JD 1988 Illusion and well-being: a social psychological perspective on mental health. Psychological Bulletin 103:193–210
79 Ley P, Spelman MS 1967 Communicating with the patient. Stables Press, London
80 Wienfield HR 1994 The nature and elicitation of social support: Some implications for the helping professions. Behavioral Psychotherapy 12:318–30
81 Raeburn JM, Atkinson JM, Dubignon JM, McPherson M, Elkind GS 1993 'Unstress': a low-cost community psychology approach to stress management: An evaluated case study from New Zealand. Journal of Community Psychology 21:113–23
82 Sallis JF, Trevorrow TR, Johnson CC, Hovell MF, Kaplan RM 1987 Worksite stress management: a comparison of programmes. Psychology and Health 1:237–55
83 Lazarus RS 1993 Coping theory and research: past, present and future. Psychosomatic Medicine 55:324–47

CHAPTER CONTENTS

11

Nutrition: pivotal in prevention and treatment of disease and promotion of health

Sandra Goodman

INTRODUCTION: THE VAST RESEARCH DATABASE IN NUTRITION

The last 50 years have seen a vast accumulation of scientific research on nutrition in all areas of health and disease. This research literature includes in vitro studies using cell and tissue cultures, animal research as well as considerable epidemiological and clinical studies in humans. The research encompasses a wide expanse of methodologies, ranging from determining the optimal dosage of single nutrients such as vitamins, minerals and fatty acids upon diseases such as arthritis, cancer and tardive dyskinesia, to discovering their potential cytotoxic effects upon cancerous cells. A considerable body of epidemiological research has been ongoing for decades involving large cohorts of people in many parts of the world including Europe, North America, Australia, Japan and China. These studies have investigated the potentially therapeutic and preventive effects of various dietary components — fruits, vegetables, red meat, fat, antioxidant vitamins — upon the major diseases afflicting the majority of 'developed' populations — cancer, heart disease and aging. This burgeoning research literature includes a large variety of clinical trial methodologies; randomized, single and double-blind, placebo-controlled and crossover studies researching the effect of single or multiple dietary or nutritional components in the treatment of disease.

Searching this international body of research for the nutritional aspects of any one health topic — cancer, heart disease, aging, diabetes — leads to the discovery of thousands or even tens of thousands of published papers. This is quite apart from the huge body of research published regarding the surgical, pharmacological and general medical aspects of these diseases. For example, a search of MedLine targeting published research in the field of nutrition and cancer from 1983–1993 uncovered 5000 published records including the key words of nutrition, diet, vitamins, minerals and fatty acids. This research literature was compiled into what became the Bristol Cancer Help Centre Nutrition and Cancer Database[1]. Further analysis of this particular database revealed that much of this research had been carried out in prestigious academic and government-funded laboratories around the world, headed by the finest scientists, clinicians and oncologists. Furthermore, the overwhelming majority of the nutrition and cancer research had been published in respected, peer-reviewed medical and scientific journals, including the *Lancet, British Medical Journal, Cancer, Journal of the American Medical Association, American Journal of Epidemiology, American Journal of Clinical Nutrition, Journal of the National Cancer Institute* and so on. A compendium of this nutrition and cancer research, detailing the effects of each nutrient in prevention and treatment of various cancers was published in book form by the author[2].

The expanse of nutritional research is not confined to investigating the effects of single nutrients in single diseases. There is a large body of evidence detailing the multi-nutrient, multidisciplinary approach in most illnesses. As it is impossible within the space constraints of a single chapter to reproduce a comprehensive listing of nutritional research across the entire domain of illnesses, a small sample of recently published research articles is listed below, demonstrating the existence of a considerable body of evidence-based nutritional research (see Box 11.1).

Box 11.1 Effects of nutritional ingredients on health and illness

- Retinoid and carotenoid effects in cancer[1–5], heart disease[6–9], diabetes[10], candidiasis[11], HIV[12], arthritis[13–14], infectious disease[15], and smoking-related pulmonary dysfunction[16].
- B Vitamins effects on: learning[17], memory and behavior[18], and cancer[19–20].
- Vitamin C's effect on: cancer[1–4,21–25], heart disease[6,9,26–29], asthma[29–31], allergies[29], diabetes[10,32], critical illness[33], aging[34–36], and respiratory disease[37–38].
- Vitamin E's effect on: cancer[1–4,39–41], heart disease[6,8,27,42–48], asthma[30,49], cystic fibrosis[50–54], diabetes[10,55–58], aging[36,45,59–60], athletic performance[61], and arthritis[13].
- Selenium's effect on: cancer[62–65], heart disease[66–69], muscular dystrophy[70], aging[59–60,71], athletic performance[72], respiratory disease[73], arthritis[13,74–75], cystic fibrosis[52,76].
- Essential Fatty Acid's effect on: cancer[22,77–79], heart disease[80–83], intestinal disease[84–87], psoriasis and dermatitis[88–91], rheumatoid arthritis[92], and infant early development[93].
- Coenzyme Q10 effect on: antioxidant function[94,95], aging[96–98], cardiovascular diseases[99–104], sperm quality[105–106], skin protection[107], cancer[108–109], tooth and gum disease[110], neurodegenerative disease[111] and athletic performance[112–113].

NUTRITIONAL RESEARCH IN SELECTED ILLNESSES

Today's physicians receive little training in nutritional approaches to medicine and may therefore be unaware of potential underlying nutritional factors contributing to particular conditions, or of possible nutritional treatment approaches which have been shown to be therapeutically effective in treating a variety of illnesses. As detailed above, there is considerable published and ongoing research into preventive nutritional approaches as well as research investigating nutrition as a treatment. Some of this literature is described in greater detail below, with the intent of stimulating greater clinical interest among physicians who may be searching for treatment options which do not have the side effects of many drug treatments.

Arthritis

Antioxidants

Heliovaara et al. (1994)[13] conducted a case control study to determine whether antioxidant status is a factor in rheumatoid arthritis (RA). Some 1400 adults were followed for 20 years of whom 14 people developed RA. Two controls were individually matched for each case. Serum levels of vitamin E, beta-carotene and selenium were measured and an antioxidant index calculated.

Low levels of vitamin E, beta-carotene and selenium were associated with an elevated risk of RA, although these associations were not significant. However, a low antioxidant index was significantly associated with an elevated relative risk for RA, which was 8.3 between lowest and highest tertiles[13].

Fish oil

Lau et al. (1993)[92] in a double-blind placebo-controlled study, studied whether fish oil (omega-3 fatty acids) supplements could reduce arthritis patients' requirement for non-steroidal anti-inflammatory drugs (NSAIDS). Sixty-four RA patients took either fish oil capsules containing n-3 fatty acids or placebo capsules for 1 year, following which all took placebo capsules for 3 months. Patients were instructed to slowly reduce their NSAID dosage providing symptoms did not worsen and were clinically reviewed every 3 months.

At 3 months, the patients taking fish oil capsules significantly reduced their NSAID usage — 71% compared with the placebo group's 89.7%. After 12 months, the reduction was maximal — 40.6% for the fish oil group, compared with 84.1% for the placebo group. This trend was maintained to month 15 — 44.7% for the fish oil group, compared with 60.5% for the placebo group[92].

Vitamin C

McAlindon et al. (1996)[114] investigated whether an increased antioxidant intake was associated with decreased rates of osteoarthritis (OA) in the knees, a common age-related disorder. Knees were evaluated by radiography between 1983–1985 and between 1992–1993 and were classified following clinical evaluation as either being without OA, having progressive OA at follow-up, or having cartilage loss or osteophyte growth. Dietary intake was assessed using the Food Frequency Questionnaire. The association of vitamins C, E and beta-carotene intake, ranked in sex-specific tertiles with OA incidence and progression, was compared with non-antioxidant vitamins B_1, B_6, niacin and folate. The lowest dietary tertile was used as the referent category. Odds ratios (OR) were adjusted for age, sex, body mass index, weight change, knee injury, physical activity, energy intake, and health status.

Of the 640 participants who received complete assessments, incident and progressive OA occurred in 81 and 68 knees, respectively. There was no significant association of incident OA with any nutrient. However, a three-fold reduction in risk of OA progression was found for both the middle and highest tertile of vitamin C intake, which related predominantly to a reduced risk of cartilage loss. Those people with high intake of vitamin C also had a reduced risk of developing knee pain. Reductions in risk of OA progression were also seen for beta-carotene and vitamin E intake, although these were less consistent. No significant associations were found for the non-antioxidant nutrients[114].

Asthma

Vitamins C and E

Britton et al. (1995)[31] studied the relation between lung function and dietary intake of antioxidant vitamins C and E, in over 2600 adults aged 18–70 years. Clinical measurements included respiratory functions, forced vital capacity (FVC), forced expiratory volume (FEV), allergen skin sensitivity to grass pollen, cat fur and house dust mite and smoking history. Dietary intake of vitamins C and E was determined by semi-quantitative food questionnaire.

Following adjustments for age, sex, height, mean allergen skin diameter and smoking history, significant and independent relationships were found for both FEV1 and FVC and vitamin C intake. Moreover, a standard deviation higher vitamin C intake (40 mg/day) was related to a 25 ml higher FEV1 and a 23.3 ml higher FVC. Additionally, vitamin E intake was positively related to lung function, and a standard deviation (2.2 mg) higher intake was related to a 20.1 ml higher FEV1 and a 23.1 ml higher FVC. Vitamin C and E intakes were significantly correlated, however, after allowing for the effects of vitamin C, there was no additional independent effect of vitamin E upon FEV1 or FVC[31].

Troisi et al. (1995)[30] evaluated the associations between dietary factors and the incidence of asthma in adults, hypothesizing that the pathophysiology of asthma may be mediated by altered immune or antioxidant activity. Throughout a 10-year period, almost 78 000 women between ages 34–68 completed a semi-quantitative food frequency questionnaire.

The results showed that the women with the highest vitamin E dietary (not supplements) intake had just over half (0.53) the risk of developing asthma compared with women with the lowest intake. However, when the vitamin E contribution from nuts was removed the risk difference decreased to 0.74. Positive associations were also found for vitamin C and E supplements, although these may be explained by women, at high risk of developing asthma, commencing vitamin supplements prior to diagnosis. There was also a non-significant inverse association with beta-carotene intake[30].

Bierlory and Gandhi (1994)[29] carried out a comprehensive search and review of the literature regarding the role of vitamin C in the treatment of asthma and allergy. Increased vitamin C intake has been shown to produce positive effects on pulmonary function, bronchoprovocation challenges with methacholine, histamine or allergens, improvements in white blood cell function and motility and a decrease in respiratory infections. However, several studies did not support a beneficial role for vitamin C.

The authors concluded that the role of vitamin C in the treatment of asthma and allergy is not well defined, since the majority of studies were short-term, and only assessed the immediate effects of vitamin C supplementation. The long-term or delayed effects of vitamin C supplementation have yet to be investigated and such research will be required in order to define the role of vitamin C in allergic disease[29].

Fish oil

Arm et al. (1994)[115] reviewed the literature (60 references) describing the role that fish oil may play in inhibiting the inflammatory action of leukotrienes which contribute to allergic asthma. The two major polyunsaturated fatty acids in fish oil are eicosapentanoic acid (EPA) and docosahexanoic acid (DCHA) which inhibit leukotriene synthesis and substitute fatty acids as alternatives to arachidonic acid in leukotriene synthesis. Both EPA and DCHA inhibit the conversion of arachidonic acid by the cyclooxygenase pathway to prostanoid metabolites (inflammatory products) and also reduce production of platelet-activating factor (PAF)[115].

All cancers

Vitamins A, C, E and carotene

Eicholzer et al. (1990)[3] investigated the health of 2974 men working in Basel Switzerland. The plasma levels of vitamins C, E, A and carotene in this cohort had been measured in 1971–1973. During the 17 years of follow-up, 290 men died from cancer, including 87 of lung, 30 of prostate, 28 of stomach and 22 of colon cancer.

The overall cancer mortality was associated with low plasma carotene and vitamin C levels. Lung and stomach cancers were particularly associated with low plasma carotene levels. In addition, low levels of plasma carotene and lipid-adjusted vitamin A levels were associated with a significantly increased mortality risk for all cancers, particularly lung, when all deaths during the first 2 years of follow-up were excluded. Furthermore, low levels of plasma vitamin C and lipid-adjusted vitamin E were also associated with a significantly increased risk of lung cancer. Low levels of vitamin E in smokers were also related to an increased risk of prostate cancer.

These data clearly demonstrated that low plasma levels of vitamins A, C, E and carotene are related to increased risk of dying from all cancers, particularly lung, and vitamin E levels in smokers are related to an increased risk of death from prostate cancer[3].

Breast cancer

Fruit and vegetables

Freudenheim et al. (1996)[4] have suggested that the international variations in the incidence of breast cancer and the changes in incidence among migrant populations may be due to dietary factors. Thus diet may be a significant risk factor for breast cancer. Numerous published studies have demonstrated that a diet high in the consumption of vegetables and fruits protects against breast cancer.

The authors conducted a case-control study evaluating supplement consumption and the risk of premenopausal breast cancer. This involved just under 300 premenopausal women diagnosed with breast cancer and followed from 1986 through to 1991. Controls, matched to cases on the basis of age and county of residence, were randomly selected from New York State Department of Motor Vehicles records. The study evaluated intake of vegetables and fruits, vitamins C, E, folic acid, individual carotenoids and dietary fiber. Interviews included detailed assessments of individual's daily diet during the 2 previous years.

The results demonstrated that high intake of certain nutrients was associated with a reduction in risk. Using the lowest intake quartile as the referent, the adjusted odds ratios (ORs) for the highest quartile of intake for specific nutrients are shown in Box 11.2 below.

No association was found for beta-cryptoxanthin, lycopene or grain fiber and only a weak association was found between risk reduction and fruit consumption. The strong inverse association found between risk of breast cancer and total vegetable intake (OR, 0.46) was independent of vitamins C, E, folic acid, dietary fiber and alpha-carotene, although it was somewhat attenuated by adjustments for beta-carotene and lutein plus zeaxanthin. No association was found between breast cancer risk and the intake of vitamins C, E and folic acid supplements.

In contrast, vegetable intake reduced the risk of premenopausal breast cancer in this population of women, but there did not appear to be any single dietary factor to account for this. It is possible that the multiple components found in vegetables may exert a synergistic effect upon breast cancer. Alternatively, there may be other 'unmeasured factors' within these foods which may influence risk[4].

Box 11.2 Odds ratio risk of breast cancer

Vitamin C	0.53
Vitamin E	0.55
Folic acid	0.50
Alpha-carotene	0.67
Beta-carotene	0.46
Lutein and zeaxanthin	0.47
Total vegetable intake	0.46
Dietary fiber from fruit and vegetables	0.48

Colon cancer

Multiple nutrients

La Vecchia et al. (1996)[22] estimated the percent population attributable risk (PAR) for colorectal cancer in northern Italy, from a case-control study conducted between 1985–1992 on 828 colon and 498 rectal cancer cases and more than 2000 control patients. PAR for colorectal cancer was estimated in relation to beta-carotene and vitamin C as markers of a diet rich in fruit and vegetables. In addition, other factors such as red meat and seasoning fat intake, daily meal frequency and family history of the disease were evaluated.

A low intake of beta-carotene accounted for 39% of all the cases, a low intake of vitamin C accounted for 14%, based upon multivariate odds ratios, adjusted for total calorie intake. These two micronutrients together explained 43% of all colorectal cancer cases within this population. A high frequency of red meat consumption accounted for 17%; a high score of seasoning fats, 4% and higher daily meal frequency, 13%. These five dietary factors together explained 63% of colorectal cancer cases within this population.

Family history of colorectal cancer accounted for 4% of cases. Despite the limitations of the dietary data and the somewhat arbitrary assumptions underlying the PAR estimates, about two-thirds of all colorectal cancers in this population could be accounted for in terms of a handful of dietary risk factors. Management of these few dietary factors could potentially prevent a large percentage of the more than 18 000 deaths from colorectal cancer occurring each year in Italy[22].

Prostate cancer

Multiple nutrients

Rohan et al. (1995)[116] conducted a case-control study in order to investigate the relationship between prostate cancer risk and dietary intake of energy, fat, vitamin A and other nutrients. The study involved 207 men with recent, histologically confirmed diagnoses of prostate cancer and 207 age-matched controls. Dietary intake information was obtained by quantitative diet history.

Results demonstrated a positive relationship between energy intake and risk of prostate cancer. Men in the uppermost quartile energy intake levels had a 75% increased risk. However, there was no clear relationship between the non-energy effects of total fat or mono-unsaturated fat intake and prostate cancer risk. The evidence for an inverse correlation with saturated fat intake was irregular. The authors also found a weak, statistically non-significant correlation between polyunsaturated fat intake and risk of prostate cancer. High levels of vitamin A intake correlated with reduced risk. There was no correlation between dietary beta-carotene intake and risk[116].

Lung cancer

A case control study was conducted by Garcia et al. (1995)[117] to investigate the association between carotenes, vitamin A intake and lung cancer. This study involved 61 male lung cancer patients and 61 controls, matched for age, sex and smoking history.

The results showed that men with lung cancer consumed fewer winter vegetables — chard, beet, chicory, spinach and cabbage — than controls. No differences were found between carotene and vitamin A consumption[117].

Cancer biology

Lupulescu (1994)[118] reviewed the experimental evidence (78 studies), for the role of vitamins A, C and E and beta-carotene in cancer cell biology and metabolism. Such molecular biological studies may provide important information on the role of vitamins in cancer treatment.

Vitamins A, C and E have been strongly implicated as regulatory factors of cancer cell differentiation, regression, membrane biogenesis, DNA, RNA, protein and collagen synthesis. In addition, there is good evidence that they may play a central role in the transformation of precancerous into cancer cells. These vitamins also exert cytotoxic and cytostatic effects and may cause the cancer cells to regress to a normal phenotype. The interaction of vitamins A, C and E with oncogenes and growth factors is of considerable importance to cancer cell biology. The data summarized present new insights into the potential anti-carcinogenic mechanisms of vitamins and provide a logical rationale for their use in cancer chemo-prevention and treatment programs[118].

A study was carried out by Sagar and Das (1995)[77] on the effects of n-3 and n-6 fatty acids (FAs) on the growth of human cervical cancer (HeLa) cells.

Of all the FAs evaluated, docosahexanoic acid (DHA) and eicosapentanoic acid (EPA) had the most potent cytotoxic action upon HeLa cells. The order of potency of various FAs in their cytotoxic action, in decreasing potency is:

1. DHA
2. EPA
3. dimono-gamma-linolenic acid (DGLA) = gamma-linolenic acid (GLA)
4. linoleic acid (LA)
5. arachidonic acid (AA)
6. alpha-linolenic acid (ALA).

The data demonstrate that free radicals whose formation is calmodulin-dependent modulate the cytotoxic action of unsaturated fatty acids, specifically, lipoxygenase products, which are believed to be the main tumoricidal action faction of fatty acids[77].

Selenium

Oh et al. (1995)[65] evaluated the chemoprotective effect of dietary selenium on mouse skin tumors, induced by topical application of tumor initiator 2′-(4-nitrophenoxy)oxirane (NPO) and tumor promoter 12-*O*-tetradecanoylphorbol-13-acetate (TPA). The basal diet was supplemented using sodium selenite or Se-rich eggs (0.3 ppm to 0.07 ppm Se).

The results indicated that selenium supplementation as sodium selenite or Se-rich eggs reduced papilloma formation, 12 weeks following NPO treatment, by 40 or 37% respectively. Dietary supplementation to the basal diet with Se-rich eggs reduced the incidence and multiplicity of papillomas during the early promotion phase (11 weeks); however anti-tumor activity declined thereafter. This result suggested that the accumulation of tissue selenium above saturation level may not be beneficial. Concentrations of selenium in blood, liver and skin tissue of mice fed the basal diet plus the 0.3 ppm supplementation increased significantly. Glutathione peroxidase activity in the blood of the group fed the basal diet plus selenium supplementation increased significantly. In addition, liver and skin tissue enzyme activity was increased by the 0.3 ppm, but not by the further 1.0 ppm supplementation.

Hence, moderate levels of dietary selenium (0.3 ppm) exerted a chemoprotective effect at the promotional stage of cancer and dietary selenium-rich egg as well as dietary selenite exerted anti-tumor activity[65].

Combination therapy: radiation plus vitamins

An investigation was carried out by Taper et al. (1996)[23] on the effect of pretreatment with vitamins C and K3 upon solid mouse tumors treated with a single dose of radiotherapy.

The results demonstrated that pretreatment with vitamins C and K3 resulted in a statistically significant potentiation of the effects of 20–40 Gy of radiotherapy. The combination of vitamins C and K3 constitutes a redox-cycling system producing hydrogen peroxide and other active oxygen species. Cancer cells are particularly sensitive to such oxidative attack due to their frequent deficiency in free radical defense systems. The introduction of this, and other non-toxic and selective potentiation procedures, into classical human cancer therapy protocols would appear to be generally accessible and without any additional risk for patients[23].

Crohn's disease

Fish oil

Belluzzi et al. (1996)[119] hypothesized that because fish oil has anti-inflammatory actions, it could reduce the frequency of relapses in patients with Crohn's disease. However, its unpleasant taste and gastrointestinal side effects mean that it is often poorly tolerated. The authors conducted a 1-year, double-blind, placebo-controlled study to investigate the effects of a new fish oil preparation in maintaining remission in 78 patients with Crohn's disease with high risk of relapse. Patients received either nine fish oil capsules containing a total of 2.7 g of n-3 fatty acids or nine placebo capsules each day. A special coating protected the capsules against gastric acidity for at least 30 minutes.

Of the 39 patients in the fish oil group, 11 (28%) suffered relapses, four dropped out due to diarrhea and one withdrew for other reasons. In marked contrast, from the 39 patients taking placebo capsules in whom 27 (69%) suffered relapses, one dropped out due to diarrhea and one withdrew for other reasons. The difference in replase rate was 41%. After 1 year of treatment with fish oil 23 patients (59%) remained in remission, compared with 10 patients (26%) in the placebo group. Logistic-regression analysis indicated that only fish oil predicted the relapse rate, age, sex, previous surgery, duration of disease or smoking habit had no effect. The odds ratio (OR) for the placebo group compared with the fish oil group was 4.2. These results suggested a new enteric-coated fish oil preparation may be effective in reducing the rate of relapse of patients with Crohn's disease in remission[119].

Antioxidants

Buffinton and Doe (1995)[120] investigated the effects of antioxidants in gastrointestinal inflammation. Antioxidant defenses, against reactive oxygen and nitrogen species produced by the inflammatory cell infiltrate in inflammatory bowel disease (IBD), are seldom considered. The authors measured total peroxyl radical scavenging capacity and levels of urate, glutathione, vitamin E and ubiquinol-10 in paired non-inflamed and inflamed mucosal biopsies from people with inflammatory bowel disease.

Their results revealed that substantial changes in antioxidant defenses in inflamed tissue compared to paired non-inflamed mucosa (see Table 11.1).

These data support earlier findings of decreased vitamin C levels in inflamed IBD mucosa and demonstrate that the loss of antioxidant defenses affects virtually all aspects of inflammation. Diminished antioxidant defenses may severely compromise the inflamed mucosa, rendering it more susceptible to oxidative damage hindering mucosal recovery and cellular integrity. The loss of antioxidant defenses provides a strong rationale for the development of novel antioxidant therapies for treating inflammatory bowel disease[120].

Cystic fibrosis

Selenium

An investigation was carried out on the use of selenium in patients with cystic fibrosis (CF) by Kauf et al. (1995)[52]. The antioxidative/oxidative balance in cystic fibrosis patients is chronically disturbed, free radicals are generated by bronchial infection, and antioxidants like vitamin E and selenium are often deficient. Selenium is an essential component of the glutathione peroxidase antioxidant enzyme system and therefore selenium supplementation should theoretically be useful in airway inflammation. In Kauf's study, patients with CF were given sodium selenite (4 µg per kg per day) for 3 months.

After 3 months of therapy a number of therapeutic results were apparent:

- **Metabolic:** normalized plasma selenium and glutathione peroxidase activity.
- **Hormonal:** enhanced thyroid hormone efficacy, increased IgF-1, reduced LDL cholesterol.
- **Clinical:** enhanced cardiac output.

Side effects were noted in three patients, including anorexia, nausea and mild hair loss. Long-term sodium selenite, with only 60 µg/day for 1 year, maintained the favorable outcome without the side effects. The authors recommended sodium selenite therapy, preferably in combination with vitamin E, for cystic fibrosis patients[52].

Table 11.1 Antioxidant defenses in inflamed and non-inflamed colonic mucosa

	Crohn's disease	Ulcerative colitis
Urate	62.2%	47.3%
Glutathione	–	59%
Total glutathione	–	65.2%
Ubiquinol	75.7%	90.5%

Total peroxyl radical scavenging capacity decreased 55%.
Mean vitamin E content was unchanged.

Vitamin E

Winklhofer-Roob et al. (1996)[50] reported that low levels of vitamin E and plasma lipids are frequently found in CF patients. The authors measured the response to a single oral dose of all-rac-alpha-tocopheryl acetate (100 mg/kg body wt) over 25 hours in 25 CF patients with pancreatic insufficiency and in 23 healthy controls. Patients received pancreatic enzymes along with the vitamin E dose.

The results demonstrated that at baseline, plasma alpha-tocopherol concentrations correlated with cholesterol concentrations and were lower in patients than in controls. From 3 and 6 hours onward, plasma and red blood cell alpha-tocopherol concentrations were significantly higher than baseline levels and peaked at 6 and 12 hours respectively. Maximum increases and alpha-tocopherol concentrations were smaller in patients than in controls. Patients were shown to respond as effectively as controls when ratios of plasma alpha-tocopherol to cholesterol or red blood cell alpha-tocopherol concentrations were applied. Thus vitamin E supplementation corrected the low plasma lipid clinical status.

Based on these data, the authors recommend that CF patients should receive vitamin E supplements in high enough doses to achieve a comparable level to that found in healthy individuals. These supplements should be taken with appropriate amounts of pancreatic enzymes. It is possible that much lower doses than those used in the above study may be sufficient for long-term supplementation[50].

Winklhofer-Roob et al. also investigated which one of three types of vitamin E preparations was most effective in optimizing vitamin E status in CF. Twenty-nine CF patients (aged 0.7–29.8 years) were randomly assigned to receive 400 IU of either RRR-alpha-tocopherol (A: 268 mg, n=10), or racemic alpha-tocopheryl acetate, which is fat-soluble (B: 400 mg, n=10) or a water-miscible preparation (C: 400 mg, n=9). Patients were followed for 6 weeks.

The results indicated that plasma alpha-tocopherol concentrations increased from baseline (10.5 µmol/L) to 3 weeks (25.7 µmol/L), but did not increase any further between 3 and 6 weeks. Concentrations at 3 and 6 weeks were not different from age-matched control subjects, and there was no significant difference in the increase from baseline to 6 weeks among preparations A, B or C. There was no significant difference in the increase in plasma alpha-tocopherol concentrations between patients with CF-associated liver disease and those without liver disease. Any one of these three vitamin E preparations at 400 IU/day is an efficient supplement in CF patients, and can increase levels of vitamin E to that found in healthy control subjects[51].

Heart disease

Antioxidant vitamins

Stephens et al. (1996)[121] have suggested that vitamin E (alpha-tocopherol) plays an important role in prevention of atherosclerosis by inhibiting the oxidation of low-density lipoprotein (LDL). A number of epidemiological studies have demonstrated an association between high dietary intake or high serum concentrations of vitamin E and reduced rates of ischemic heart disease. The authors tested the hypothesis that treatment with a high dose of vitamin E would reduce subsequent risk of myocardial infarction (MI) and cardiovascular death in patients with established ischemic heart disease.

They conducted a double-blind, placebo-controlled study with stratified randomization with 2002 patients with angiographically proven coronary atherosclerosis, who were enrolled and followed up for a median of 510 days. A total of 1035 patients were given vitamin E capsules — 546 patients took 800 IU daily, the remainder took 400 IU daily; 967 patients received identical placebo capsules. The primary endpoints were cardiovascular death and non-fatal MI.

Plasma vitamin E concentrations rose in the active treatment group but were unchanged in the placebo group. Vitamin E treatment significantly reduced the risk of the primary trial endpoint of cardiovascular death and non-fatal MI — 41 vs. 64 events; relative risk (rr) 0.53. The beneficial effects were due to a significant reduction in the risk of non-fatal MI (14 vs. 41: rr = 0.23); however there was a non-significant excess of cardiovascular deaths in the vitamin E group (27 vs. 23; rr = 1.18). All-cause mortality was 36 of 1035 vitamin E-treated patients and 27 of 967 placebo patients.

The authors conclude that vitamin E treatment substantially reduced the rate of non-fatal MI, with beneficial effects apparent after 1 year of treatment, in patients with angiographically proven symptomatic coronary atherosclerosis. The effect of vitamin E treatment on cardiovascular deaths requires further study[121].

The efficacy of antioxidant vitamins was investigated by Singh et al. (1996)[6] in 63 patients with acute myocardial infarction and 62 controls. The randomized, double-blind placebo-controlled trial compared the effects of treatment with antioxidant vitamins A (50 000 IU/day), C (1000 mg/day), E (400 mg/day) and beta-carotene (25 mg/day) for 28 days.

Compared with the placebo group, the mean infarct size was significantly less in the antioxidant-treated group. Analysis of cardiac enzymes post infarction showed a decrease in AST by 45.6 IU/dl in the antioxidant group versus 25.8 IU/dl in the placebo group, while LDH increased slightly in the antioxidant group compared with the placebo group. Antioxidant vitamin administration also increased serum levels compared with placebo (see Table 11.2).

In addition, serum lipid peroxides decreased by 1.22 pmol/ml in the antioxidant group compared with 0.22 pmol/ml in the placebo group. Angina pectoris, arrhythmic events and poor left ventricular function occurred less often in the antioxidant patients and cardiac end points were also significantly less in the antioxidant group.

These data suggest that treatment of patients who have recently suffered an acute myocardial infarction with a combination of antioxidant vitamins A, E, C and beta-carotene may protect against cardiac muscle necrosis and may be beneficial in preventing post infarct complications and further cardiac events[6].

PROTECTIVE MECHANISMS

Cellular adhesion

Weber et al. (1996)[122] studied the effects of cigarette smoking and vitamin C on endothelial adhesion in a model of atherogenesis. They compared monocyte-endothelial adhesion in non-smokers and smokers prior to and following supplementation with vitamin C using a monocyte adhesion assay.

Monocyte adhesion increased by 150% in people who smoked one to two packs of cigarettes per day, mediated by the integrin CD11b/CD18. Vitamin C plasma levels were reduced by 30% in smokers compared with non-smokers, but no significant differences were found in levels of vitamins A, E or beta-carotene. This confirmed that the free radical scavenger vitamin C is consumed by the oxidative stress induced by cigarette smoking. Supplementation with vitamin C (2 g per day for 10 days) raised plasma levels in smokers to above those in non-smokers, and reduced monocyte adhesion to the level seen in non-smokers. However, vitamin C supplementation did not affect monocyte adhesiveness in non-smokers, despite increasing plasma levels.

These data indicate that cigarette smoking increases CD11b-dependent monocyte adhesiveness in humans. Restoring reduced plasma vitamin C levels in smokers by oral supplementation reduced monocyte adhesion to levels found in non-smokers[122].

Table 11.2 Changes in serum level after antioxidant vitamin administration

	Vitamin group (μmol/L)	Placebo (μmol/L)
Vitamin E	8.8	2.2
Vitamin C	12.6	4.2
Beta-carotene	0.28	0.06
Vitamin A	0.36	0.12

LDL oxidation

Panzetta et al. (1995)[123] demonstrated that oxidized low-density lipoproteins (LDL) play an important role in the pathogenesis of atherosclerosis. The authors state that is still unclear whether the positive effects of fish oil depend mainly upon its polyunsaturated fatty acid content, or whether other factors, such as the addition of antioxidants may play a role. Their study evaluated the effects of fish oil supplementation — 20 ml containing vitamin E (20 IU) as antioxidant for 30 days and vitamin E (50 IU) for another 30 days — on lipid metabolism and susceptibility of LDL to oxidation in vitro (lag phase).

In hemodialysis patients, the lag phase and vitamin E concentration were significantly reduced. Following fish oil and vitamin E supplementation, the length of the lag phase and vitamin E concentration increased significantly; plasma lipids were significantly reduced. These results demonstrated that LDL susceptibility to oxidation is enhanced in hemodialysis patients. Thus there may be a relationship between excessive LDL peroxidation and accelerated atherosclerosis. The increased susceptibility of LDL to in vitro oxidation may be partially explained by a reduced LDL vitamin E concentration. Because fish oil increased the lag phase to the same extent as vitamin E supplementation, the positive effect of fish oil may be partly due to its antioxidant content[123].

SIDE EFFECTS

Kidney stones

The possibility that high vitamin intake was associated with an increased risk of renal calculi has been investigated by Curhan et al. (1986)[124]. In a prospective study involving 45 251 men aged 40–75 years with no history of renal calculi, the vitamin C and B_6 intake from foods and supplements was assessed using a semi-quantitative food frequency questionnaire.

During 6 years of follow-up, 751 cases of kidney stones were documented. The results showed that neither vitamin C nor vitamin B_6 intake was significantly associated with the risk of stone formation. With respect to vitamin C, the age-adjusted relative risk was 0.78 for men consuming 1500 mg daily or more compared with less than 250 mg daily. For vitamin B_6, the age-adjusted relative risk was 0.91 for men consuming 40 mg daily or more compared with less than 3 mg daily. After adjusting for other potential stone risk factors the relative risks did not change significantly.

These data do not support any association between high daily intake of vitamin C or vitamin B_6 and the risk of kidney stone formation, even when consumed in large doses[124].

NUTRITION: A WELL-KEPT SECRET

Over the past few decades, there has been a huge investment of research funds into nutritional research in health and disease, and large, internationally renowned teams of expert scientific and medical personnel have conducted and published research in nutritional medicine. The compelling results of all this work on the importance of nutrition would appear to be a well-guarded secret, known mainly to those scientists and researchers who read the scientific literature.

The evidence from the published nutritional literature would suggest that physicians should consider offering their patients nutritional treatment in conjunction with other standard treatments for many of the most common ailments — allergies, asthma, arthritis, heart disease, even cancer. However, despite the existence within the medical professional of a branch called 'Nutritional Medicine', nutrition appears to be a subject of which the majority of physicians admit to a glaring ignorance.

It is not clear why there is such a vacuum of knowledge despite the huge evidence base for nutritional medicine, published in a wide variety of journals right around the world.

Nutrition is overlooked in the majority of medical school curricula. As a result the extent of nutritional knowledge gleaned by the general physician is often confined to a few outmoded notions about what constitutes a 'balanced diet', recommended daily allowances (RDAs) of certain vitamins, and the levels required to prevent deficiency diseases such as beri beri and scurvy. Considering that health-promoting nutrition is such a basic and fundamental requirement for good health, and that every person must eat to remain alive, the omission of this most universal medical tool from the physician's armament of knowledge and experience is a tragic wasted opportunity.

Consequently, the general and specialist practitioner is rarely informed about nutritional approaches to health and disease and is therefore unable to accurately inform his patients about the possible therapeutic efficacy of nutritional interventions. The inadequate dissemination of this evidence base to health professionals has led the author to establish and publish a journal for practitioners devoted to disseminating recently published research regarding nutrition and other non-drug approaches to health[125].

Furthermore, nutritional approaches to illnesses such as cancer, heart disease, diabetes and cystic fibrosis are rarely mentioned in the written or broadcast media. Numerous television programs which have been devoted to illnesses such as cancer have overflowed with advice about lifestyle, stress reduction, even massage, in addition to the approved treatments — surgery, radiotherapy or chemotherapy, but nutrition is rarely mentioned. Any mention of nutritional approaches to cancer is often framed in a derogatory manner, with suggestions of 'quackery' or faddish and bizarre practices.

Various dietary regimes which may have a role in the treatment of some cancers, including vegetarian, raw food, fruit, macrobiotic, or the Gerson regime are marginalized and defamed, and practitioners daring to suggest a dietary approach may be subjected to criminal litigation or may even be struck off the medical registers. It is astonishing that hard evidence demonstrating that low blood levels of vitamins A, C, E and carotene are related to increased risk of cancer mortality is rarely broadcast[1–3]. Similarly, the evidence demonstrating that the risk of premenopausal breast cancer is more than halved in women whose diet is high in vegetables and fruits[4], and that two-thirds of all colorectal cancer cases in Italy can be attributed to five dietary risk factors — low beta-carotene and vitamin C intake, red meat consumption, seasoning fat intake and increased daily meal frequency, is not widely known[22].

The situation with respect to cardiovascular diseases — heart attack, stroke, hypertension — is similarly dominated by medical, surgical and pharmacological approaches. There is much discussion and reporting of cholesterol-lowering drugs, ACE inhibitors, aspirin and triple-bypass surgical techniques, whereas the significant effects of dietary and lifestyle changes in cardiovascular disease are normally overlooked or omitted altogether. Techniques such as EDTA chelation[125–129] (the intravenous infusion of a combination of antioxidant and anti-atherogenic nutrients) which has been successfully performed for decades, are rarely mentioned, let alone offered by the majority of physicians.

It must be remembered that what is published today in the research literature regarding the positive therapeutic effects of antioxidants, essential fatty acids and coenzyme Q10 is frequently the results of decades of intensive research. Twenty-five years ago, eating a diet high in organically grown fruits and vegetables, pulses and taking vitamins was considered by society-at-large to be an aberrant or fringe lifestyle. Today major national and international health organizations and governments espouse exactly such practices[130]!

ACTION ON NUTRITION: THE WAY FORWARD

Today there exist a variety of non-mainstream nutritional therapeutic practices — various dietary regimes, fasting, colon cleansing, herbal regimes — espoused by a variety of practitioners which may be scorned by the general medical community, but which, if subjected to serious and concerted research, may reveal significant therapeutic efficacy. Today's marginal practice may become tomorrow's mainstream clinical protocol. Integrating known knowledge on nutritional medicine will require a number of specific initiatives in education, research and health policy (see Box 11.3).

CONCLUSION

The urgency for immediate action is highlighted by the data placing the UK almost at the top of the mortality league table for heart disease. Elevated mortality from heart disease in the UK, and Scotland in particular, has been linked with a high-fat, low fiber diet and a conspicuous lack of fresh fruit and vegetables.

The proportion of overweight or obese adults in the UK is approaching 50%, due to

Box 11.3 Recommendations for the promotion of nutritional medicine

- The urgent addition of nutrition into the medical school curriculum.
- The improved communication of published research to physicians and the systemic and comprehensive integration of published findings into clinical practice.
- The requirement of open and vigorous debate about fundamental precepts such as RDAs, balanced diet and the use of supplements.
- The necessity for serious research about the many and varied dietary regimes currently being advocated and used by many tens of thousands of people, who claim efficacy, particularly for cancer — vegetarian, frugivore, raw food, macrobiotic, Gerson diet, fasting.
- The identification and research of components within vegetables and other foods which appear to protect against cancer and heart disease.
- Research of anti-estrogen foods such as soybeans and their preventive effects in cancer.
- Research of nutritional and herbal alternatives to HRT for menopausal women.

the consumption of high-fat and protein, low fiber diets and sedentary lifestyle. These trends, taken together, add up to a lethal cocktail of ill health, disease and suffering into the next millenium. The prescription needed to reverse these trends is well known and relies upon the simple nutritional practices of consuming a diet replete with fresh fruits and vegetables, whole grains, restraining alcohol overconsumption, taking moderate exercise and managing stress. This is not to say that adoption of the above measures will prevent or cure all cancers and heart disease, as clearly such diseases are multifactorial in nature, but the published nutritional research clearly points the way to better health and the prevention of much disease in the general population.

However, campaigns for the implementation of a more healthy diet have frequently run aground for a variety of reasons. There have been attacks in the media about the 'food police', and sarcastic sniping at food scares — to protests from the food industry over reports that nutrients such as sugar may be detrimental to health. Popular food programs on television have attacked, ridiculed and over-emphasized the dangers of taking nutritional supplements, while regaling their viewers with recipes for high-fat meat dishes, desserts cooked with large quantities of fat and sugar, and the obligatory gustatory tasting of wines.

People's reluctance to adopt healthier dietary and lifestyle practices is a major impediment to achieving better health. However, the disastrous events over the past decade which have posed serious dangers to public health — salmonella, listeria, BSE and CJD and the development of super-resistant bacteria — and which appear to have arisen from intensive agricultural and livestock handling techniques, have struck deep into the public psyche, and may be powerful allies in enabling the implementation of better dietary and nutritional habits. It is sincerely hoped that physicians will be leading the way in this campaign.

REFERENCES

1 Bristol Cancer Help Centre (BCHC) Nutrition and Cancer Database. For information about how to search the database for specific clinical topics, please contact Bristol Cancer Help Centre, Grove House, Cornwallis Grove, Clifton Bristol, BS8 4PG. Tel: 0117 980 9500

2 Goodman S 1995 Nutrition and cancer: state-of-the-art. Green Library, London, UK

3 Eichholzer M et al. 1996 Prediction of male cancer mortality by plasma levels of interacting vitamins: 17-year follow-up of the prospective Basel study. International Journal of Cancer 66(2):145–50

4 Freudenheim JL et al. 1996 Premenopausal breast cancer risk and intake of vegetables, fruits and related nutrients. Journal of the National Cancer Institute 88(6):340–8

5 Levy J et al. 1995 Lycopene is a more potent inhibitor of human cancer cell proliferation than either alpha-carotene or beta-carotene. Nutrition and Cancer 24(3):256–66

6 Singh RB et al. 1996 Usefulness of antioxidant vitamins in suspected acute myocardial infarction (the Indian experiment of infarct survival-3). American Journal of Cardiology 77(4):232–6

7 Kardinaal AF et al. 1995 Association between beta-carotene and acute myocardial infarction depends on polyunsaturated fatty acid status. The EURAMIC Study. European Study on Antioxidants, Myocardial Infarction, and Cancer of the Breast. Arteriosclerosis and Thrombosis Vascular Biology 15(6):726–32

8 Levy Y et al. 1994 Relationship between plasma antioxidants and coronary artery disease. Harefuah 127(5–6):154–7

9 Gey KF et al. 1993 Poor plasma status of carotene and vitamin C is associated with higher mortality from ischemic heart disease and stroke: Basel Prospective Study. Clinical Investigations 71(1):3–6

10 Cotter MA et al. 1995 Effects of natural free radical scavengers on peripheral nerve and neurovascular function in diabetic rats. Diabetologia 38(11):1285–94

11 Mikhail MS et al. 1994 Decreased beta-carotene levels in exfoliated vaginal epithelial cells in women with vaginal candidiasis. American Journal of Reproductive Immunology 32(3):221–5

12 Coodley GO et al. 1993 Beta-carotene in HIV infection. Journal of Acquired Immune Deficiency Syndrome 6(3):272–6

13 Heliovaara M et al. 1994 Serum antioxidants and risk of rheumatoid arthritis. Annals of Rheumatic Diseases 53(1):51–3

14 Potapova AA et al. 1993 The effect of beta-carotene on the development of adjuvant arthritis and interleukin-1 production in rats. Biulleten Eksperimentalnoi Biologii Meditsing 116(12):611–3

15 Rumore MM 1993 Vitamin A as an immunomodulating agent. Clinical Pharmacology 12(7):506–14

16 Van Antwerpen VL et al. 1995 Plasma levels of beta-carotene are inversely correlated with circulating neutrophil counts in young male cigarette smokers. Inflammation 19(4):405–14

17 Benton D 1992 Vitamin-mineral supplementation and the intelligence of children: a review. Journal of Orthodox Medicine 7:31–8

18 Zeisel S, Blusztajn J 1994 Choline and human nutrition. Annual Review of Nutrition 14:269–96

19 Butterworth CE Jr. 1992 Effect of folate on cervical cancer. Synergism among risk factors. Annals of the New York Academy of Sciences 669:293–9

20 Poydock ME 1991 Effect of combined ascorbic acid and B-12 on survival of mice with implanted Ehrlich carcinoma and L1210 leukemia. American Journal of Clinical Nutrition 54(6 Suppl):1261S–5S

21 Goodman S 1991 Vitamin C — The master nutrient. Keats Connecticut

22 La Vecchia C et al. 1996 Attributable risks for colorectal cancer in northern Italy. International Journal of Cancer 66(1):60–4

23 Taper HS et al. 1996 Potentiation of radiotherapy by nontoxic pretreatment with combined vitamin C and K3 in mice bearing solid transplantable tumor. Anticancer Research 16(1):499–503

24 Nunez-Martin C, Ortiz de Apodaco y Ruiz A 1995 Ascorbic acid in the plasma and blood cells of women with breast cancer. The effect of the consumption of food with an elevated content of this vitamin. Nutricion Hospitalaria 10(6):368–72

25 Cohen M, Bhagavan HN 1995 Ascorbic acid and gastrointestinal cancer. Journal of the American College of Nutrition 16(6):565–78

26 Retsky KL, Freeman MW, Frei B 1993 Ascorbic acid oxidation product(s) protect human low density lipoprotein against atherogenic modification. Anti- rather than prooxidant activity of vitamin C in the presence of transition metal ions. Journal of Biological Chemistry 268(2):1304–9

27 Slattery ML et al. 1995 Dietary antioxidants and plasma lipids: the Cardia Study. Journal of the American College of Nutrition 14(6):635–42

28 Howard PA, Meyers DG 1995 Effect of vitamin C on plasma lipids. Annals of Pharmacotherapy 29(11):1129–36

29 Bielory L, Gandhi R 1994 Asthma and vitamin C. Annals of Allergy 73(2):89–96

30 Troisi RJ, Willett WC et al. 1995 A prospective study of diet and adult-onset asthma. American Journal of Respiratory Critical Care Medicine 151(5):1401–8

31 Britton JR et al. 1995 Dietary antioxidant vitamin intake and lung function in the general population. American Journal of Respiratory Critical Care Medicine 151(5):1383–7

32 Nakajima H et al. 1993 Effects of ascorbic acid on trace element metabolism in the choroid-retina of streptozotocin-induced diabetic guinea pigs. Nippon Ganka Gakkai Zasshi 97(3):340–5

33 Schorah CJ et al. 1996 Total vitamin C, ascorbic acid, and dehydroascorbic acid concentrations in plasma of critically ill patients. American Journal of Clinical Nutrition 63(5):760–5

34 Gale CR et al. 1996 Cognitive impairment and mortality in a cohort of elderly people. British Medical Journal 312(7031):608–11

35 Moustafa SA et al. Effects of ageing and antioxidants on glucose transport in rat adipocytes. Gerontology. 41(6):301–7

36 Azhar S et al. 1995 Alteration of the adrenal antioxidant defense system during aging in rats. Journal of Clinical Investigation 96(3):1414–24

37 Hemila H, Herman ZS 1995 Vitamin C and the common cold: a retrospective analysis of Chalmers' review. Journal of the American College of Nutrition 14(2):116–23

38 Khaw KT, Woodhouse P 1995 Interrelation of vitamin C, infection, haemostatic factors, and cardiovascular disease. British Medical Journal 310(6994):1559–63

39 Torun M et al. 1995 Serum beta-carotene, vitamin E, vitamin C and malondialdehyde levels in several types of cancer. Journal of Clinical Pharmacy and Therapeutics 20(5):259–63

40 Dimitrov NV et al. 1994 Some aspects of vitamin E related to humans and breast cancer prevention. Advances in Experimental Medicine and Biology 364:119–27

41 Yano T et al. 1994 Effect of vitamin E on 4-nitroquinoline 1-oxide-induced lung tumorigenesis in mice. International Journal of Vitamin and Nutrition Research 64(3):181–4

42 HOPE study investigators 1996 The HOPE (Heart Outcomes Prevention Evaluation) Study: the design of a large, simple randomised trial of an angiotensin-converting enzyme inhibitor (ramipril) and vitamin E in patients at high risk of cardiovascular evens. Canadian Journal of Cardiology 12(2):127–37

43 Prasad K, Kalra J 1993 Oxygen free radicals and hypercholesterolemic atherosclerosis: effect of vitamin E. American Heart Journal 125(4):958–73

44 Mantha SV et al. 1993 Antioxidant enzymes in hypercholesterolemia and effects of vitamin E in rabbits. Atherosclerosis 101(2):135–44

45 Burton GW 1994 Vitamin E: molecular and biological function. Proceedings of the Nutrition Society 53(2):251–62

46 Kushi LH et al. 1996 Dietary antioxidant vitamins and death from coronary heart disease in post-menopausal women. New England Journal of Medicine 334(18):1156–62

47 Regnstrom J et al. 1996 Inverse relation between the concentration of low-density-lipoprotein vitamin E and severity of coronary artery disease. American Journal of Clinical Nutrition 63(3):377–85

48 Carpenter KL et al. 1995 Depletion of alpha-tocopherol in human atherosclerotic lesions. Free Radical Research 23(6):549–58

49 Boljevic S et al. 1993 Changes in free radicals and possibility of their correction in patients with bronchial asthma. Vojnosanitetski Pregled 50(1):3–18

50 Winklhofer-Roob BM et al. 1996 Response to a single oral dose of all-rac-alpha-tocopheryl acetate in patients with cystic fibrosis and in healthy individuals. American Journal of Clinical Nutrition 63(5):717–21

51 Winklhofer-Roob BM et al. 1996 Long-term oral vitamin E supplementation in cystic fibrosis patients: RRR-alpha-tocopherol compared with all-rac-alpha-tocopheryl acetate preparations. American Journal of Clinical Nutrition 63(5):722–8

52 Kauf et al. 1995 The value of selenotherapy in patients with mucoviscidosis. Medizinische Klinik 90(Suppl 1):41–5

53 Nasr SZ et al. 1993 Correction of vitamin E deficiency with fat-soluble versus water-miscible preparation of vitamin E in patients with cystic fibrosis. Journal of Pediatrics 122(5 Pt 1):810–2

54 Wilfond BS et al. 1994 Severe hemolytic anemia associated with vitamin E deficiency in infants with cystic fibrosis. Implications for neonatal screening. Clinical Pediatrics 33(1):2–7

55 Kuznetsov NS et al. 1994 The comparative evaluation of the efficacy of tocopherol acetate in the combined treatment of patients with hypertension and diabetes mellitus. Vrachebnoe Delo (9–12):133–6

56 Paolisso G et al. 1993 Daily vitamin E supplements improve metabolic control but not insulin secretion in elderly type II diabetic patients. Diabetes Care 16(11):1433–7

57 Caballero B 1993 Vitamin E improves the action of insulin. Nutrition Review 51(11):339–40

58 Gerster H 1993 Prevention of platelet dysfunction by vitamin E in diabetic atherosclerosis. Zeitschrift für Ernahrungswissenschaft 32(4):243–61

59 Congy F et al. 1995 Study of oxidative stress in the elderly. Presse Medicale 24(24):1115–8

60 Roy M et al. 1995 Supplementation with selenium restores age-related decline in immune cell function. Proceedings of the Society of Experimental Biology and Medicine 209(4):369–75

61 Rokitzki L et al. 1994 Alpha-tocopherol supplementation in racing cyclists during extreme endurance training. International Journal of Sport Nutrition 4(3):253–64

62 Haradell L et al. 1995 Levels of selenium in plasma and glutathione peroxidase in erythrocytes in patients with prostate cancer or benign hyperplasia. European Journal of Cancer Prevention 4(1):91–5

63 Lou H et al. 1995 Relation between selenium and cancer of uterine cervix. Chung Hua Chung Liu Tsa Chih 17(2):112–4

64 Burguera JL et al. 1995 Gastric tissue selenium levels in healthy persons, cancer and non-cancer patients with different kinds of mucosal damage. Journal of Trace Elements and Medical Biology 9(3):160–4

65 Oh SH et al. 1995 Evaluation of chemopreventive effect of dietary selenium-rich egg on mouse skin tumor induced by 2′-nitrophenoxy)oxirane and 12-O-tetradecanolyphorbol-13-acetate. Carcinogenesis 16(12):2995–8

66 Thiele R et al. 1995 Selenium level in patients with acute myocardial infarct and in patients with severe angina pectoris without myocardial infarct. Medica Klinica 90(Suppl 1):45–8

67 Vinceti M et al. 1994 Changes in drinking water selenium and mortality for coronary disease in a residential cohort. Biological Trace Elements Research 40(3):267–75

68 Nyyssonen K et al. 1994 Increase in oxidation resistance of atherogenic serum lipoproteins following antioxidant supplementation: a randomised double-blind placebo-controlled clinical trial. European Journal of Clinical Nutrition 48(9):633–42

69 Luomo P et al. 1995 High serum alpha-tocopherol, albumin, selenium and cholesterol, and low mortality from coronary heart disease in Northern Finland. Journal of Internal Medicine 237(1):49–54

70 Yamaguchi T 1996 Selenium concentration in blood and Duchenne-type progressive muscular dystrophy. Nippon Rinsho 54(1):134–40

71 Foster HD, Zhang L 1995 Longevity and selenium deficiency: evidence from the People's Republic of China. Science of the Total Environment 170(1–2):133–9

72 Tessier F et al. 1995 Selenium and training effects on the glutathione system and aerobic performance. Medicine and Science in Sports and Exercise 27(3):390–6

73 Darlow BA et al. 1995 The relationship of selenium status to respiratory outcome in the very low birth weight infant. Pediatrics 96(2 Pt 1):314–9

74 Wang WC et al. 1995 Effect of nationwide selenium supplementation in Finland on selenium status in children with juvenile rheumatoid arthritis. A ten-year follow-up study. Analyst 120(3):955–8

75 Wang WC et al. 1995 Effect of nationwide selenium supplementation in Finland on selenium status in children with juvenile rheumatoid arthritis. A ten-year follow-up study. Analyst 120(3):955–8

76 Portal B et al. 1995 Effect of double-blind cross-over selenium supplementation on lipid peroxidation markers in cystic fibrosis patients. Clinica Chimica Acta 234(1–2):137–46

77 Sagar PS, Das UN 1995 Cytotoxic action of cis-unsaturated fatty acids on human cervical carcinoma (HeLa) cells in vitro. Protaglandins Leukotrienes and Essential Fatty Acids 53(4):287–99

78 Hendrickse CW et al. 1995 Dietary omega-3 fats reduce proliferation and tumor yields of colorectal anastomosis in rats. Gastroenterology 109(2):431–9

79 Caygill CP, Hill MJ 1995 Fish, n-3 fatty acids and human colorectal and breast cancer mortality. European Journal of Cancer Prevention 4(4):329–32

80 Skuladottir GV et al. 1995 Plasma fatty acids and lipids in two separate, but genetically comparable, Icelandic populations. Lipids 30(7):649–55

81 Siscovick DS et al. 1995 Dietary intake and cell membrane levels of long-chain n-3 polyunsaturated fatty acids and the risk of primary cardiac arrest. JAMA 274(17):1363–7

82 Howe PR 1995 Can we recommend fish oil for hypertension? Clinical Experimental Pharmacology and Physiology 22(3):199–203

83 McDougall J et al. 1995 Rapid reduction of serum cholesterol and blood pressure by a twelve-day, very low fat, stricly vegetarian diet. Journal of the American College of Nutrition 14(5):491–6

84 Greenfield SM et al. 1993 A randomised controlled study of evening primrose oil and fish oil in ulcerative colitis. Alimentary Pharmacology and Therapeutics 7(2):159–66

85 Ross E 1993 The role of marine fish oils in the treatment of ulcerative colitis. Nutrition Review 51(2):47–9

86 Chawla A et al. 1995 Effect of N-3 polyunsaturated fatty acid supplemented diet on neutrophil-mediated ileal permeability and neutrophil function in the rat. Journal of American College of Nutrition 14(3):258–63

87 Buhner S et al. 1995 Ileal and colonic fatty acid profiles in patients with active Crohn's disease. Gut 35(10):1424–8

88 Collier PM et al. 1993 Effect of regular consumption of oily fish compared with white fish on chronic plaque psoriasis. European Journal of Clinical Nutrition 47(4):251–4

89 Tollesson A, Frithz A 1993 Transepidermal water loss and water content in the stratum corneum in infantile seborrhoeic dermatitis. Acta Dermato-Venereologica 73(1):18–20

90 Grimminger F et al. 1993 A double-blind, randomized placebo-controlled trial of n-3 fatty acid based lipid

infusion in acute, extended guttate psoriasis. Rapid improvement of clinical manifestations and changes in neutrophil leukotriene profile. Clinical Investigations 71(8):634–43

91 Henneicke-von-Zepelin HH et al. 1993 Highly purified omega-3-polyunsaturated fatty acids for topical treatment of psoriasis. Results of a double-blind, placebo-controlled multicentre study. British Journal of Dermatology 129(6):713–7

92 Lau CS et al. 1993 Effects of fish oil supplementation on non-steroidal anti-inflammatory drug requirement in patients with mild rheumatoid arthritis — a double-blind placebo controlled study. British Journal of Rheumatology 32(11):982–9

93 Nettleton JA 1993 Are n-3 fatty acids essential nutrients for fetal and infant development? Journal of the American Dietetic Association 93(1):58–64

94 Crane FL, Navas P 1995 Dynamic antioxidant action of coenzyme Q. Proceedings of the National Academy of Sciences of the USA 92:4887

95 Niki E et al. 1996 Mechanism and dynamics of antioxidant action of coenzyme Q. 9th International Symposium on Biomedical and Clinical Aspects of Coenzyme Q, Ancona, Italy

96 Sohal RS 1996 Relationship between coenzyme Q homologues, mitochondrial free radical generation and aging. 9th International Symposium on Biomedical and Clinical Aspects of Coenzyme Q, Ancona, Italy

97 Alho H et al. 1996 Uniquinone and total peroxyl radical trapping capacity of LDL lipoproteins during aging: the effect of Q_{10} supplementation. 9th International Symposium on Biomedical and Clinical Aspects of Coenzyme Q, Ancona, Italy

98 Linnance AW 1996 The universality of bioenergetic disease an amelioration therapy: Coenzyme Q_{10} and analogues. 9th International Symposium on Biomedical and Clinical Aspects of Coenzyme Q, Ancona, Italy

99 Yamamoto Y, Yamashita S 1996 Simultaneous detection of ubiquinol and uniquinone as a marker of oxidative stress. 9th International Symposium on Biomedical and Clinical Aspects of Coenzyme Q, Ancona, Italy

100 Stocker R 1996 Inhibition of radical-initiated LDL oxidation by ubiquinol-10. A protective role for coenzyme Q in atherogenesis? 9th International Symposium on Biomedical and Clinical Aspects of Coenzyme Q, Ancona, Italy

101 Alleva R et al. 1996 Oxidation of LDL and their subfractions: kinetic aspects and CoQ_{10} content. 9th International Symposium on Biomedical and Clinical Aspects of Coenzyme Q, Ancona, Italy

102 Mortensen SA 1996 Coenzyme Q clinical overview: potential roles in prevention and as adjunctive therapy of cardiovascular disease. 9th International Symposium on Biomedical and Clinical Aspects of Coenzyme Q, Ancona, Italy

103 Langsjoen PH, Willis R, Folkers K 1996 Treatment of hypertrophic cardiomyopathy with coenzyme Q10. 9th International Symposium on Biomedical and Clinical Aspects of Coenzyme Q, Ancona, Italy

104 Soja AM, Mortensen SA CoQ_{10} in the treatment of congestive heart failure: a meta-analysis of randomized controlled trials. 9th International Symposium on Biomedical and Clinical Aspects of Coenzyme Q, Ancona, Italy

105 Lewin A 1996 The effect of coenzyme Q_{10} on sperm motility. 9th International Symposium on Biomedical and Clinical Aspects of Coenzyme Q, Ancona, Italy

106 Alleva R et al. 1996 Protective role of uniquinol content against hydroperoxide formation in human seminal fluid. 9th International Symposium on Biomedical and Clinical Aspects of Coenzyme Q, Ancona, Italy

107 Podda M, Packer L 1996 Uniquinol: a marker of oxidative stress in skin. 9th International Symposium on Biomedical and Clinical Aspects of Coenzyme Q, Ancona, Italy

108 Lockwood K et al. 1994 Partial and complete remission of breast cancer in patients in relation to dosage of coenzyme Q_{10}. Biochemical Biophysical Research Communications 199:1504–8

109 Lockwood K et al. 1996 Progress on therapy of breast cancer with coenzyme Q_{10} and the regression of metastases. 9th International Symposium on Biomedical and Clinical Aspects of Coenzyme Q, Ancona, Italy

110 Nylander M 1996 Coenzyme Q_{10}: a therapeutic adjuvant in periodontal disease. 9th International Symposium on Biomedical and Clinical Aspects of Coenzyme Q, Ancona, Italy

111 Beal FM 1996 Neuroprotective effects of coenzyme Q in models of neurodegenerative diseases. 9th International Symposium on Biomedical and Clinical Aspects of Coenzyme Q, Ancona, Italy

112 Salonen JT et al. 1996 Coenzyme Q_{10} supplementation and lipoprotein oxidation resistance: a randomized placebo-controlled double-blind study in marathon runners. 9th International Symposium on Biomedical and Clinical Aspects of Coenzyme Q, Ancona, Italy

113 Battino M et al. 1996 Metabolic and antioxidant markers in plasma of sportmen from a mediterranean town performing not agonist activity. 9th International Symposium on Biomedical and Clinical Aspects of Coenzyme Q, Ancona, Italy

114 McAlindon TE et al. 1996 Do antioxidant micronutrients protect against the development and progression of knee osteoarthritis? Arthritis and Rheumatism 39(4):648–56

115 Arm JP et al. Leukotrienes, fish-oil and asthma. Allergy Proceedings 15(3):129–34

116 Rohan TE et al. 1995 Dietary factors and risk of prostate cancer: a case-control study in Ontario, Canada. Cancer Causes and Control 6(2):145–54

117 Garcia J et al. 1995 Dietary carotene intake and lung cancer among men from Santiago. Revista Medica Chile 123(1):51–60

118 Lupulescu A 1994 The role of vitamins A, beta-carotene, E and C in cancer cell biology. International Journal of Vitamin and Nutrition Research 64(1):3–14

119 Belluzzi et al. 1996 Effect of an enteric-coated fish-oil preparation on relapses in Crohn's disease. New England Journal of Medicine 334(24):1557–60

120 Buffinton GD, Doe WF 1995 Depleted mucosal antioxidant defences in inflammatory bowel disease. Free Radical Biology and Medicine 19(6):911–8

121 Stephens NG et al. 1996 Randomised controlled trial of vitamin E in patients with coronary disease: Cambridge Heart Antioxidant Study (CHAOS) 347(9004):781–6

122 Weber C et al. 1996 Increased adhesiveness of isolated monocytes to endothelium is prevented by vitamin C

intake in smokers. Circulation 93(80):1488–92
123 Panzetta O et al. 1995 Increased susceptibility of LDL to in vitro oxidation in patients on maintenance hemodialysis: effects of fish oil and vitamin E administration. Clinical Nephrology 44(5):303–9
124 Curhan GC, Willett WC et al. 1996 A prospective study of the intake of vitamins C and B_6, and the risk of kidney stones in men. Journal of Urology 155(6):1847–51
125 Positive Health. Positive Health Publications Ltd., 51 Queen Square, Bristol BS1 4LJ. Tel: (0117) 983 8851; Fax: (0117) 908 0097
126 Perry W 1989 Protocol of the American College of Advancement in Medicine for the Safe and Effective Administration of EDTA Chelation Therapy
127 Chappell LT 1994 Bibliography on Mechanisms of Action of EDTA. Townsend Letter for Doctors 130:475
128 Chappell LT, Stahl JP 1993 The correlation between EDTA chelation therapy and improvement in cardiovascular function: a meta-analysis. Journal of Advancement in Medicine 6:2
129 Hancke C, Flytlie K 1993 Benefits of EDTA chelation therapy in arteriosclerosis: A retrospective study of 470 patients. Journal of Advancement in Medicine 6(3):161–71
130 1992. The Health of the Nation. Government White Paper, HMSO

CHAPTER CONTENTS

12

Substance misuse

Patricia D. Culliton
Tacey Ann Boucher
Gregory A. Carlson

INTRODUCTION

Acupuncture as a method of treating illness dates back well over 3000 years. Herbal remedies and nutritional therapies were used to treat disease long before the Hippocratic oath was conceptualized. Today these and other therapies are often labeled 'alternative' modalities, 'defined through a social process as those practices that do not form part of the dominant system for managing health and disease'[1].

The use of 'alternative modalities' to treat problems of substance misuse dates back at least to the turn of the century when peddlers sold 'remedies' for every ailment imaginable. However, it has only been in the past two or three decades that researchers have taken an active role in exploring the efficacy of alternative therapies for the treatment of substance misuse. Because the scope of both addiction medicine and alternative medicine is broad and ever changing, the work has hardly begun.

This chapter summarizes the current state of addiction medicine and gives an overview of what alternative therapies have been used to treat addiction. We will review conventional treatment modalities, and addiction methodology and research. Our critique of the conventional will lead us into our overview of alternative medicine, and a review of current research. Finally, we will provide directions for future research.

Statement of the problem

The consequences of addiction vary depending upon the substance(s), patterns of use, and characteristics of the users themselves. The physiological consequences of addiction are extensive and can be devastating. In addition, substance misuse has been shown to increase the risk of violence, sexually transmitted disease, chronic ailments, and traumatic injury. Alcohol, in particular, is a primary contributor to the number of unintentional injuries, drowning, motor vehicle crashes, and violent acts such as homicide or suicide[2].

The economic and social costs of substance misuse are high. One estimate placed the total expenditures on US health care, related to drug and alcohol abuse, at $14 billion. Another estimate placed the total costs of tobacco, alcohol and illicit drug use for the US economy including health care and lost productivity at more than $238 billion in 1990[3]. The costs to the criminal justice system are also high with over 60% of incarcerated individuals in the USA there on drug-related offenses. The negative impacts of misuse can be measured in every social institution including the community, the workplace, the schools, and the family. Meanwhile, 'crack' cocaine and amphetamines, with severe consequences of dependence, threaten to increase worldwide illegal drug use[4].

RECENT HISTORY OF SUBSTANCE MISUSE

Substance misuse is an issue of great complexity. Though literature is abundant, consensus over definitions, diagnosis, and treatment is lacking. Models of addiction and abuse still contain elements of both medical and moral explanations, and attribute misuse to biochemical, behavioral, social, and genetic causal determinants[5]. The consequences of misuse vary widely depending upon the user's social environment and pattern of use, but may result in a wide variety of physiological ailments and include any number of social costs.

Concern over increasing drug use in Europe and the USA led to the development of clinical conceptions of addiction in the late 1870s[6], even though the psychological and physical effects of many drugs had been noted for centuries. In the late 19th Century, a number of behaviors, including drug misuse, were no longer seen as moral failings, and the medical profession identified addicts as chronically ill and in need of physician care. However, in the USA during the 1920s, the medical perspective was replaced with a punitive model which treated addicts as hedonists and degenerates who needed to be punished[7].

The New York Society of Medicine was a pioneer in the battle to have addiction recognized as a disease. The states of California and New York were early leaders in the formation of the disease model. However, in the USA not until 1966 did the American Medical Association formally recognize alcoholism as a disease; drug addiction was not defined as a disease until 1988. This designation was an attempt to incorporate users into the treatment community by influencing physician attitudes towards users as well as to encourage providers of insurance to cover treatment services[8].

In the 1920s, the Department of Health in the UK stated that addiction was a health problem and recommended that addicts be seen as patients. Thus medical treatment for substance misuse was legitimized and the administration of narcotics to patients was legalized. This stance differed markedly from the US position at the time and had significant social and legal consequences. Even when legislation and enforcement practices were altered decades later, the UK maintained a uniform system for the diagnosis and treatment of dependence and abuse[9]. Despite the consistency of the UK approach, the UK and the USA are confronted with similar problems today, and neither system seems to have had a significant impact on the prevalence of misuse.

DEPENDENCE VS. ABUSE

To date, there has not been a clear-cut, universally accepted definition of substance misuse.

Criteria have varied significantly by discipline. The medical model assumes a unitary disease entity having a prescribed physical origin while psychiatric and psychological definitions assume that use disorders are rooted in mental or behavioral disorders. Scientific definitions have ranged from cognitive-behavior approaches, which focus on observations of the user's behavior, to pharmacological definitions which emphasize criteria of tolerance and physical dependence. All of these conflict with legal definitions which incorporate moral and physiological causes, and sociological concepts which may emphasize the importance of cultural definitions and labeling in the identification of physical illness or mental and behavioral disorders. Yet despite the lack of standardization most agree that misuse includes the consumption of psychoactive substances which often results in intoxication or impairment[8].

Classification of types of use are also contested. There seems to be some agreement over the distinction between substance dependence, substance abuse, and harmful use of a substance. Such a distinction is made in the most popular diagnostic tools, the Diagnostic Statistical Manual of Mental Disorders (DSM) and the International Classification of Disease (ICD). The World Health Organization (responsible for the creation of the ICD) defines substance abuse as 'persistent or sporadic excessive use inconsistent with or unrelated to acceptable medical practice'[9]. The WHO also introduced the term 'harmful use' which refers to 'a pattern of psychoactive drug use that causes damage to health, either mental or physical' as well as to family, community, and the larger society. These two terms differ from dependence which incorporates the preoccupation with obtaining the substance, and persistent use. The WHO recognizes that the determinants and consequences may be biological, psychological, or social and are difficult to isolate[9].

The difficulties in defining and differentiating dependence/addiction, abuse and harmful use can create confusion in the literature when the purpose or intent of an intervention is unclear. We have thus selected a term which encompasses both issues of abuse and dependence to be used throughout this review, 'substance misuse.' Where chemical dependency or substance abuse may only refer to one aspect of the topic being discussed, substance misuse or substance use disorders incorporate the entire range of use patterns. The terms 'abuse' and 'dependence' will be used in accordance with the DSM and ICD, or when use of the terms in the literature being discussed cannot be inferred.

Operational definitions/diagnostic tools

The classification of a disorder universally precedes treatment, yet the method for classifying any ailment is far from universal. Substance misuse is certainly no exception. Despite the WHO definitions, there are no uniform cross-cultural standards by which to evaluate addiction. Even the methods and instruments of diagnosis utilized by health care systems in the UK and the USA differ significantly. While US treatment facilities and physicians rely heavily upon the DSM III-R and IV, and the ICD 9 and 10, the British incorporate a much broader range of criteria including life histories in an attempt to more accurately define the severity or dimension of the problem.

US organizations have concentrated on the DSM as the result of two primary factors: first, the DSM serves to improve communication about substance use among clinicians, researchers, and the public and second, it serves an administrative function for chemical dependency centers by regulating access to and financing of treatment programs particularly in respect to insurance coverage[8,10]. The DSM has also helped standardize data collection and has facilitated the creation of theories about etiology and the natural history of substance misuse[10].

In contrast to US practices, the UK system requires a more thorough method of assessment, especially in drug dependence treatment units (DDTUs) where the evaluation process may take weeks. Insurance is not the primary concern of the UK system. Rather, due to the popularity of methadone maintenance programs, specialists must be certain that program attendees truly are in need of a prescription and do not obtain one for other purposes[9].

Effectiveness of diagnosis

Despite the prevalence of available tools and methods, studies indicate that 'only about 10% of patients who meet research diagnostic criteria for substance abuse ... are recognized by primary care providers'[11]. Two factors which contribute to this low rate of identification are the types of substances utilized as well as patient demographics. First, the majority of discussions about addictions relate to problems involving illicit substances (heroin, cocaine, opium) or legal substances such as alcohol and nicotine. Addictions to over the counter and prescription medications are often viewed as unrelated or less serious.

Second, certain providers of care have less success identifying substance abusers and addicts within social demographic groups such as the elderly, business people, and physicians. Studies have reported that employed, married, white, insured, or female patients misusing substances are unlikely to be identified[12]. Even when abuse is suspected, intervention may be delayed. Often a diagnosis is not made until the user displays physical and psychiatric complications during a late stage of addiction[11]. Due to the difficulties and bias underlying the diagnosis of substance misuse, it has been suggested that whenever patients present to physicians, substance misuse should be considered as a causal or contributing factor in every case until deemed otherwise[13].

CAUSES OF SUBSTANCE MISUSE

We still do not have answers to many of the questions concerning substance misuse. While we know that the majority of humans use psychoactive drugs (including nicotine, caffeine and alcohol), the majority of users never misuse substances[14]. Why? The causes of addiction are complex and varied. Explanations derive from five perspectives which in turn have numerous subsets: systemic, sociological, psychological, physiological, and pharmacological. Each strand of thought implies a certain response or mode of treatment.

Perhaps one of the most obvious causes is systemic and pertains to the availability of the drug. Quite simply if the substance is unavailable it cannot be misused. This has become a basic tenet of many law enforcement agencies with regard to illicit substances. Still, most enforcement agencies have been unable to significantly reduce the flow of illegal drugs to date, and legal substances such as alcohol, tobacco, and over the counter medications are readily available to most populations. Yet in some Eastern localities where alcohol is not readily available and its use is prohibited by law or religious precepts, alcoholism is virtually unknown[15]. Asian countries with severe penalties and social sanctions against drug use also report few drug problems.

Sociologists have taken a myriad of approaches to the issue of substance abuse and dependence but have traditionally focused on the environment or social interactions[14]. Some have focused upon external and inhibitory factors resulting from daily activities, rapid social changes, various cultural expectations, as well as social organizations such as the family, religion, the legal system, the media, and the educational system[16]. Others have focused on the dominant ideologies pertaining to substance use, the inequalities of the social system, and the impact of labeling upon diagnosis and recovery[8]. Sociologists have highlighted the group functions associated with psychoactive drugs. Substance use in religious ceremonies or rituals has been frequent across cultures and time, from the use of alcohol in Jewish and Christian ceremonies to the use of peyote by the Native American Church or opium at certain Hindu marriages[17].

Though psychoanalytic, family therapy, and cognitive-behavioral explanations differ, psychiatric or psychological models of substance misuse typically implicate the mental or behavioral disorders associated with physical and environmental factors as causing addiction and abuse. For example, individuals suffering from an underlying psychological conflict and experiencing difficulties in interpersonal relationships, or behavioral responses modified and reinforced by antecedent conditions and consequences may then discover that substance use helps them achieve relief from this suffering or stimulates distraction[8,17]. Recently psychiatrists have also branched towards more physiological approaches and turned their attention to the role of neurotransmitters in the etiology and maintenance of addiction[14].

Physiological explanations

Numerous physiological causes of substance misuse have been contemplated in the literature and overlap with pharmacological discussions. Included in this discussion are genetic and neurochemical explanations. Thus far genetic explanations have shown great promise for both male and female substance abusers and dependents[18–20]. Researchers have mapped out the genetic influences related to alcohol-metabolizing enzymes, personality traits, as well as relevant neurochemical receptors for alcoholism. Alcoholism has been more extensively studied than other forms of misuse, but the evidence suggests that physiological explanations may be applicable for other substances[15].

Advances in neurochemistry and molecular biology have generated considerable enthusiasm over the past decade as well. Newer research methods and techniques, such as PET scanning of the brain continue to yield new findings. Of particular interest to researchers interested in substance misuse is that related to dopamine and serotonin activity in the brain[15,21–23].

A recent review by Nutt[23] outlined the treatment implications of this research. The neurochemical data suggest that misused drugs are neuroactive and alter excitatory and inhibitory neurochemical receptive and transmitter functions. The better a drug is at producing its neuropharmacological effect, the greater its addiction potential and street value. Fortunately, the molecular pharmacology of most drugs of misuse has now been characterized and is providing valuable insights into the roles of neurotransmitters in addiction[23]. In the next decade research will surely uncover links to neurotransmitters other than dopamine, GABA, serotonin and the endogenous opioids, but these have been most intensely studied to date.

Most mood altering drugs increase dopamine levels and higher steady state levels are established with chronic use such that when the drug is stopped dopamine levels decrease below normal and the user experiences the 'crash'. Research has implicated dopamine as a prime mediator of alcoholic delirium tremens, and has also suggested that cocaine globally decreases brain metabolic activity[23].

Serotonin (5-HT) has numerous behavioral effects including some related to addiction, such as increased appetite, impulsivity, and craving. Synaptic levels of 5-HT can be augmented with the use of selective serotonin reuptake inhibitors (SSRIs). Use of the SSRIs has been studied for treatment of cocaine addiction and more recently has been correlated with voluntary reduction in alcohol consumption in heavy social drinkers[24].

Endogenous opioids are involved in regulating the body's appetite, and response to pain and stress. The effects of natural opioids are mimicked by misused opioids such as heroin. The potency of illicit opioids enables endogenous opioid production to generate exaggerated behavior and perceptual responses. The production of endogenous opioids may decline and desire for the illicit opioids may result. Craving may also result from other neurochemical deficits involving the dopaminergic, GABA-ergic or serotonergic system. These deficits may be genetically induced or result from long-term stress or heavy drinking.

An increasingly active area of research involves what is known as 'residual effects'[25]. This refers to impairments in neurobehavioral responses, including perception and cognition, which remain after detoxification. Such residual effects may also hold valuable clues for researchers. For example, repeated withdrawal may help to explain brain damage found among heavy drinkers. The amino acids GABA and glutamate are the major excitatory and inhibitory transmitters in the brain. Alcohol and barbiturates block some glutamate receptors, resulting in an upregulation in receptor numbers. During withdrawal this increase in receptor numbers contributes to cellular hyperexcitibility state, and the neurotoxic effects of excessive glutamate activity may result in brain damage[26].

Behavioral manifestations of substance use differ cross-culturally, which lends some researchers to argue that molecular structure has less to do with the behavioral effects of drug dependence than does the environment[27]. However, recent neurochemical and molecular findings provide strong evidence for a physiological model of dependence.

ADDICTION TREATMENT

Historical issues

During the first half of this century treatment for addictive disorders was largely limited to public or exclusive private residential settings which employed somatic therapies and abstinence enforced via institutionalization[28]. Turn-of-the-century treatment for morphinism specialized in 'hot baths and electro-therapy' (Fig. 12.1). Fifty years later state-of-the-art treatment of alcoholism had progressed little; generally limited to residential-based, medically managed withdrawal and referral to Alcoholics Anonymous. The 'disease model' of alcoholism was not widely accepted by medical professionals at the time. While the relative success of this approach is unknown, it is believed to have been highly ineffective and in part responsible for the growth of the anti-medical, anti-professional self-help movement and the eventual recognition by the medical community that detoxification did not constitute treatment. Addictionologists of the day reasoned that since this approach provided sufficient treatment 'intensity' (i.e. full inpatient services, 24-hour nursing care, etc.), its ineffectiveness must be due to its short duration. Treatment programs were initiated which emphasized long duration, low intensity services, typically last-

WALNUT LODGE HOSPITAL

HARTFORD, CONNECTICUT

Organized in 1880 for the Special Medical treatment of

Alcohol and Opium Inebriates

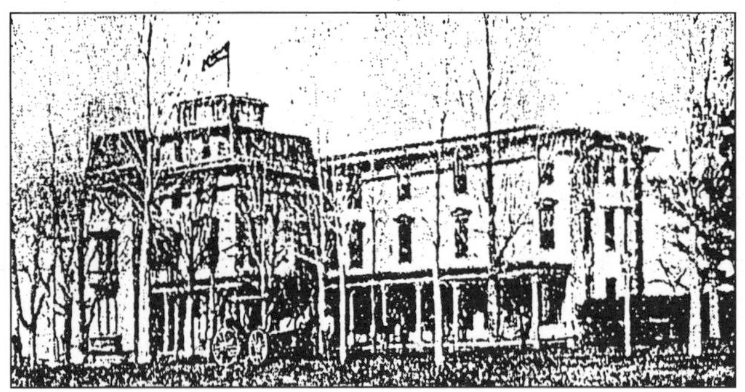

Elegantly situated in the suburbs of the city, with every appointment and appliance for the treatment of this class of cases, including Turkish, Roman, Saline and Electric Baths. Each case comes under the direct personal care of the physician. This institution is founded on the well-recognized fact that Inebriety is a disease and curable and all these cases require rest, change of thought and living, with every means known to science and experience to bring about this result. Applications and all inquiries should be addressed.

T. D. CROTHERS, M. D., Sup't, Walnut Lodge, HARTFORD, CONN.

Figure 12.1 'Hot baths and electro-therapy'

ing 6 months and often in treatment settings for the chronically mentally ill. Treatment interventions included enforced abstinence and individual or group psychotherapy. Unfortunately, this duration-based, enforced abstinence treatment approach was also ineffective; relapse rates from Public Health Service narcotic treatment hospitals at Lexington, KY and Fort Worth, TX were as high as 96% at 6 months post discharge[29].

By the early 1960s experiments in 'high intensity, short duration' treatment were under way. Wilmar State Hospital and Hazelden Treatment Center in Minnesota were among the first residential settings to incorporate the disease concept of alcoholism and the principles of Alcoholics Anonymous[30–32]. Patients completing 6 to 10 weeks of this treatment approach and who became active in regular aftercare (Alcoholics Anonymous) appeared to achieve and maintain significant periods of abstinence. However, patients not participating in ongoing mutual self-help groups post discharge were believed to fare no better than those receiving long duration, low intensity treatment. A number of studies[33–35] have found a strong relationship between abstinence and participation in mutual assistance groups such as Alcoholics Anonymous and Narcotics Anonymous, although a cause and effect relationship has not been definitely established. (It is important to note that in the USA only about 15% of recovering persons actively participate in self-help groups.) More recent studies[36] have concluded that it is not intensity or duration of treatment alone, but rather the amount of treatment received over time that is associated with outcome of abstinence. Economics have played a significant role in the shift of treatment from primarily inpatient to primarily outpatient settings. A number of researchers in the late 1980s precipitated a revolution in treatment funding by establishing that for the majority of patients outpatient was as effective as inpatient, and at greatly reduced per-patient costs. In fact, at least one researcher found that access to inpatient treatment was inversely related to the need for such treatment[37]. Aside from the need for detoxification, it appears that in the USA the vast majority of addicts can be treated in outpatient settings more cost-effectively than in inpatient settings, particularly hospital-based settings. This has had the effect of focusing attention instead on the relative effectiveness of individual treatment methods and interventions.

Treatment methods and interventions

In contrast to past treatment approaches which were unidimensional and characterized by 'one size fits all' approaches, most contemporary US treatment programs attempt to incorporate eclectic, holistic, and highly individualized approaches. Currently there is an emphasis on identifying treatment/patient matching technologies which maximize patient outcome. Treatment techniques and components found in the majority of US treatment programs are briefly summarized below:

Comprehensive assessment

Contemporary treatment approaches emphasize comprehensive evaluation by a multidisciplinary team which may include physicians, psychiatrists, nurses, chemical dependency counselors, social workers, occupational therapists, and psychologists. The effects of substance abuse on functioning in addition to psychiatric and medical problems are determined via structured clinical interviews, self-rating instruments, and interviews with family members. Special assessment services include work evaluation, physical medicine and rehabilitation, neuropsychological testing, and special psychological assessments.

Medical services

Includes physical examination and assessment of the need for medical treatment. This may include, but is not necessarily limited to, detoxification from substances of abuse, routine health monitoring, diagnosis and treatment of minor medical disorders, consultation and referral for co-existing medical conditions or disease, nutritional counseling, and access to wide range of medical services.

Sociotherapies

Patients in most treatment programs participate in a therapeutic milieu based on a 'recovering community' concept in which group therapy provides peer-based confrontation, support, education, and role-modeling. Involvement in mutual assistance and self-help groups is usually mandatory. Treatment activities include 'first-step' presentations, alumni testimonials, chemical health groups, audio-visual exercises, group treatment review, affirmation presentations, relapse prevention exercises, weekend planning and 'check-in' groups.

Pharmacotherapies

In contrast to historical 'anti-medication' sentiments, pharmacotherapies are currently emerging in the USA as a integral component of treatment and a consideration in all treatment plans. Agents include narcotic agonist and antagonist therapies, nausea aversion therapies (disulfiram), somatic treatments for affective disorders, tricyclic and SSRI antidepressant medications, anti-anxiety and anti-mania medications, neuroleptics, somatic treatment, etc. Naltrexone, an opiate antagonist, is showing promise in helping to maintain alcohol abstinence. In treatment settings patients are often required to demonstrate medication compliance by ingesting medication in the presence of staff or in group therapy.

Psychosocial education

Information regarding substance abuse, mental illness, and associated health problems is provided along with education about the diagnosis, treatment and recovery principles involved in treating substance misuse. These are usually provided in the form of a didactic lecture, individual sessions, video/audio tapes, book and article readings, and tutorial study guides. Educational programs may be provided by chemical health education groups, physicians or nurses, nutritionists, experts in wellness, or outside speakers.

12-Step work

Structured individual and group exercises based on the principles of Alcoholics Anonymous are used extensively in almost all treatment programs and usually require that patients complete a least the first five 'steps' of AA/NA prior to completion of the program. Variations and modifications of AA/NA such as Rational Recovery (RR) are becoming very popular with recovering persons not accepting of traditional self-help philosophy.

Relapse prevention

Most programs include relapse prevention education and self-monitoring, self-review techniques based on extensive relapse studies and prevention techniques (i.e. Marlott and Gorden).

Cognitive therapies

Cognitive restructuring techniques including Rational-Emotive Therapy (RET), Cognitive-Behavioral Therapy (CBT) and brief motivational analysis (Motivational Interviewing) is provided on an individual or group basis and in primary and continuous care settings.

Psychotherapies

Individual and group psychotherapies including both dynamic oriented approaches (analytic, Rogerian, Jungian, etc.) and non-verbal psychotherapies (art therapy, music therapy, etc.) are also utilized. These services are usually provided through trained, licensed program staff or outside therapists, but are generally viewed as an adjunctive to primary treatment.

Behavioral therapies

Behavioral criteria and measures are used to provide feedback and therapeutic focus to patients and staff in many treatment programs. These treatment services include routine toxicology (urine-drug) screening, behavioral oriented treatment planning, medication monitoring, individual treatment review sessions, contingency contracting, token economies (point system), coping catalogs, relaxation therapy, and movement therapy.

Family therapy

Involvement in the recovery process of the patient's significant other(s), family, and supportive social network is emphasized in most traditional treatment programs. Structured and Strategic Family Therapy principles are most often used. Included is an initial assessment interview followed by education, intervention, and recovery maintenance sessions. These sessions typically include family of origin and generation, but may also include substitute 'family' members including other health care providers involved in the patient's recovery.

Occupational therapy

These services include assessment of functioning skills, abilities, and exposure to recovery resources. Program modules include daily living/independent living skills assessments, leisure/vocational skills assessment, prevocational/vocational skills assessment, psychosocial/community-social skills assessment, basic living skills group, orientation to recovery resources (via in-program presentations or field trips), and leisure/vocational activities.

Brief interventions/case management

Brief interventions, usually in the office practice of a certified physician addictionologist, and ongoing case management approaches are increasing in popularity for medically ill or chronically addicted persons.

It is important to note that traditional treatment methods and interventions have included a variety of alternative medicine elements (i.e. relaxation, meditation, nutritional counseling, etc). At present, the degree to which these elements contribute to treatment outcome is unknown, but believed to be significant.

Treatment effectiveness

In a classic review by Holder et al.[38] the relative effectiveness of contemporary approaches to the treatment of alcoholism in the USA were evaluated and, based on existing studies in the literature, categorized by their efficacy (Box 12.1). Modalities were evaluated by examining controlled studies which had been conducted looking at outcome data on levels of consumption and relative effectiveness of treatment (to controls, placebos, and other established modalities). Studies were then established as either positive or negative, and each modality was ranked using a weighted evidence index, so that modalities with one positive and one negative study would not be ranked the same as modalities with five positive and five negative studies ((P–N) + (1 for every P over 2) — so if 2 negative and 3 positive studies: 3–2+1=+2).

Box 12.1 Evaluation of treatment effectiveness

- **No evidence for effectiveness**
  Antianxiety medications
  Confrontational interactions
  Educational lectures/films
  Electrical aversion therapy
  General counseling
  Group therapies
  Insight-oriented psychotherapies
  Nausea aversion therapies
  Residential milieu therapies
- **Insufficient evidence (fewer than three studies)**
  Alcoholics Anonymous (AA)
  Minnesota model of residential treatment
  Halfway houses
  Acupuncture
- **Indeterminate evidence of effect**
  Cognitive therapy
- **Good evidence for effectiveness**
  Behavioral marital therapies
  Brief motivational counseling
  Community reinforcement approach
  Self-control training
  Social skills training
  Stress management

Adapted from Holder et al., 1991

This list provides a starting point for resource allocation for alcoholism. Unfortunately a similar list has not yet been constructed for the treatment of other drug use disorders. However, Gerstein[39] reviewed methadone maintenance programs, therapeutic communities, outpatient non-methadone treatment, chemical dependency treatment, and correctional treatment programs. Results were varied though he concluded that methadone treatment for opioid-dependent individuals was more effective than no treatment at all. Furthermore, most therapeutic community patients stop using illicit drugs while in residence and graduates from treatment programs perform better after discharge; however, dropout rates range between 75% and 85%. The efficacy of outpatient non-methadone treatments are similar to therapeutic communities, although the rate of attrition is even higher. There is insufficient evidence by which to evaluate chemical dependency treatment though there is reason to believe this method of treatment is less effective for drugs other than alcohol. Finally, while some correctional treatment programs may reduce rearrest rates, relapse rates are generally unknown[39].

ADDICTION RESEARCH: METHODOLOGICAL PROBLEMS

There is no question that substance abuse is a serious problem. In the USA, it is estimated that alcoholism alone results in costs greater than the combined costs resulting from all cancers and respiratory diseases[40]. However the methods used to study drug problems are complex, and the lack of standardization hinders comparative analysis. We have compiled a list of the major criticisms confronting addiction research and will look at each one in detail (Box 12.2):

1. Preparation of research protocol
2. Selecting subjects and treatment assignments
3. Treatment comparisons
4. Analysis and outcomes.

Box 12.2 Common difficulties in chemical dependency research

- **Difficulties in designing a research protocol:**
  1. *Inadequate definition of the problem**.
  2. Selective and incomplete reviews of the literature.
  3. Inadequate accounting of motivation for treatment.
- **Pitfalls in selecting subjects and assigning them to treatment groups:**
  4. *Inadequate choice of diagnostic criteria for selecting subjects**.
  5. Studies compromised by opt-out options or self-assignment to treatment group.
  6. Unclear treatment assignment rules.
- **Difficulties of study comparisons of treatment effects:**
  7. *Lack of uniform standards in the evaluation of treatment efficacy**.
  8. Inappropriate choice of, or omission of, treatment comparison groups.
  9. The use of non-comparably trained and dedicated therapists in the treatment groups.
  10. The use of treatments that are comparably time and therapist-intensive.
  11. Failure to equate the credibility of treatments under comparison.
  12. The generalization of treatment effects to all substances of abuse.
- **Errors in the analysis and evaluation of outcomes:**
  13. *Inadequate length of follow-up**
  14. Failure to account for placebo and non-specific treatment effects.
  15. Failure to measure treatment compliance.
  16. Failure to include an appropriate, multidimensional range of outcomes (such as social and family outcomes, employment and psychological status) in addition to cocaine use.
  17. Use of outcomes of dubious validity (self-reports unverified by collateral information).
  18. Failure to include cost analyses of treatment and outcomes.
  19. Inadequate handling of dropout data.
  20. Failure to distinguish statistical vs. clinical significance.

**Items in italics are discussed in more detail in text*

Inadequate definition of the problem

Difficulties first arise when researchers attempt to define the parameters of their study. How do they differentiate between acceptable use and misuse of various substances? When is a subject abusing a substance and when are they addicted? Quite frequently these issues are not addressed in published research. The problem of definition becomes apparent when comparing studies cross-culturally as patterns of acceptable use vary widely[41]. Several standardized measurement tools have been developed which can help clarify these issues such as the DSM and ICD discussed earlier, as well as the Addiction Severity Index (ASI), the Alcohol Dependence Scale (ADS), the Timeline Follow Back (TLFB), and the Michigan Alcohol Screening Test (MAST). Despite the availability of such standards, use is not uniform making comparisons between studies more difficult. In addition, while there does seem to be some agreement between the DSM and ICD, most scales have not been comparatively evaluated further complicating analysis.

Inadequate choice of diagnostic criteria for selecting subjects

Selecting subjects for inclusion in a study is a potential source of difficulties. For example, some diagnosed alcoholics have been drinking for less than a year while others are severe recidivists, yet researchers often do not differentiate between the two. Patient characteristics are a source of complexity and difficulty. Many individuals in the subject pool use more than one substance regularly[42] and these people are usually excluded from research so their use of the second substance will not bias the research results. Many studies also exclude dually diagnosed patients, those patients diagnosed with both substance use disorders and mental health problems[43,44]. Individuals who use multiple substances and the dually diagnosed make up a large percentage of the substance using community. While their exclusion is understandable methodologically due to the need for controlled research, the exclusions result in the decreased generalizability of findings to large segments of the treatment seeking population.

Issues of treatment efficacy and the relationship to gender, race and ethnicity have also been neglected. While there have been accusations that treatment centers neglect the diversity of cultural beliefs and differential experience and there has been a demand for centers which cater to specific populations, there is a paucity of comparative data on outcomes. Harrison et al. did do some preliminary work on treatment programs for women. They compared the retention rates in Minnesota for women treated in mixed gender programs (*N*=8776) and those women treated in women-only programs (*N*=1576). The findings did not substantiate improvements in length of stay for either program type, and researchers did not examine the efficacy of the treatments for either group[45]. Clearly, opportunities for research are abundant.

Lack of uniform standards in the evaluation of treatment efficacy

Further problems arise in the analysis of treatment efficacy as a wide variety of measures have been used to proclaim success or failure. Researchers have determined treatment efficacy using a myriad of measures including abstinence, decreased use, decreased cravings, decreased depression, improved outlook, and increased productivity, among others. Some studies report on one criteria, others use two or more. However the distinction between criteria is critical as abstinence, for example, most certainly differs from reduced cravings. For example, in one study 95% of subjects had a relapse to alcohol dependence during a 3 year follow-up, yet 100% of patients achieved at least 6 months of abstinence. In this study a majority of patients could be considered both treatment successes and treatment failures[40]. Apparent discrepancies can often be explained by selected definitions. For example, the Rand report boldly proclaimed that 67% of patients who enter publicly funded alcohol treatment centers improve, while Gordis states that only a minority of patients who enter treatment are helped to long-term recovery[40]. These statements could both be accurate as improvement could be determined by criminality and social relationships, while recovery may be determined by abstinence.

Inadequate length of follow-up

Finally, the majority of studies lack adequate long-term follow-up. This is largely due to constraints of time and budget. The majority of studies follow patients for 3 months to 12 months. A controlled study by Lambe of hypnosis and smoking cessation demonstrated significant differences at the 3-month follow-up when 21% of hypnosis patients had quit smoking compared to only 6% of controls. However at the 1-year mark there were no significant differences between groups (22% vs. 20%)[46]. Six to 18 months after treatment the majority of treated alcoholics will drink less and function better than during the month prior to admission. Yet like a chronic illness, alcoholism will ebb and flow and this improvement may well be the natural course of the disorder[40]. Longitudinal studies of 2 years or more examining the nature and progression of substance misuse must be conducted if we are to fully understand the impact of treatment and be able to determine what constitutes adequate follow-up.

CRITIQUE OF CONVENTIONAL TREATMENTS

Conventional treatment approaches to substance misuse have been criticized on a number of levels. Dropout rates from most treatment programs are extremely high; rates of 50% or more are common for alcohol misuse and 75 to 85% for cocaine or crack cocaine addiction[40, 47–49]. Some facilities do not include dropout rates in their outcome assessments and significantly inflate their rates of success and misrepresent their capabilities to the general public. A 25% overall success rate (success measured as abstinence) is typical within conventional treatment facilities. Furthermore, despite the substantial amount of time, energy, and money expended by conventional treatment facilities there has been scant assessment of the impact of their programs on costs to society or reduction in arrest rates.

Critics have also pointed out that treatment facilities are often not available or accessible to special populations and the high rate of dropout and recidivism of these special populations suggests that their needs are not being met. In addition, critics question whether current programs are able to handle the full scope of physiological, sociological, and psychological problems of clients, all of which must be addressed during recovery. The increasing treatment unity, such as the reliance in the USA on the Minnesota model and the prominence of the 12-step groups (AA, NA, CA, etc.) despite the lack of controlled research demonstrating the efficacy of these programs has been severely questioned[38,50,51].

One way to combat these deficiencies would be to increase the frequency, intensity, and/or types of treatment services offered. Many studies have indicated that increasing the number of modalities provided increases rates of treatment success[49]. In this context alternative medicine (AM) approaches promise to expand and enrich the treatment continuum and improve overall treatment outcome.

ALTERNATIVE MEDICAL TREATMENTS

The number of patients seeking alternatives to allopathic medicine has significantly increased in recent years. Interest extends around the world and seemingly has no limits in regards to social class, education level, age, or sex[52–55].

Physician willingness to utilize complementary or alternative medicine (CAM) does appear to be related to both the ailment and the modality. Physicians appear more willing to refer patients to CAM practitioners when the patient is suffering from non-specific complaints. Substance misuse is no exception. Since the appearance of crack cocaine in the 1980s, treatment programs in the USA have desperately searched for an effective cure. As a result many centers embraced modalities such as acupuncture.

Integrative nature of addiction medicine

Alternative therapies have been integrated into addiction medicine, perhaps more so than in any other field of medicine. Therapies which already play a major role in the management of addiction in many conventional treatment facilities, such as group therapy, or the 12-step program which is dependent upon spiritual awareness, would be considered highly alternative for the treatment of cancer or HIV. While such approaches may be taught in some medical schools, covered by some insurance companies, and widely available to individuals seeking treatment, their conventional status is tentative at best. However, the use of acupuncture, hypnosis, and nutrition therapy is becoming commonplace in the treatment of substance misuse, though research on the efficacy of these treatment modalities lags behind. With the use of acupuncture and CAM approaches to addiction increasing, distinctions and broad generalizations about conventional and alternative treatment become difficult. Furthermore, treatment programs increasingly use a combination of methods from within both treatment frameworks. For example, acupuncture treatments may be delivered in conjunction with 12-step programs and individual counseling.

In the absence of substantial evidence on the efficacy of alternative therapies, we must remain open-minded about their use and their place in conventional treatment programs. While a high percentage of people struggling with substance misuse are still not being reached and standard therapies remain largely unsuccessful, we must not exclude any approaches that may improve outcome. The goal should not be to discover which is superior — alternative or conventional treatments — rather we should focus on integrative programs and attempt to identify the most effective solutions.

Alternative medicine methodology

The history of medicine is replete with treatments initially applied with enthusiasm but later discovered to be ineffective[56]. This history has established a justifiable skepticism of all new treatments. Thus, controlled research is an integral part of the process of confirmation or refutation. Alternative approaches to addiction must be subjected to this process. However, such research can only be conducted by individuals with an understanding of the common methodological problems inherent in CAM research in addition to the methodological difficulties of addiction research already discussed.

Both individual and institutional barriers have contributed to the dearth of research on the efficacy of alternative modalities. In particular, controlled research of alternative modalities has been sparse due to lack of funding and professional pressure. In the USA and Europe many professionals who have stepped into the alternative arena have found themselves ostracized by the medical community, their professional integrity questioned and their license to practice at risk. The American Medical Association has been one of the harshest opponents of alternative medicine usually dismissing it out of hand as quackery[57], though recently a bulletin was released asking physicians to participate in research of alternative modalities when presented with the opportunity.

The majority of alternative medicine research still consists of retrospective and prospective case studies, and clinic data. Such findings are rarely generalizable and of course lack adequate assurances of reliability and validity. Claims of alternative medicine practitioners, especially with regards to substance abuse, may include grandiose success rates of 75 to 95%. However, no follow-up studies have ever been able to substantiate such claims and raise questions about practitioner and researcher neutrality.

Some researchers and practitioners claim that it is nearly impossible to accurately assess alternative medicine using conventional western research standards. They argue that alternative medicines' philosophical standpoints and individualized treatment make it impossible to randomize patients in a double-blind controlled trial, and appropriate placebo controls are difficult to design. However, these problems are not insurmountable and if alternative modalities are going to be integrated into the mainstream and if the antipathy of many physicians is to be reduced, methodologically sound controlled studies must be conducted[58].

Placebo effect

Numerous debates over the relationship of alternative medicine to the placebo effect have taken place throughout the past decades, however to what extent the effects of modalities like acupuncture are the result of a placebo and to what extent the results are due to physiological changes produced by the technique is still unclear. Classically defined, a placebo effect is an effect that occurs after the administration of a therapeutically inactive substance. Non-specific effects are effects that occur after a treatment, that are known to be due directly to that treatment. Non-specific can also be used to describe treatments whose effects are brought about by some, as yet unexplained, mechanism. For example, in conventionally treated alcoholics, non-specific treatments such as information, evaluation only, advice, encouragement, and exhortation have been shown to have salutary effects[59–62].

The concern is of more than academic interest, since variously defined placebo and non-specific treatments have been shown to be as effective as certain forms of surgery, influence the effectiveness and action of medications and hypnosis analgesia in dentistry, enhance tolerance of pain, increase survival rates in the elderly, reduce post-surgical length of stay and requests for pain medication, and, in certain individuals and cultures, cause death[63–67]. Jerome Frank's work[68] on the role of persuasion in healing has been followed by many reviews of the topic indicating its importance in any form of treatment delivery[69,70].

Shapiro et al. have developed reasonably reliable and valid measures of placebo response, and have found, for example, in a study of psychotropic medications, non-specific factors (such as liking the therapist and preference for type of treatment) accounted for more of the variance in treatment outcome than did the medication[56].

Early accusations that the therapeutic effect of alternative therapies such as acupuncture were attributable to suggestibility stimulated experimentation on animals and an investigation of the inhibitory effects of naloxone on humans under hypnosis. Both lines of inquiry indicated that the effects of acupuncture were not explained by suggestion. The role of non-specific effects in addiction, acupuncture treatment for addiction, or other alternative approaches to addiction has not been studied.

Acupuncture

The use of acupuncture and electro-acupuncture (EA) increased significantly during the 1980s and has been widely integrated into US treatment facilities in contrast to other alternative therapies. There is an abundance of literature on the use of acupuncture for substance misuse, yet the evidence is still insufficient to fully determine efficacy[38,51]. Not surprisingly, believers find minimal supporting evidence as very encouraging, while debunkers dismiss the value of any preliminary findings[71–74].

The connection between acupuncture and substance abuse was first reported by Wen in 1973[75]. It was noted that opium addicts being treated with post-surgical analgesic EA reported relief from withdrawal symptoms. Subsequent research combining naloxone with EA yielded a drug-free rate of 51% at the 1-year follow-up (although these data have been questioned)[76]. The importance of Wen's research lies in his recognition of the distinction between craving and abstinence, and between detoxification and subsequent psychosocial rehabilitation[75,77,78].

In the 1970s, stimulation of various acupuncture points on the body was shown to promote the release of endorphins and enkephalins in animals and humans. Similarly, auricular acupuncture has been associated with changes in endorphin levels in rodents. Blockade of analgesic effects by opiate antagonists further supported the link with the endorphin system. Interestingly, one hypothesis underlying naltrexone's effectiveness in alcoholism is that it also increases beta endorphin levels[79]. In addiction research, Pomeranz reports five successful replications of Wen's findings, but indicates that the underlying mechanism remained unclear. For example, acupuncture increased the total brain beta endorphin level in mice undergoing opiate withdrawal in addition to reducing withdrawal symptoms. Similarly, CSF metenkephalin levels in human addicts were changed following acupuncture compared with normal subjects[80]. Steiner reported that acupuncture has been shown to alter levels of other central neurotransmitters, including serotonin and norepinephrine, and also to affect regulation of other hormones, including prolactin, oxytocin, thyroid hormone, corticosteroid, and insulin[81].

Current theory suggests that exogenous opiates bind endogenous endorphin sites and down regulate the production and action of natural endorphins[186]. Acupuncture may enhance the production of endogenous endorphins, which then compete for receptor sites from which they had been displaced. In alcohol addiction, endogenous opioid receptor sites can be occupied by alcohol metabolites such as tetrahydroisoquinolines.

While a number of randomized controlled studies have been conducted, there are numerous variations in protocol and methodological flaws in the literature making comparison of studies difficult. The number and location of needle placement vary. The type of acupuncture also varies including staples, needles, lasers and stitches, with and without electrical stimulation. The frequency and duration of treatments are not comparable. Studies that use a total of two or three treatments on a once per week schedule may be subtherapeutic. The definition of 'placebo' has varied to include treatments that are known to have therapeutic effects for other forms of substance abuse (sham acupuncture, self-monitoring). While some articles find patient characteristics to be important in terms of treatment outcome, others do not differentiate severity of smoking behavior, personality, or motivational characteristics. Outcome measures vary, and many studies have relied on self-report surveys. Follow-up times have also varied from study to study, but have generally been inadequate. Sample sizes have also varied considerably, and the statistical power of the analyses has not usually been considered[81–88].

Early clinical trial research on heroin and alcohol addiction set the stage for greater standardization of treatment, improved control over treatment assignment, and improved outcome measurement[89–92]. However, gaping holes in our current knowledge impair discussions of treatment effectiveness. Nevertheless, despite the lack of conclusive evidence in support of the efficacy of acupuncture for the treatment of substance abuse, interest has continued to rise. For example, the National Acupuncture Detoxification Association was founded in 1985 and by 1994 reported a membership of 4000[5].

Opiates

The first published study of acupuncture for addictions was authored by Wen and Cheung and appeared in the 1970s. This study suggested EA was effective in alleviating opiate withdrawal symptoms. Several studies followed which also described the efficacy of acupuncture and EA for treating opiate addiction[93]. However, methodological difficulties such as lack of adequate controls have cast a shadow of doubt over these findings. Around this time, several studies of opiate withdrawal were conducted on rats and mice. A review of all five studies done showed a significant decrease in symptoms of morphine withdrawal in the treatment groups. Four of the studies used naloxone to induce withdrawal, and in the fifth study withdrawal was naturally induced. One of the studies stimulated acupuncture points in the paw, the other four used points on the ear.

Subsequent human studies have compared the success of acupuncture or methadone in managing withdrawal symptoms. Acupuncture produced comparable detoxification success rates which implies that acupuncture is effective in the treatment of opiate withdrawal symptoms since methadone is generally accepted as effective. However, Brewington et al.[93] have pointed out that there is no evidence to indicate that acupuncture is effective in the prevention of relapse, and may only be useful as a detoxification regimen for the alleviation of withdrawal symptoms.

Alcohol

The first two controlled studies on acupuncture and alcoholism were conducted by Bullock et al.[94,95]. Both studies were placebo-controlled studies using true and sham acupuncture and a single-blind design with independent assessment (the patient and the follow-up interviewers did not know of the treatment assignment). Bullock et al. utilized the Smith auricular acupuncture method and obtained promising results[94]. In the first study, the effects of acupuncture on 54 chronic 'skid row' alcoholics were evaluated. Subjects were randomized into two arms, true acupuncture and placebo acupuncture. Subjects receiving true acupuncture had significantly better program attendance and significantly less self-reported need for alcohol. This study also found that after 3 months there were significant differences in self-reported drinking episodes, subjects' desire to drink, and the number of subjects admitted to a local detoxification unit.

The study was repeated with 80 subjects using galvanometric identification of acupuncture points and a 6-month follow-up period[95]. This replication confirmed the original findings, and they found that placebo subjects self-reported over twice the number of drinking episodes and had twice the number of admissions to the local hospital detoxification unit compared with subjects treated with acupuncture at each follow-up.

A third controlled study by Worner which is sometimes referred to as a replication of the Bullock et al. studies despite the differences in treatment protocol and analysis[5] has been conducted. This study involved 56 alcoholics and showed no significant differences between three treatment groups in attendance, completion of treatment, or relapses and concluded that fixed point specific standardized acupuncture did not improve outcomes. Despite the results of this third trial the balance of the evidence suggests that acupuncture could be a viable method for the treatment of alcohol misuse.

Cocaine

The use of acupuncture for the treatment of cocaine addiction is relatively recent. There have been a number of large-scale clinical trials performed. Smith, in particular, has reported positive outcomes in open clinical trials of acupuncture for the abuse of cocaine, 'crack' cocaine, and other substances in 1500 volunteers in New York City[96]. To date no studies have been published that have formal, controlled research designs and employed randomization to treatments, placebo controls, and long-term follow-up. However Bullock, Culliton, and Kiresuk have conducted such a trial and are currently analyzing their results.

Although a preliminary model has been developed to explain the effect of acupuncture on pain, opiate, and alcohol addiction, there are no explanations for acupuncture's mode of action in the treatment of cocaine abuse. Wise has described the relationship between opioids and the dopaminergic reward system[97]. While this relationship may provide the conceptual connection to the early reports of acupuncture in the treatment of cocaine abuse, the connection has not been explicitly formulated.

Smoking

Generally, the literature regarding the use of acupuncture for smoking appears to be similar to the rest of the literature on the use of acupuncture for substance abuse. The several articles which have been published can be characterized by their emotional tone and evident, prior beliefs. The studies are not comparable and have not been replicated; their results are inconclusive.

Electro-acupuncture

In electro-acupuncture (EA), the acupuncture needle delivers mild electricity to the acupuncture site. A similar procedure delivering mild electricity using direct contact to the skin rather than needles is discussed later in this text as CES. Studies to date of the clinical and neurophysiologic effects of EA in animals and humans have been exploratory; more systematic research is required. The early findings suggest that EA may alleviate symptoms associated with addiction to various substances[75,77,78,98,99] and may be responsible for various neurophysiologic changes observed[100,101]. No significant negative side effects have been reported. However, there are no systematic, placebo-controlled studies of EA for the treatment of substance misuse in humans. The use of EA for the treatment of substance misuse is growing in popularity, despite the lack of controlled research.

Biofeedback

Research on the effects of biofeedback for substance misuse has been varied and the outcomes used have been questionable. While there have been several impressive case studies focused on abstinence presented in the literature[102,103] controlled studies have been inconsistent at best. Recently Taub[104] concluded that there is support for the use of biofeedback in the prevention of relapse in alcoholics. This study was a 2-year follow-up of 70 transient alcoholics who had been treated in a residential facility. Patients treated with biofeedback significantly increased their percentage of non-drinking days. Another controlled study of 82 alcoholic males, who had completed six or more biofeedback sessions in an inpatient treatment center, showed that symptom relief for anxiety was positively correlated with sobriety[105]. These findings are not contingent upon biofeedback as a treatment modality and lack specificity.

Another study concluded that the amount of biofeedback received has a significant impact on abstinence.[106] Denny et al. looked at 233 male veterans 3, 6, and 12 months post discharge from an inpatient alcoholic rehabilitation unit and found that those who had received biofeedback training had a higher frequency of sobriety than those who received no training. There was a dose effect (eight or more sessions of biofeedback correlated with greater frequency of sobriety) but only at the 3 month follow-up. Finally, a double-blind study using biofeedback and a pseudo-biofeedback control group was conducted on opiate users. All patients were stabilized on a study dose of methadone, and while both groups showed improvement on several variables the differences were not group specific[107].

Thus there is evidence to suggest that biofeedback may be useful in the prevention of relapse[102,103], however on balance it seems that biofeedback is not useful for the reduction of withdrawal symptoms. Furthermore, research has been conducted which shows that the use of alcohol or nicotine results in poor performance during biofeedback sessions. The ability of smokers to modulate blood pressure is restricted when compared to non-smokers[108] and the ability to manipulate skin temperature appears to be greatest in non-smokers and impossible for people who smoke just prior to the biofeedback session[109]. Seven alcoholics who were unable to succeed in four biofeedback trials immediately after hospitalization returned for a fifth session approximately 4 months later. The six patients who had not relapsed were immediately successful in the exercise, but the one patient who had relapsed was still unable to control his brain potentials successfully[110].

Nutrition/vitamins

Nutrition therapy, including orthomolecular treatments, are once again gaining popularity for the treatment of alcohol misuse. Few methodologically sound studies have been conducted to determine the efficacy of nutrition therapy. Nutritional remedies are appealing to the public because intuitively the efficacy of such treatments seems plausible. Advocates of nutritional therapy emphasize that one in four deaths among people who have been treated for alcoholism is due to suicide, and the majority of these deaths occur within a year of treatment[111]. In addition, abstinent alcoholics have been known to suffer from anxiety, tremors, memory dysfunction, and other ailments long after treatment[112]. Advocates of nutritional therapy attribute the depression and other ailments to nutritional deficits, undiagnosed hypoglycemia, and unidentified food allergies which when diagnosed can be treated through special diets, exercise, and vitamin and mineral supplements[112–114].

Some research has produced promising results. In the early 1980s, Guenther studied patients at a VA treatment center. One group received individual and family counseling, and attended 12-step meetings, while the second group also added a whole-food diet, nutritional supplements, and nutritional education. A total of 81% of the nutrition group compared with 38% of the control group were sober after 6 months. A second study by Beasely ran a 28 day program, involving both counseling and nutrition and after 1 year 74% of those treated remained sober[113]. A third study by Mathews-Larson and Parker followed up 100 patients who had received 6 weeks of outpatient nutritional therapy and counseling and reported an 81.3% abstinence rate after 6 months[112].

While the impressive differences between Guenther's treatment and control groups may be attributed to the added attention and time spent with the nutritional group rather than the therapy, and the studies by Beasely and Mathews-Larson had no controls, there seems to be enough evidence to warrant further investigation of nutritional therapies. Such research should also extend to other substance use disorders.

Hypnosis

Few controlled studies have been conducted using hypnosis as a treatment for substance misuse, and the results have varied making analysis of hypnosis as a treatment option difficult. Several case studies have reported stunning successes using both self-hypnosis[115] and hypnotherapy[116]. One study involving 168 subjects compared the efficacy of hypnosis, health education, and behaviour modification groups for smoking cessation. They found no significant differences between the three approaches at the 6-month follow-up[117]. A controlled study compared the effects of hypnosis, focused smoking, attention placebo, and a waiting list control group. Results were analyzed using self-monitoring and blood analysis of thiocyanate levels. While the three treatment groups showed improvement over the control, there were no significant differences between the groups at the 3– and 6-month follow-ups[118]. Another controlled study by Lambe et al.[46] reported that 21% of hypnosis patients had quit smoking at the 3-month follow-up compared with 6% of the control group. However, at the 1-year mark 22% of the treatment group and 20% of the control group were abstinent. This highlights the importance of long-term follow-ups in similar studies. Although the rate at which smokers quit appeared to have been accelerated by hypnosis, it offered no long-term benefit[46].

While many advertisements profess cure rates of 95%, no studies have come close to verifying such claims[119]. Though hypnotherapy has been used to treat substance misuse for over a century and is accepted by the AMA, most modern practitioners believe that hypnosis alone provides no cure[120]. Rather hypnosis may enhance other modalities[119,120]. Researchers also feel that aversive posthypnotic suggestion is the least effective use of hypnosis[120].

Outcomes of 93 men and 93 women who completed a 2-week program which combined hypnosis and aversion therapy showed abstinence in 92% of men and in 90% of women. Three months later 86% of both groups maintained abstinence[121]. Another psychiatrist studying 616 smokers combined one session of psychotherapy with hypnosis and then did a follow-up study. Results showed that 35% of the subjects had stopped smoking for 1 year (non-respondents counted as failures). When Pederson et al., in a small study of 17 smokers, added group counseling to a single hypnosis session, they raised the quit rate to 53%[122]. Another study combined restricted environmental stimulation (REST) (vide infra) with hypnosis and reported a 47% abstinence rate at 4 months. Serious methodological flaws reduce our confidence in the majority of these studies, though the findings suggest a need for further research on the efficacy of hypnosis.

Transcendental meditation (TM)

The majority of research on transcendental meditation (TM) has produced positive results for the treatment of substance use disorders. However, most of the studies have lacked rigorous methods and appropriate controls. Most recently, Taub[104] conducted a study comparing a control group receiving AA and counseling to three groups receiving the control conditions plus either TM, biofeedback, or electric neurotherapy. The TM and biofeedback groups significantly increased their number of non-drinking days as compared with the electric neurotherapy and control groups after a 2-year follow-up. However, the percentage of non-drinking days is a much less robust measure than an assessment of abstinence and makes it difficult to interpret these findings.

Gelderloos et al.[123] reviewed 24 studies on TM and the treatment and prevention of substance misuse. The authors, affiliated with the Marharishi University, positively evaluated all 24 studies despite often serious methodological flaws. Studies have infrequently controlled for type of drug(s) used, the length of time subjects have used the drug, or the severity of misuse, and few were prospective, randomized, controlled, or blind. For ten of the studies success rates were listed as percentages and ranged from 65% in a controlled study of skid row recidivist alcoholics (with 2-year follow-up) to 98% in a retrospective analysis of drug use among TM program participants. Despite the multitude of studies on TM and substance abuse[124], further methodologically sound study should be conducted by researchers not affiliated with the programs.

Restricted environmental stimulation (REST)

A number of studies have been conducted demonstrating the effectiveness of restricted environmental stimulation therapy (REST) for the modification of smoking behavior, though little has been done on REST and drug misuse. Reduced stimulation environments are likely to decrease arousal and include chamber REST and flotation REST. Monotonous stimulation environments are more likely to increase arousal and have not been used in the treatment of substance misuse.

Flotation REST consisting of a pool of water supersaturated with Epsom salts enclosed in a sound attenuated and lightproof room has not been found effective in smoking cessation research; however there is some evidence that flotation REST can diminish the psychotic-like symptoms of people on PCP and LSD and may be useful for the treatment of drug withdrawal symptoms[125].

Two studies using a 2×2 design found significant effects using chamber REST for smoking cessation. The four groups were REST interrupted with anti-smoking messages, REST alone, messages alone, and a treatment control group. The first study found that subjects in both the REST plus messages group, and the REST alone group showed mean smoking reductions of 40% after 3 months, but no message effect was found. The second study used more elaborate anti-smoking messages and used subjects who had expressed a desire to quit smoking. They found mean smoking reductions of 50% in the two REST groups after 24 months, again finding no message effect[126–128].

Studies combining REST with other modalities often result in even higher rates of abstention. Barabasz et al.[129] studied 307 smokers given one of six treatment options. They found that hypnosis by an experienced clinician combined with REST resulted in 47% abstinence at 4 months. Tikalsy[130] conducted a 6-month follow-up of a program which combined REST, self-management, and social support and reported an 88% rate of abstention. In contrast, combining aversion therapy with REST has not resulted in significant smoking reductions[125].

Little research has been done on alcohol consumption and REST. Ten self-proclaimed alcoholics rated their experience with REST more positively than their normal life, however records of alcohol consumption were not clearly documented. A study of students in a prodromal stage of alcoholism received 2.5 hours of chamber REST with a stop drinking message and showed a 30% decrease in alcohol consumption at 2 weeks while controls showed little or no change. A duplicate study also showed an immediate decrease in consumption which was maintained at the 6-month follow-up[125]. Barabasz and Dyer found that the amount of time spent in REST had an impact on outcome with subjects who had received 24 hours of REST maintaining a significant decrease in consumption after 6 months. While chamber REST shows promise for smoking cessation, it has not been adequately tested for the treatment of alcohol misuse, nor for the misuse of other substances.

Transcranial neuroelectric stimulation (CES)

Transcranial neuroelectric stimulation, or cranial electric stimulation (CES), has been the subject of a number of studies related to substance misuse, but the results have not been promising. CES involves the placement of surface electrodes in the mastoid region (behind the ear) and infusing them with low amperage and frequency alternating current. Gariti et al.[131] conducted a randomized, double-blind study of opiate and cocaine users. Subjects were hospitalized for 12 days and 88% completed the study. While both opiate and cocaine groups claimed improvement and a comfortable detoxification, the active and placebo groups did not differ significantly.

Brewington et al.[93] discussed several CES studies in their 1994 review of acupuncture and electro-acupuncture. Although suffering from methodological flaws, Gossop's research (1984) found that the CES group actually manifested more withdrawal symptoms than the control group. Elmoghazy et al. (1990) found support for the use of CES but only after excluding drop outs from the final analysis, the majority of which were from the CES group. Overall it appears that CES fails to suppress opiate or cocaine withdrawal symptoms.

Studies designed to decrease the amount of anxiety and depression in alcoholics have been flawed or have generated no clear support for CES[93]. Furthermore, when CES was used as an arm in a research project by Taub et al.[104], results did not support the usefulness of CES for the treatment of alcoholism, even when coupled with AA and counseling.

Homeopathy

Homeopathic remedies for substance abuse appear to be more frequently utilized in Europe than the USA. The classical homeopath prescribes one remedy per patient, while the pluralist uses several remedies simultaneously. Often combinations of remedies designed for a specific purpose, such as detoxification, are sold over the counter. While these standardized tinctures may be appealing to the public or to researchers wanting to conduct controlled clinical trials, classical critics of the pluralist approach would say these groupings violate the basic principles of homeopathy (treatment of the individual; not of a symptom), are untested and possibly dangerous[132].

Recently a controlled clinical double-blind study of homeopathy for polydrug misuse was conducted in the USA (N=703). While the results have yet to be published, preliminary results indicate that patients treated homeopathically received a significantly better prognosis at discharge, an 88% abstinence rate at 6 months, and maintained a 68% abstinence rate (self-report confirmed by urine testing) at 18 months compared with 32% and 30% for placebo and control groups respectively[133]. Homeopathy appears to show promise for the treatment of substance misuse, and this study could serve as a model for future research.

Kudzu/Radix puerarieae/other herbs

Foliage in the Southern USA has long been plagued by the kudzu plant. However, the plant may turn out to be useful after all. The American Journal of Hospital Pharmacy[134] reported that Radix puerarieae (extract from the kudzu plant) has the potential to moderate alcohol abuse. A tea made from various parts of the kudzu plant have long been used by Chinese herbal doctors for the treatment of both intoxication and alcoholism[135].

Research by Keung et al.[136,137] has demonstrated the putative antidipsotropic effect of Radix puerarieae. The research was conducted on Syrian golden hamsters, but the model has high predictive validity. The hamsters voluntarily decreased or discontinued their ethanol intake after the Radix puerarieae was administered. Keung et al.[138] have isolated two isoflavones from the kudzu extract, daidzein and daidzin, which curb ethanol intake. Despite claims of predictive validity, no human studies have been conducted to measure the impact of Radix puerarieae, or kudzu.

While various other herbs and herbal mixtures have been touted for their ability to reduce craving and assist in the process of detoxification[139,140] virtually no work has been done to assess their efficacy. Many herbal remedies are safe with few side effects, however some can be toxic if administered incorrectly.

Relaxation training

Relaxation training carries an underlying assumption that substance users consume drugs, including alcohol and tobacco, for their tranquilizing effects. Yet researchers have commented that many drugs may be consumed for their euphoric effects[141,142], which calls into question the validity of relaxation training as a treatment for substance abuse. Furthermore, the majority of studies examining the efficacy of relaxation training for the treatment of substance abuse have yielded little support. Biofeedback[104] and cue exposure[143] have both been shown to be more effective for treating substance disorders than relaxation training, as measured by abstinence rates and length of follow-up.

One study of 76 smokers explored the impact of 3 months of guided relaxation imagery upon smoking recidivism and did show positive outcomes[144]. Significant changes in variables, including abstinence, were noted for the treatment group. Other studies, with less intensive interaction and time requirements, do not mirror these findings. The impact of anxiety management and relaxation training was examined in two groups at an Alcohol Treatment Unit[145]. Dependent variables studied were anxiety levels and alcohol consumption. While the study found a reduction in anxiety there was no impact on levels of consumption.

Ibogaine

Ibogaine is a psychoactive indole alkaloid found in the root bark of Tabernanthe iboga, a West African shrub[146]. Anecdotal observations and animal research have led some researchers to hypothesize that ibogaine may interrupt dependency on opiates, cocaine, amphetamine, alcohol, and nicotine[147,148].

A stimulant, ibogaine has been used in ritualistic settings by various indigenous populations. In small doses it has also been used to help hunters and warriors stay awake while motionless for long periods. In high doses users have reported experiencing high states of excitement, mental confusion, and even hallucinations. Extremely high doses can be fatal[148]. Currently ibogaine is classified as a Schedule I substance by the US Food and Drug Administration (all non-research use forbidden), but is accessible through much of the European community[148]. Individuals dependent on various substances may even receive ibogaine-based treatment in countries such as Holland[149].

Multiple studies have documented the effects of ibogaine on various animal populations including rodents, dogs, cats, and primates. Ibogaine has been shown to attenuate the alcohol intake of alcohol-preferring rats[146], and results in the reduction of cocaine preference and the attenuation of cocaine-induced ambulatory and stereotypical activity in mice[147]. Numerous other animal studies have studied the effect of ibogaine on dopaminergic systems, opioid systems, serotonergic systems, intracellular calcium regulation, cholinergic systems, δ-aminobutyric acidergic systems, voltage-dependent sodium channels, glutamatergic systems, s receptors, and adrenergic systems (see Popik et al., 1995 for review)[148]. The response of subjects to ibogaine does seem to be dose, setting, sex, and species specific indicating the need for further information on its effects in both animals and humans.

The anecdotal evidence supporting the anti-addictive nature of ibogaine is impressive, as is the case with numerous new or alternative therapies. Preliminary published case studies in humans using single doses of 700 to 1800 mg have shown promise, but have been largely inconclusive. One subject in a seven subject trial relapsed to opiate use after 2 days, two after a number of weeks, one reverted to intermittent heroin use, and three were drug free after 14 weeks or more[149]. Perhaps more impressive was the lack of opiate withdrawal symptoms displayed by participants at the end of the 24–38 hour psychoactive period induced by the drug. Currently there are no controlled clinical data to support the claims that ibogaine has anti-addictive properties.

LSD

In the 1960s and 1970s another illicit drug, LSD, was touted to be a viable treatment for alcoholism. A review of controlled human trials found that while existing studies were few, the findings were remarkably similar[150]. Three different LSD treatment conditions were compared with numerous drug therapies including ephedrine, amphetamine, ritalin, and librium. The majority of studies reported no difference between treatment groups, and all differences vanished by the 6-month follow-up in the remaining two studies. Furthermore in many cases the 'no therapy' controls demonstrated more impressive outcomes, and findings suggest that LSD may even possess some antitherapeutic effects[150].

Cue exposure

In a two-arm controlled trial, Drummond et al.[143] evaluated the efficacy of cue exposure for the treatment of alcohol dependence, and concluded that cue exposure is a potentially useful treatment for addiction. However, the control group was treated using relaxation training, therefore the study showed only that cue exposure was a more effective treatment than relaxation control. Thus the findings of this study are questionable.

Staiger and White[151] have stressed the importance of individualized cue programs and evaluations rather than standardized approaches. Tobena et al.[152] believed that the effects of cue exposure treatments are limited due to the unstable after effects of drug use. Other researchers suggest that the conditioning theory on which cue exposure is based at least provides a useful hypothesis for the study of relapse[153]. Some studies have shown a relationship between cue exposure and a reduction in cravings[154], however the questionable correlation between cravings and substance use sheds some doubt on the conditioning hypothesis. Drummond et al. conclude that a correlation between conditioned responses to cues and relapse to alcohol has not been demonstrated[153], and the efficacy of cue exposure is still in question.

While cue exposure research has focused primarily upon the use of alcohol, one controlled study used cue exposure to prevent relapse in opiate addiction. The authors found no significant effects immediately after treatment, nor at a 2-month follow-up[155].

Eye movement desensitization and reprocessing (EMDR)

Eye movement desensitization and reprocessing (EMDR) is a relatively new psychological methodology that practitioners believe could be a useful addition to the treatment of substance abuse. EMDR may be used at all stages of treatment though optimal effects occur when the client has been abstinent long enough to prevent withdrawal symptoms[156]. The professional community has conducted numerous trials on the efficacy of EMDR for the treatment of the psychological consequences of traumatic incidents such as sexual assault, combat, or grief[156–158].

Treatment using EMDR seems to increase clients' sense of self-worth and self-efficacy. It can assist substance abusers in confronting their denial and distortions thus aiding the recovery process. However, the use of EMDR assumes an underlying history of mental trauma. Therefore those substance misusers without such traumas may not be helped by the use of EMDR[156]. While EMDR enjoys some popularity for the treatment of the consequences of traumatic incidents, its efficacy for the treatment of substance abuse has not yet been researched.

Yoga/Tai-chi

Yoga has long been seen as a positive form of exercise for conditioning and increasing flexibility. However, according to Kapur[159] yoga and Indian systems of medicine may have great potential in the prevention and treatment of addictions and their related consequences. In 1993 the Office of Alternative Medicine funded a small pilot study exploring yoga for the treatment of opiate misuse[160]. The study followed 59 men and women for 5 months at a methadone maintenance program. Participants were randomized into either a traditional psychodynamic group or a hatha yoga group; all subjects received daily doses of methadone. Shaffer and LaSalvia found no significant differences between treatment groups, though the authors felt that both treatments assisted in significantly reducing drug use and criminal activity. The authors also noted that longer length of stays were positively correlated with reduced drug use and reduced criminal activity. Shaffer et al. concluded that further research is necessary to expand and clarify their findings.

Tai-chi, widespread in China, has become increasingly popular in the USA. Tai-chi is seen as a form of exercise to increase flexibility, improve breathing, and help with conditioning by stimulating a person's energy fields, or Qi. However, some suspect Tai-chi may assist individuals in the process of withdrawal and relapse prevention. Interestingly, legend states that Tai-chi was introduced to the masses in China in an attempt to combat opium addiction. No research has been published on the effectiveness of Tai-chi for the treatment of substance use disorders.

Light therapy

Light therapy is one of the modalities used to treat seasonal affective disorders (SADs). Research indicates that SADs may be the result of serotonin deficits, the neurotransmitter most frequently linked with alcoholism. Though previous studies looking for seasonal patterns among alcoholic-related treatment admissions have produced contradictory findings[161–163], several case studies have suggested a connection between SAD and some cases of substance abuse[164,165]. For patients with seasonal patterns of abuse, researchers feel that light therapy may complement conventional treatment. While the treatment seems plausible, no controlled research has been conducted on the efficacy of this modality for the treatment of alcoholism, nor for the dependence or abuse of any other substance.

Flower essence/aromatherapy

There is some indication that flower essence is being used for the treatment of addiction. Elixirs are created by floating flowers in a bowl of water so the water molecules absorb the 'energy resonance' of the flowers. Practitioners claim the elixirs have no biochemical impact, thus are free from the unpleasant side effects associated with other medications such as antidepressants. Rather, the flower essence adjusts the vibrational frequency of a person's cells for gentle healing[166].

Aromatherapy, a branch of herbal medicine, is also being used in some locations for the treatment of substance abuse. Fragrant essential oils of various plants are inhaled, applied to the skin, or ingested orally for the prevention and treatment of disease. One theory states that the small molecular size of the oils allows them to penetrate bodily tissues easily, and their chemical makeup provides for a variety of desirable pharmacological properties[167]. While a few case studies have been conducted, no methodologically sound research is available on either of these modalities for the treatment of any phase of substance misuse.

Electromagnetic fields

Some therapists have begun to pay attention to the impact of electromagnetic fields on abuse and addiction. Therapists believe that daily we are exposed to numerous electromagnetic currents, and chemicals in food and the environment which throw our bodies out of balance[168]. The effects can vary but sometimes result in addiction to any number of substances. Through manipulation of a client's electromagnetic currents, therapists attempt to restore the body's natural balance. However, other than case testimonials from several patients, there has been no verification of the efficacy of this modality.

Altered states of consciousness (ASC)

It has been proposed that addictions are in part caused by an individual internal need to achieve altered states of consciousness (ASCs)[169]. From the time we are children, in holding our breath or spinning until we are dizzy, we attempt to fulfill this need; however the lack of socially acceptable means available to adults may lead some to try unapproved methods such as drugs. Socially acceptable methods of achieving altered states include relaxation, meditation, art, physical activities, cognitive therapy, hypnosis, biofeedback, and prayer, and the authors assert that treatment of substance misuse should incorporate these programs. They believe that relapse can be attributed in part to the failure of treatment to provide alternative methods to achieve altered states[169]. No research has been conducted on the validity of this theory, despite research done on several of the modalities named.

Spirituality/prayer

Recent research alludes to the healing power of prayer[170,171] and discussions of prayer have become more mainstream. While no direct research has been done on prayer as a treatment for substance misuse, the use of prayer has impacted mainstream approaches. One researcher reports that in working with clients who are reshaping their lives, 'most clinicians in the field agree that issues of religiosity or spirituality are worth exploring'[172]. It should be noted that 12-step programs, the most commonly used intervention for alcoholism in the USA, involve a spiritual component and the successful completion of steps four and five require members to turn their life over to God or some higher power, and religious involvement is the third major source of help for people trying to change involuntary habits[173].

Cultural forms of healing

While traditional Chinese medicine has become a buzz word among alternative practitioners, the field has generally failed to recognize the presence of other cultural forms of healing. This is particularly true in the field of substance abuse. While authors have become increasingly aware of variations in patterns of drug use and treatment outcomes between populations[174–180], the few articles focused on culturally specific healing modalities are usually qualitative or descriptive and have not empirically considered treatment efficacy[181–185].

A significant portion of the culturally specific modalities for the treatment of substance abuse seem to be based upon spirituality, or upon a philosophy which emphasizes community health[181,183,184]. It appears that treatments are often quite complex, consisting of combinations of modalities and ritual. These treatment systems may include faith healers, shamans, or spiritual counselors, and may utilize everything from group counseling sessions and meditation to hallucinogenic agents and sweat lodges. Researchers wishing to make their mark on the field of addictions would do well to consider evaluating the efficacy of cultural healing forms for a variety of populations.

CONCLUSION

Research on the use of alternative medicine for substance misuse is in its infancy. Despite the multitude of alternative modalities being used to treat individuals at various stages of substance misuse, few have been adequately tested.

The lack of standardized research protocols and difficulties integrating alternative treatment paradigms into rigorous scientific methodology have also interfered with current efforts to compare existing studies.

Remedies such as nutrition therapies, biofeedback, homeopathy, acupuncture, and hypnosis are widely used in the USA and Europe for addictions and provide numerous opportunities to conduct small controlled trials on a variety of populations in divergent settings.

Practitioners using alternative modalities must be responsible to their patients and their profession. While anecdotal case studies may provide interesting leads, practitioners need to begin collecting standardized outcomes data on the populations they treat. Such findings can be used to fuel future proposals and inform research. At this juncture the dissemination of information should be of primary importance.

REFERENCES

1 NIH 1996 Dr. Jonas Addresses Advisory Council. Complementary and Alternative Medicine at the NIH 3(1):1–2
2 Minnesota Department of Health 1995 Alcohol use in Minnesota: extent and cost. Minneapolis, MN
3 Josiah Macy, Jr. Foundation 1995 Training about alcohol and substance abuse for all primary care physicians. New York, NY Phoenix, AZ, October 2
4 Frances R, Miller S 1991 Addiction treatment: the widening scope. In: Frances R, Miller S (eds) Clinical textbook of addictive disorders. Guilford Press, New York
5 Culliton P Kiresuk T, 1996 Overview of substance abuse acupuncture treatment research. Journal of Alternative and Complementary Medicine 2(1): 149–159
6 1981 Morgan H W (ed) Drugs in America: a social history, 1800–1980. Syracuse University Press, Syracuse, New York
7 Miller R 1974 Towards a sociology of methadone maintenance. In: Winick C (ed) Sociological aspects of drug dependence. CRC Press, Cleveland, OH
8 Babor T 1990 Social, scientific, and medical issues in the definition of alcohol and drug dependence. In: Edwards G, Lader M (eds) The nature of drug dependence. Oxford Medical Publications, New York
9 Ghodse H 1995 Drugs and addictive behavior: a guide to treatment. Blackwell Science, Cambridge, Mass
10 Skinner HA 1990 Validation of the dependence syndrome: have we crossed the half-life of this concept. In: Edwards G, Lader M (eds) The nature of drug dependence. Oxford Medical Publications, New York
11 Caulker-Burnett I 1994 Primary care screening for substance abuse. [Review]. Nurse Practitioner 19(6):42–8
12 Schottenfeld R 1994 Assessment of the Patient. In: Galanter M, Kleber H (eds) The American Psychiatric Press textbook of substance abuse treatment. American Psychiatric Press, Washington, DC
13 Beasley J 1990 Diagnosing and managing chemical dependency. Essential Medical Information Systems, Dallas, TX
14 Kalant H 1989 The nature of addiction: an analysis of the problem. Molecular and cellular aspects of the drug addictions. Springer-Verlag, New York
15 Winger G, Hofmann FG, Woods JH 1992 A handbook on drug and alcohol abuse: the biomedical aspects. Oxford University Press, New York, NY
16 Goldstein A 1989 Introduction. Molecular and cellular aspects of the drug addictions. Springer-Verlag, New York
17 Westermeyer J, Lyfoung T, Westermeyer M, Neider J 1991 Opium addiction among Indochinese refugees in the US: characteristics of addictions and their opium use. American Journal of Drug and Alcohol Abuse 17(3):267–77
18 Kendler K, Neale M, Heath A, Kessler R, Eaves L 1994 A twin-family study of alcoholism in women. American Journal of Psychiatry 151(5):707–15
19 Kendler KS, Kessler RC 1992 A population-based twin study of alcoholism in women. JAMA 268(14):1877–82
20 Goodwin D 1987 Genetic influences in alcoholism. Advances in Internal Medicine 32:283–97
21 Pomerleau O 1992 Nicotine and the central nervous system: biobehavioral effects of cigarette smoking. American Journal of Medicine 93(Supplement 1A): pp 2s–7s
22 Cold Spring Harbor Laboratory Press 1990 Banbury Report 33: Genetics and biology of alcoholism. Cold Spring Harbor
23 Nutt D 1996 Addiction: brain mechanisms and their treatment implications. Lancet 347:31–6
24 Sellers E, Higgins G, Sobell M 1992 5-HT and alcohol abuse. TIPS 13:69–75
25 Spencer JW 1990 Why evaluate for residual drug effects. In: Spencer JW, Boren JJ (eds) Residual effects of abused drugs on behavior. U.S. Department of Health and Human Services, Rockville, MD
26 Litten R, Allen J 1993 Reducing the desire to drink. pharmacology and neurobiology. Recent Developments in Alcoholism 11:325–44
27 Higgins ST 1995 Comments. In: Onken LS, Blaine JD, Boren JJ (eds) Integrating behavioral therapies with medications in the treatment of drug dependence. U.S. Department of Health and Human Services, Rockville, MD
28 Courtwright D 1982 Dark paradise: opiate addiction in America before 1940. Harvard University Press, Cambridge, MA
29 Martin WR, Isbell H (eds) 1979 Drug addiction and the US Public Health Service. NIDA, Rockville, Maryland

30 Anderson D 1981 Perspectives on treatment: the Minnesota Experience. Hazelden Foundation, Center City, MN
31 Laungergan J 1982 Easy does it: alcoholism treatment outcomes: Hazelden and the Minnesota Model. Hazelden Foundation, Duluth, MN
32 Cook C 1988 The Minnesota Model in the management of drug and alcohol dependency: miracle, method or myth? Part I, The philosophy and the programme. British Journal of Addiction 83:625–34
33 Emrick C 1987 Alcoholics Anonymous: affiliation processes and effectiveness as treatment. Alcoholism (NY) 11:416–23
34 National Council of Alcoholism 1965 Alcoholics Anonymous: pathway to recovery: a study of 1058 members of the AA fellowship in New York City, New York
35 Edwards G, Hensman C, Haukes A, Williamson V 1967 Alcoholism Anonymous, the anatomy of a self-help group. Social Psychiatry 1:195
36 Jorquez J 1983 The retirement phase of heroin users' careers. Journal of Drug Issues 13(3):343–65
37 Miller W, Hester R 1986 Inpatient alcoholism treatment: who benefits? American Psychologist 41:794–805
38 Holder H, Longabaugh R, Miller W, Rubonis A 1991 The cost effectiveness of treatment for alcoholism: a first approximation. Journal of Studies on Alcohol 52(6):517–40
39 Gerstein D 1994 Outcome research: drug abuse. In: Galanter M, Kleber H (eds) The American Psychiatric Press textbook of substance abuse treatment. American Psychiatric Press, Washington, DC
40 Vaillant G, Clark W, Cyrus C, Miloffsky E, Kopp J, Wulsin V, Mogielnicki N 1993 Prospective study of alcoholism treatment: eight year follow-up. American Journal of Medicine 75:455–63
41 Cottler L, Robins L, Grant B, Blaine J, Towle L, Wittchen H, Sartorius N 1991 CIDI-core substance abuse and dependence questions: cross-cultural and sociological Issues. British Journal of Psychiatry 159:653–8
42 Thoreson R 1995 Overview of the National Drug and Alcoholism Treatment Unit Survey (NDATUS), 1992 and 1980–1992. Substance Abuse and Mental Health Services Administration, US Dept of Health and Human Services, Rockville, Maryland, Advance Report #9 (published on the Internet)
43 Saitz R, Mayo-Smith M, Roberts M, Redmond H, Bernard D, Calkins D 1994 Individualized treatment for alcohol withdrawal: a randomized double-blind controlled trial. Journal of the American Medical Association 272:519–23
44 Baumgartner G, March RR 1991 Transdermal clonidine versus chlordiazepoxide in alcohol withdrawal: a randomized, controlled clinical trial. Southern Medical Journal 84(3):312–21
45 Minnesota Department of Human Services, Chemical Dependency Division 1995 Research News. St. Paul, MN
46 Lambe R, Osier C, Franks P 1986 A randomized controlled trial of hypnotherapy for smoking cessation. Journal of Family Practice 22(1):61–5
47 Chappel J 1993 Long-term recovery from alcoholism. Recent Advances in Addictive Disorders 16(1):177–87
48 Mammo A, Weinbaum D 1991 Some factors that influence dropping out from outpatient alcoholism treatment facilities. Journal of Studies on Alcohol 54:92–101
49 Hoffman J, Caudill B, Koman J, Luckey J, Flynn P, Hubbard R 1994 Comparative cocaine abuse treatment strategies: enhancing client retention and treatment exposure. Journal of Addictive Diseases 13(4):115–128
50 Chiauzzi E, Liljegren S 1993 Taboo topics in addiction treatment. An empirical review of clinical folklore. [Review]. Journal of Substance Abuse Treatment 10(3):303–16
51 Hester R 1994 Outcome research: alcoholism. In: Galanter M, Kleber H (eds) The American Psychiatric Press textbook of substance abuse treatment. American Psychiatric Press, Washington, DC
52 Anderson E, Anderson P 1987 General practitioners and alternative medicine. Journal of the Royal College of General Practitioners 37:52–5
53 Hadley C 1988 Complementary medicine and the general practitioner: a survey of general practitioners in the Wellington area. New Zealand Medical Journal 101:766–8
54 Visser G, Peters L 1990 Alternative medicine and general practitioners in The Netherlands: towards acceptance and integration. Family Practice 7(3):227–32
55 Eisenberg D, Kessler R, Foster C, Norlock F, Calkins D, Delbanco T 1993 Unconventional medicine in the United States: prevalence, costs, and patterns of use. New England Journal of Medicine 328(4):246–52
56 Shapiro A, Morris L 1978 Placebo effects in medical and psychological therapies. Handbook of psychotherapy and behavior change. Wiley, New York
57 Hafner AW, Zwicky JF, Barrett S, Jarvis WT 1993 Reader's guide to alternative health methods. American Medical Association, Milwaukee, WI
58 Lewith GT, Kenyon JN, Lewis PJ 1996 Complementary medicine: an integrated approach. Oxford University Press, Oxford
59 Miller W, Hester R 1980 The addictive behaviors: treatment of alcoholism, drug abuse, smoking and obesity. Treating the problem drinker: modern approaches. Pergamon Press, Oxford
60 Miller W, Baca L 1983 Two-year follow-up of Bibliotherapy and therapist-directed controlled drinking training for problem drinkers. Behavior Therapy 14:441–50
61 Powell B, Penick E, Read M, Ludwig A 1985 Comparison of three outpatient treatment interventions: a twelve-month follow-up of men alcoholics. Journal of Studies on Alcohol 46(4):309–12
62 McLellan A, Luborsky L, Cacciola J, Griffith J, Evans F, Barr H, O'Brien C 1985 New data from the addiction Severity Index. Reliability and validity in three centers. Journal of Nervous and Mental Diseases 172:412–23
63 Ader R, Cohen N 1975 Behaviorally conditioned immunosuppression. Psychosomatic Medicine 37:333–40
64 Justice B 1987 Who gets sick: thinking and health. Peak Press, Houston
65 Lefcourt H 1973 The functions of illusions of control and freedom. American Psychologist 28(3):417–25
66 Mumford E, Schlesinger H, Glass G 1982 The effects of psychological intervention on recovery from surgery

and heart attacks: an analysis of the literature. American Journal of Public Health 72(2):141–51

67 Richter C 1957 On the phenomenon of sudden death in animals and man. Psychosomatic Medicine 19(3):191–8

68 Frank J 1973 Persuasion and healing. Johns Hopkins University Press, Baltimore

69 Kiresuk TJ 1988 The placebo effect: public policy and knowledge transfer. Knowledge: Creation, Diffusion, Utilization 9(4):435–75

70 Shapiro A, Struening E, Shapiro E 1980 The reliability and validity of a placebo test. Journal of Psychiatric Research 55:253–90

71 Yongren W 1981 The effect of acupuncture in curing the smoking habit, 210 cases. Journal of Traditional Chinese Medicine 1(1):65–6

72 Choy D, Lutzker L, Meltzer L 1983 Effective treatment for smoking cessation. American Journal of Medicine 75(6):1033–6

73 Anon 1990 Many points to needle. Lancet 335:20–21

74 Skrabanek P 1984 Point of view: acupuncture and the age of unreason. Lancet 1(8387):1169–71

75 Wen H, Cheung S 1973 Treatment of drug addiction by acupuncture and electrical stimulation. Asian Journal of Medicine 9:138–41

76 Whitehead P 1978 Acupuncture in the treatment of addiction: a review and analysis. International Journal of Addictions 13(1):1–16

77 Wen H, Teo S 1975 Experience in the treatment of drug addiction by electro-acupuncture. Modern Medicine in Asia 11:23–24

78 Wen H 1979 Acupuncture and electrical stimulations (AES) outpatient detoxification. Modern Medicine in Asia 15:39–43

79 Kosten TR, Kreck MJ, Ragunath J, Kleber HB 1986. A preliminary study of beta-endorphin during chronic naltrexon maintenance treatment in ex-opiate addicts. Life Science 31(1):55–9

80 Pomeranz B 1987 Scientific basis of acupuncture. Acupuncture: textbook and atlas. Springer-Verlag, Berlin

81 Steiner RP, May DL, Davis AW 1982 Acupuncture therapy for the treatment of tobacco smoking addiction. American Journal of Chinese Medicine 10(1–4):107–21

82 Clavel F, Benhamou S, Flamant R 1987 Nicotine dependence and secondary effects of smoking cessation. Journal of Behavioral Medicine 10(6):555–8

83 Cottraux J, Schbath J, Messy P, Mollard E, Juenet C, Collet L 1986 Predictive value of MMPI scales on smoking cessation programs outcomes. Acta Psychiatrica Belgica 86(4):463–9

84 Fuller J 1982 Smoking withdrawal and acupuncture. Medical Journal of Australia 1(1):28–9

85 LaCroix J, Besancon F 1977 Tobacco withdrawal: efficacy of acupuncture in a comparative trial. Annales de Medicine Interne 128(4):405–8

86 Lamontagne Y, Annable L, Gagnon M 1980 Acupuncture for smokers: lack of long-term therapeutic effect in a controlled study. Canadian Medical Association Journal 122(7):787–90

87 MacHovec F, Man S 1978 Acupuncture and hypnosis compared: 58 cases. American Journal of Clinical Hypnosis 21(1):45–7

88 Martin G, Waite P 1981 The efficacy of acupuncture as an aid to stopping smoking. New Zealand Medical Journal 93(686):421–3

89 Shakur M, Smith M 1979 The use of acupuncture in the treatment of drug addiction. American Journal of Acupuncture 7(3):223–8

90 Smith MO, Khan I 1988 An acupuncture programme for the treatment of drug-addicted persons. Bulletin on Narcotics 40(1):35–41

91 Smith M 1985 Chinese theory of acupuncture detoxification. American Journal of Acupuncture 12(4):386–7

92 Smith M, Squires R, Aponte J, Rabinovitz N, Bonilla-Rodriguez R 1982 Acupuncture treatment of drug addiction and alcohol abuse. American Journal of Acupuncture 10(2):161–3

93 Brewington V, Smith M, Lipton D 1994 Acupuncture as a detoxification treatment: An analysis of controlled research. Journal of Substance Abuse Treatment 11(4):289–307

94 Bullock ML, Umen AJ, Culliton PD, Olander RT 1987 Acupuncture treatment of alcoholic recidivism: a pilot study. Alcoholism, Clinical and Experimental Research 11(3):292–5

95 Bullock ML, Culliton PD, Olander RT 1989 Controlled trial of acupuncture for severe recidivist alcoholism. Lancet 1(8652):1435–9

96 Smith MI 1988 Acupuncture treatment for crack: clinical survey of 1500 patients treated. American Journal of Acupuncture 16(3):241–7

97 Wise RA 1984 Neural mechanisms of the reinforcing agent of cocaine. NIDA Research Monograph 50:15–33

98 Patterson M 1975 Acupuncture and neuro-electric therapy in the treatment of drug and alcohol addictions. Australian Journal of Alcoholism and Drug Dependence 2(3):90–95

99 Lewenberg AI 1985 Electroacupuncture and antidepressant treatment of alcoholism in a private practice. Clinical Therapeutics 7(5):611–17

100 Sytinsky I, Galebskaya L 1979 Physiologo-biochemical bases of drug independence treatment by electro-acupuncture. Addictive Behavior 4:97–120

101 Ulett G 1992 Beyond yin and yang: how acupuncture really works. Warren H Green, Inc., St. Louis

102 Cohen MW, Masters JS, Doyle CC 1980 Relaxation-facilitated EMG biofeedback in the treatment of diazepam withdrawal syndrome: a case study. American Journal of Clinical Biofeedback 3(1):68–70

103 Fahrion SL, Walters ED, Coyne L, Allen T 1992 Alterations in EEG amplitude, personality factors, and brain electrical mapping after alpha-theta brainwave training: a controlled case study of an alcoholic in recovery. Alcoholism, Clinical and Experimental Research 16(3):547–52

104 Taub E, Steiner SS, Weingarten E, Walton KG 1994 Effectiveness of broad spectrum approaches to relapse prevention in severe alcoholism: a long-term, randomized, controlled trial of transcendental meditation, EMG biofeedback and electronic neurotherapy. Alcoholism Treatment Quarterly 11(1/2):187–220

105 Denney MR, Baugh JL 1992 Symptom reduction and sobriety in the male alcoholic. International Journal of the Addictions 27(11):1293–1300

106 Denney MR, Baugh JL, Hardt HD 1991 Sobriety outcome after alcoholism treatment with biofeedback par-

ticipation: A pilot inpatient study. International Journal of the Addictions 26(3):335–41
107 Khatami M, Woody G, O'Brien C, Mintz J 1982 Biofeedback treatment of narcotic addiction: a double-blind study. Drug and Alcohol Dependence 9(2):111–17
108 Birbaumer N, Elbert T, Rockstroh B, Kramer J, Lutzenberger W, Grossmann P 1992 Effects of inhaled nicotine on instrumental learning of blood pressure responses. Biofeedback and Self Regulation 17(2):107–23
109 Grimsley D 1990 Nicotine effects on biofeedback training. Journal of Behavioral Medicine 13(3):321–6
110 Schneider F, Elbert T, Heimann H, Welker A, Stetter F, Mattes R, Birbaumer N, Mann K 1993 Self-regulation of slow cortical potentials in psychiatric patients: alcohol dependency. Biofeedback and Self Regulation 18(1):23–32
111 Anon 1992 Seven weeks to abstinence: a practical miracle. The FELIX Letter: A Commentary on Nutrition, Berkeley, CA, #63
112 Mathews-Larson J, Parker RA 1987 Alcoholism treatment with biochemical restoration as a major component. International Journal of Biosocial Research 9(1):92–104
113 Littlefield RW 1994. Four recipes for recovery. Natural Health 24(2)
114 Colby-Morley E 1982 The reflection of hypoglycemia and alcoholism on personality: nutrition as a mode of treatment. Journal of Orthomolecular Psychiatry 11(2):132–9
115 Page R, Handley G 1993 The use of hypnosis in cocaine addiction. American Journal of Clinical Hypnosis 36(2):120–3
116 Orman D 1991 Reframing of an addiction via hypnotherapy: a case presentation [see comments]. American Journal of Clinical Hypnosis 33(4):263–71
117 Rabkin S, Boyko E, Shane F, Kaufert J 1984 A randomized trial comparing smoking cessation programs utilizing behavior modification, health education or hypnosis. Addictive Behaviors 9(2):157–73
118 Hyman G, Stanley R, Burrows G, Horne D 1986 Treatment effectiveness of hypnosis and behavior therapy in smoking cessation: a methodological refinement. Addictive Behaviors 11(4):355–65
119 Haxby D 1995 Treatment of nicotine dependence. [Review]. American Journal of Health-System Pharmacy 52(3):265–81, quiz 314–5
120 Stoil M 1989 Problems in the evaluation of hypnosis in the treatment of alcoholism. Journal of Substance Abuse Treatment 6:31–5
121 Johnson D, Karkut R 1994 Performance by gender in a stop-smoking program combining hypnosis and aversion. Psychological Reports 75(2):851–7
122 Schwartz J 1992 Methods of smoking cessation. [Review]. Medical Clinics of North America 76(2):451–76
123 Gelderloos P, Walton KG, Orme-Johnson DW, Alexander CN 1991 Effectiveness of the transcendental meditation program in preventing and treating substance misuse: a review. [Review]. International Journal of the Addictions 26(3):293–325
124 1995 Self recovery: treating addictions using trancendental meditation and Maharishi Ayur-Veda. Harrington Park Press, New York
125 Borrie R 1990 The use of restricted environmental stimulation therapy in treating addictive behaviors. [Review]. International Journal of the Addictions 25(7A–8A):995–1015
126 Suedfeld P 1990 Restricted environmental stimulation and smoking cessation: a fifteen-year progress report. International Journal of the Addictions 25:861–88
127 Suedfeld P, Ikard F 1974 The use of sensory deprivation in facilitating the reduction of cigarette smoking. Journal of Consulting and Clinical Psychology 42:888–95
128 Suedfeld P, Landon P, Pargament R, Epstein Y 1972 An experimental attack on smoking (attitude manipulation in restricted environments, III). International Journal of the Addictions 7:721–33
129 Barabasz A, Baer L, Sheehan D, Barabasz M 1986 A three-year follow-up of hypnosis and restricted environmental stimulation therapy for smoking. International Journal of Clinical and Experimental Hypnosis 34(3):169–81
130 International Congress of Psychology 1984 The effectiveness of reduced stimulation in smoking cessation programs. Acapulco, Mexico
131 Gariti P, Auriacombe M, Incmikoski R, McLellan A, Patterson L, Dhopesh V, Mezochow J, Patterson M, O'Brien C 1992 A randomized double-blind study of neuroelectric therapy in opiate and cocaine detoxification. Journal of Substance Abuse 4(3):299–308
132 Mirman JI 1994 (ed) What the hell is homeopathy? New Hope Publishers, New Hope, MN
133 Garcia-Swain S 1996 Personal conversation
134 Anon 1994 Kudzu extract shows potential for moderating alcohol abuse. American Journal of Hospital Pharmacy 51(6):750
135 Althoff S 1994 Weed for alcoholics. Natural Health Magazine 24(2)
136 Keung W, Vallee B 1993 Daidzin and daidzein suppress free-choice ethanol intake by Syrian golden hamsters. Proceedings of the National Academy of Sciences of the United States of America 90(21):10008–12
137 Keung W 1993 Biochemical studies of a new class of alcohol dehydrogenase inhibitors from Radix puerariae. Alcoholism, Clinical and Experimental Research 17(6):1254–60
138 Keung W, Vallee B 1994 Therapeutic lessons from traditional Oriental medicine to contemporary Occidental pharmacology. In: Jansson HJ (ed) Toward a molecular basis of alcohol use and abuse. Birkhauser Verlag, Boston, MA
139 Petri G, Takach G 1990 Application of herbal mixtures in rehabilitation after alcoholism. Planta Medica 56(6):692–3
140 Shanmugasundaram E, Subramaniam U, Santhini R, Shanmugasundaram K 1986 Studies on brain structure and neurological function in alcoholic rats controlled by an Indian Medicinal Formula (SKV). Journal of Ethnopharmacology 17:225–45
141 Klajner F, Hartman L, Sobell M 1984 Treatment of substance abuse by relaxation training: a review of its rationale, efficacy and mechanisms. Addictive Behaviors 9(1):41–55
142 Suraway C, Cox T 1986 Smoking behavior under conditions of relaxation: a comparison between types of smokers. Addictive Behaviors 11(2):187–91

143 Drummond D, Glautier S 1994 A controlled trial of cue exposure treatment in alcohol dependence. Journal of Consulting and Clinical Psychology 62(4):809–17

144 Wynd C 1992 Relaxation imagery used for stress reduction in the prevention of smoking relapse. Journal of Advanced Nursing 17(3):294–302

145 Ormrod J, Budd R 1991 A comparison of two treatment interventions aimed at lowering anxiety levels and alcohol consumption amongst alcohol abusers. Drug and Alcohol Dependence 27(3):233–43

146 Rezvani AH, Overstreet DH, Lee Y 1995 Attenuation of alcohol intake by ibogaine in three strains of alcohol-preferring rats. Pharmacology Biochemistry and Behavior 52(3):615–20

147 Sershen H, Hashim A, Lajtha A 1994 Ibogaine reduces preference for cocaine consumption in C57BL/6By mice. Pharmacology Biochemistry and Behavior 47:13–19

148 Popik P, Layer RT, Skolnick P 1995 100 Years of ibogaine: neurochemical and pharmacological actions of a putative anti-addictive drug. Pharmacological Reviews 47(2):235–53

149 Sheppard SG 1994 A preliminary investigation of ibogaine: case reports and recommendations for further study. Journal of Substance Abuse Treatment 11(4):379–85

150 Ludwig A, Levine J, Stark L 1970 LSD and alcoholism: a clinical study of treatment efficacy. Charles C Thomas, Springfield, IL

151 Staiger P, White J 1991 Cue reactivity in alcohol abusers: stimulus specificity and extinction of the responses. Addictive Behaviors 16(5):211–21

152 Tobena A, Fernandez-Teruel A, Escorihuela R, Nunez J, Zapata A, Ferre P, Sanchez R 1993 Limits of habituation and extinction: implications for relapse prevention programs in addictions. [Review]. Drug and Alcohol Dependence 32(3):209–17

153 Drummond D, Cooper T, Glautier S 1990 Conditioned learning in alcohol dependence: implications for cue exposure treatment. [Review]. British Journal of Addiction 85(6):725–43

154 Powell J, Gray J, Bradley B 1993 Subjective craving for opiates: evaluation of a cue exposure protocol for use with detoxified opiate addicts. British Journal of Clinical Psychology 32(Pt 1):39–53

155 Dawe S, Powell J, Richards D, Gossop M, Marks I, Strang J, Gray J 1993 Does post-withdrawal cue exposure improve outcome in opiate addiction? A controlled trial. Addiction 88(9):1233–45

156 Shapiro F, Vogelmann-Sine S, Sine L 1994 Eye movement desensitization and reprocessing: treating trauma and substance abuse. Journal of Psychoactive Drugs 26(4):379–91

157 Montgomery R, Ayllon T 1994 Eye movement desensitization across subjects: subjective and physiological measures of treatment efficacy. Journal of Behavior Therapy and Experimental Psychiatry 25(3):217–30

158 Silver S, Brooks A, Obenchain J 1995 Treatment of Vietnam War veterans with PTSD: a comparison of eye movement desensitization and reprocessing, biofeedback, and relaxation training. Journal of Traumatic Stress 8(2):337–42

159 Kapur P 1992 Yoga, family therapy and Indian systems of medicine as effective strategies in the prevention and treatment of alcohol and drug abuse. 36th International Congress on Alcohol and Drug Dependence (36eme Congres International sur l'Alcoolisme et les Toxicomanies), Glasgow, Scotland I:180–8

160 National Institute of Health 1995 Comparing methadone maintenance treatment enhanced by hatha yoga or dynamic group psychotherapy: A randomized clinical trial. NIH, Division of Alternative Medicine, Bethesda, MD

161 Eastwood M, Stiasny L 1978 Psychiatric disorder, hospital admission, and season. Archives of General Psychiatry 35:769–71

162 Poikolainen K 1982 Drug alcohol dependence. Seasonality of alcohol-related hospital admissions has implications for prevention 10:65–9

163 American Psychological Association 1988 96th Convention, Atlanta, GA

164 Satel S, Gawin F 1989 Seasonal cocaine abuse. American Journal of Psychiatry 146:534–5

165 McGrath R, Yahia M 1993 Preliminary data on seasonally related alcohol dependence. Journal of Clinical Psychiatry 54(7):260–2

166 Morrison H 1995 Nature's Prozac. Natural Health 25:3

167 Burton Goldberg Group (ed) 1993 Alternative medicine: the definitive guide. Future Medicine Publishing, Inc., Puyallup, WA

168 Alexander S 1995 Healing hands for addictions. Earth Star 15:104

169 McPeake JD, Kennedy BP, Gordon SM 1991 Altered states of consciousness therapy. A missing component in alcohol and drug rehabilitation treatment [see comments]. [Review]. Journal of Substance Abuse Treatment 8(1–2):75–82

170 Davis T 1994 The research evidence on the power of prayer and healing. Canadian Journal of Cardiovascular Nursing 5(2):34–6

171 Koenig H, George L, Meador K, Blazer D, Ford S 1994 Religious practices and alcoholism in a Southern adult population. Hospital and Community Psychiatry 45(3):225–31

172 Schuckit M 1994 Goals of treatment. In: Galanter M, Kleber H (eds) The American Psychiatric Press textbook of substance abuse treatment. American Psychiatric Press, Washington, DC

173 Vaillant GE 1993. The natural history of alcoholism. Havard University Press, MA

174 Gillis J, Mubbashar M 1995 Risk factors for drug abuse in Pakistan: a replication. Psychological Reports 76(1):99–108

175 Perez-Arce P 1994 Substance use patterns of Latinas: commentary. International Journal of the Addictions 29(9):1189–99

176 Greberman S, Wada K 1994 Social and legal factors related to drug abuse in the United States and Japan. [Review]. Public Health Reports 109(6):731–7

177 Seale JP, Muramoto ML 1993 Substance abuse among minority populations. Primary Care, Clinics in Office Practice 20(1):167–80

178 Babor TF 1986 Taking stock: method and theory in cross-national research on alcohol. Alcohol and Culture: Comparative Perspectives From Europe and America. New York Academy of Sciences

179 Westermeyer J, Peake E 1983 A ten-year follow-up of alcoholic native Americans in Minnesota. American Journal of Psychiatry 140(2):189–94
180 Westermeyer J, Peng G 1977 Opium and heroin addicts in Laos. The Journal of Nervous and Mental Disease 164(5): 346–54
181 Hall RL 1986 Alcohol treatment in American Indian populations: an indigenous treatment modality compared with traditional approaches. Alcohol and culture: comparative perspectives from Europe and America. New York Academy of Sciences
182 Babor TF, Mendelson JH 1986 Ethnic/religious differences in the manifestation and treatment of alcoholism. Alcohol and culture: comparative perspectives from Europe and America. New York Academy of Sciences
183 Brady M 1991 Drug and alcohol use among aboriginal people. The health of Aboriginal Australia. Harcourt, Brace, Jovanovich, Sydney, Orlando
184 Singer M, Borrero MG 1984 Indigenous treatment of alcoholism: the case of Puerto Rican spiritism. Medical Anthropology 8(4):246–73
185 Westermeyer J, Bourne P 1978 Treatment outcome and the role of the community in narcotic addiction. Journal of Nervous and Mental Disease 166(1):51–8
186 Berg BJ, Volpicelli JR, Alterman AI, O'Brien CP 1991 The relationship between endogenous opiods and alcohol drinking: The opiod compensation hypothesis. In: Naranjo CA, Sellars EM (eds) Novel pharmacological interventions for alcoholism. Springer-Verlag, NY

CHAPTER CONTENTS

13

Mind–body approaches to successful aging

Frederic Luskin
Kathryn Newell

'Remember to cure the patient as well as the disease'.
Dr Alvan Barach (Quoted in Moyers (1993)[1]

INTRODUCTION

The number of people over the age of 65 years is rising dramatically. A brief glance at statistics prepared in 1995 by the American Association of Retired Persons (AARP) attests to some remarkable demographic changes (Box 13.1)[2].

If physicians are not already skilled in the field of geriatrics, these statistics suggest that they will need to be. As the size of the elderly population increases so will their health care requirements. In the face of such demographic changes physicians may need to re-evaluate what is considered 'normal aging' and not restrict their approach to traditional biological and disease-based models of ill health. Rather, it is necessary for physicians to take a broader, mind–body approach when dealing with the elderly. One compelling reason for adopting a mind–body approach is made clear by Dr Thomas Delbanco, Director of the Division of General Medicine and Primary Care at Beth Israel Hospital in Boston, who states[1]:

> Mind and body are inextricably woven together. Studies show that probably half the visits to us in the office are related to mind issues rather than body issues. We'd better be educated if we're going to serve those patients as well. Studies have also shown that in the elderly population, the percentage of patients seeing doctors for psychosocial reasons is even higher than 50%.

Box 13.1 Aging statistics

- Population related
  - Individuals aged 65 years or older represented 12.7% of the US population in 1994 which translates to 33.2 million people, or about one in every eight Americans. The number of individuals aged 65 years or older increased by 2.1 million or 7% since 1990, compared with an increase of only 4% for the under-65 population.
  - Individuals aged over 85 years constitute the fastest growing segment of the US population. Since 1900, the percentage of older Americans has more than tripled (4.1% to 12.7%) and the number has increased nearly eleven times (3.1 million to 33.2 million).
  - By the year 2030, there will be an estimated 70 million aged 65 years or more in the USA (20% of the population) — more than twice that of 1990.
  - Half of all older women in 1994 were widows. At age 85 there are 39 men for every 100 women.
- Health related
  - In 1993, 28% of individuals aged 65 or more stated that their health was only fair to poor.
  - 36% of all hospital stays and 48% of total days of doctor care were for individuals aged 65 or more.
  - The elderly used 36% of total health care expenditures in 1987. The cost totaled $162 billion which breaks down to $5360/year spent on older patients compared with the $1290/year spent on younger patients.
  - The most frequently occurring conditions in 1993 per/100 elders, were the chronic conditions of arthritis (49%) and hypertension (35%).

A second reason for adopting a mind–body approach derives from the need to learn and incorporate current theories about the aging process itself. There is a wealth of new and exciting information about what really happens biologically when we age that looks dramatically different from many of the traditional beliefs held about the aging process. For example, the National Institute on Aging conducted a study which showed that if the heart is free of disease, blood pumps just as efficiently in a 90-year-old as in a young adult, contrary to earlier suggestions that hearts normally pump less blood with age[3].

A third reason for adopting a broader approach than the traditional biomedical model lies with the unique needs of the elderly patient. Elderly patients, by nature, are dealing with more than just physical concerns as they approach the later part of life. They inevitably come to question the meaning of their lives, must face their own mortality and they have to deal with the imposed societal myths about aging. These, when combined with the physical challenges of aging demand a different approach if physicians truly wish to address all their elderly patient's concerns.

MIND–BODY CARE OF THE ELDERLY

Physicians who only address the biophysical aspects of aging, those uneducated about current trends in geriatric medicine and those insensitive to the unique needs of the elderly, may feel inadequately equipped to treat the complexities of their patients' needs. Both patients and physicians may feel unsatisfied with their interactions and the need to find space for healing may become a source of additional pain for both. To quote Dr Delbanco[1]:

> It's probably easier to study [the body] and that's what we learned in medical school — 95% body, and 5% mind. But I'll tell you, once you're in practice, and you're taking care of real people, it becomes much closer to 50–50.

In order to understand the importance of the mind–body link and what it means for treating elderly people it is important to be aware of, and to utilize, the vast literature which establishes the link between an individual's thoughts or emotions and the physical process of aging and disease. It is equally important to become aware of the research which documents the effect of the beliefs, practices and attitudes of the physician on the patient. In addition, in order to optimize the patient's health and enhance the relationship between the physician and the patient it is useful to study the research which investigates the mind–body link and its effect on disease.

A number of key questions have to be addressed in order to incorporate the lessons of mind–body medicine into elderly care practice:

- How does a doctor use the doctor–patient relationship to maximize the effectiveness of any treatment prescribed?
- What are the behaviors that are most conducive to help create the optimal environment for recovery in an elderly patient?
- What information from the mind–body interaction is useful in planning treatment in an elderly population?
- What beliefs and attitudes held by physicians are the most efficacious when treating the elderly?

This chapter examines and attempts to answer the key mind–body questions by focusing on four psychosocial behaviors that help a physician interact with and assist the patient in mind as well as body:

- listen to and support the patient
- encourage the patient
- be willing to evaluate one's own beliefs about aging, death and spirituality
- be receptive to the research literature which demonstrates the efficacy of specific mind–body treatment interventions.

THE VALUE OF LISTENING

The single most powerful quality a physician can offer the patient is a simple one and that is the ability to listen to the patient and by doing so offer emotional support. Listening both creates a partnership with the patient and may offer help towards the goal of optimal health. While this may sound simple, in reality it appears quite difficult. Beckman (1984)[4] showed that the average patient only speaks for 18 seconds before interruption by their doctor. That same patient, once interrupted, has only a 2% chance of completing their statement or question.

A study published in the *Journal of the American Medical Association* demonstrated that physicians' inability to listen can create an almost complete disregard for their patients' wishes[5]. In this study over 2000 physicians treating seriously ill patients were informed by a team of nurses about the specific wishes of their patients regarding areas such as medication and pain management. The nurses had extensive contact with the patients and their families and their purpose was to facilitate patient–doctor communication. The startling conclusion of the study was that the effort of the nurses failed completely. These quite ill patients were treated with no more concern for their pain or their desires than were the patients looked after by a control group of physicians who did not have the nurses to advise them.

Studies have shown that patients often know more about the present and future state of their health than their physicians, who rely largely on the results of laboratory test results to predict health. Researchers from Yale Medical School conducted a study in which 2500 men and women, aged 65 and older, were asked to rate the state of their health from poor to excellent. The patient self-reports proved to be better able to predict health outcome than could the physicians' use of evidence gained from laboratory testing. The ability of the patients to understand their health was even more predictive of health outcome than looking at the traditional risk factors such as cigarette smoking. In fact, people who smoked were twice as likely to die during the next 12 years as people who did not smoke. However, people who thought they were in 'poor health' were seven times as likely to die as those who thought they were in 'excellent health'[6].

A similar study, cited by Ornstein and Sobel (1987)[7], refers to 3500 elderly adults in Canada who were asked to rate their health on a continuum from poor to excellent. The researchers retrieved their health reports from hospitals and physicians. At the end of 7 years, the self-ratings were found to be more predictive of morbidity than the health reports. What was most interesting was that those patients shown to be in poor health by objective measures survived at a higher rate if they themselves rated their own health to be good or excellent. The only predictor more powerful than the patient's self-reports was the effect of advancing age on morbidity. That is, people died more often with each succeeding year of age.

A different kind of study conducted by Lawlis and Achterberg showed that evaluating the drawings created during a period of guided imagery with cancer patients was more predictive of disease outcome than the results of the laboratory tests. Tumor progression was directly related to the specificity, strength, vividness and clarity of the images patients were able to create during sessions of guided practice. Imagery, in this case, proved to be another way that patients could access information about their health that was unavailable to physicians who only used objective data[8].

Social support

Listening to elderly patients is not only important because they know more about their health than the physician does — it has other salutary effects. Listening offers much needed social support. Research has clearly established that level of social support is an important and independent risk factor for many diseases and is predictive of longevity by itself[9]. There are five key components to social support[10]:

- being cared for and loved
- being valued
- sharing companionship
- having access to information and guidance
- physical and material assistance.

In the Alameda, California study, 7000 people were followed for 9 years to ascertain if social support was related to morbidity and longevity. The participants were separated into two groups: those that lived lonely lives with minimal social support and those who had a full life with family and friends. Participants were assessed for other risk factors such as obesity, cigarette and alcohol consumption, and general health at the beginning of the study. After 9 years the researchers found that the common denominator that most often led to good health and long life was the amount and quality of social support a person enjoyed. For people over 60, having close ties with friends and/or relatives was the best predictor of good health and reduced mortality. For those under 60, marital status was the best predictor of health[11].

Another interesting survey of 700 elderly adults showed that their health and vitality were directly related to what they contributed to their social network rather than what they took out of it[12]. This suggests that it is health-enhancing to not only have relationships but to actively participate in those relationships. Another epidemiological study investigated the effect of social support on the incidence of heart disease. Support proved to be the critical difference between the town of Roseto, Pennsylvania and comparable towns nearby that explained the inhabitants' vastly lower rates of coronary heart disease for 15 years, from the early 1960s until the mid 1970s. The incidence of heart disease changed when the community's young people left behind some of the traditional behaviors and for the first time began to move away to other communities. By the mid-1970s the mortality and rate of heart disease in Roseto was equal to surrounding towns.

Detailed analysis of Roseto's residents during the 1960s showed that they only took an average amount of exercise, their levels of obesity, and high blood pressure were equal to those in surrounding towns, and their diets were higher in fat and meat than the average US diet. The difference was in their sense of community, their well-defined social roles and their extended network of family and friends. Interestingly, when Roseto had an intact social support network the men had only 16% the incidence of heart disease and death from heart disease compared with the US average[13]. Amazingly enough the rate for women was even lower. One of the researchers comments on how the elderly were treated in that community:

> There was a remarkable cohesiveness and sense of unconditional support within the community. Family ties were very strong. And what impressed us most was the attitude toward the elderly. In Roseto, the older residents weren't put on the shelf; they were promoted to 'supreme court' No-one was ever abandoned[9].

Change and abandonment

For the elderly in the USA change and abandonment are common occurrences. Elderly people are particularly affected by disrupted social ties. Whether because of retirement, giving up a home after the children have left, bereavement, or disability, changes in social support are quite common among the elderly. Research has shown that these changes can cause depression. However, if the elderly person has at least one close and supportive confidant the disruptive effects can be mitigated[14]. Further support for the incredible health-providing power of social support in the lives of the elderly emerges from a study described by Ornstein and Sobel (1993)[7]. In this work, 2500 elderly men and women were asked to state their level of social support. Researchers then observed those who were eventually hospitalized for a heart attack. There were substantial differences in survival rates. Only 12% of the patients with two or more sources of social support died in the hospital, while 38% of those with no reported social support died. The results applied to both men and women and were predictive even when taking into account the severity of the attack, other illnesses and other known risk factors.

While a physician clearly cannot serve as a source of primary support, listening to the elderly provides benefits in five ways. First, visits to a doctor's surgery often produce anxiety and being listened to reduces blood pressure and anxiety[15]. Second, allowing an elderly person to talk provides a modeling experience which, it is hoped, they will try to duplicate in their social world through the development of self-efficacy[16]. Third, listening is an expression of care and care is in itself therapeutic. Fourth, a physician can gain critical information about the levels of social support in the elderly person's life and can help the person find ways of increasing this if necessary. Finally, listening makes it clear to the patient that they have a role in the healing partnership. The opinion of the patient is seen as important, and they can understand that they have a responsibility to share what they know with the physician.

It is important to remember that many people go to their physician for social support in the first place. One study found that 60–90% of visits to physicians were prompted by conditions related to stress and other mind–body interactions[17]. Kroenke and Mangelsdorff reviewed the records from an internal medicine clinic of more than 1000 patients over a 3-year period. They found that fewer than 16% of the most common body complaints were organic in nature. Their conclusion was that over 70% of the symptoms reported were related to psychosocial factors[18].

Social support and immunity

Social support has been hypothesized to affect longevity because of its ability to affect the functioning of the immune system[19]. Support for this hypothesis comes from a well-known study investigating the effects of social support on the immunity of 38 elderly residents living in retirement homes. Residents were visited three times a week for 1 month by a number of volunteers, and immune function was measured throughout. After just 1 month of visits seniors showed a significant increase in their level of antibodies and natural killer cell activity suggesting improved immune functioning[20]. Similarly, in a prospective randomized control study of 60 elderly people, with a mean age of 78, it was found that the experimental group who received increased social support had increased levels of dihydroepiandrosterone (DHEA) and stable levels of growth hormones[21].

OFFERING ENCOURAGEMENT

The second psychosocial quality which the physician has to offer the elderly patient, and one that is often underutilized, is that of encouragement. The goal of encouragement is to help the patient mobilize their healing forces and to empower them to believe that they are capable of mobilizing their own resources for recovery on their own.

Encouragement can function in two ways. The first way is for the physician to commit to and believe strongly in the treatment. The power of the physician's belief augments the effectiveness of therapeutically effective treatments as well as enhancing the effect of placebos[22]. This power of belief may be one of medicine's untapped weapons in the fight against disease. Conscious advocacy for a treatment is one way a physician's belief can influence outcome. Strict adherence to the biomedical model makes it difficult for physicians to understand or harness the power of belief, and some would even suggest that encouraging belief is, in some way, cheating or unethical. The biomedical model tends to discredit and minimize the effects of belief and expectancy, choosing to focus strictly on biological processes.

The other beneficial effect of encouragement is that it supports the patient when their resources are depleted or they falter. What is remarkable is that the effects of physician advocacy may occur even when the physician's attitudes are supposedly controlled, as in double-blind experiments.

Physician as treatment

The first study to demonstrate this power of the physician to influence the outcome of treatment occurred during the late 1950s[23]. The new anxiolytic drug meprobamate, had received conflicting reports about whether or not it was clinically effective. In order to test its efficacy researchers designed a double-blind study in which one of the doctors had a skeptical attitude towards the drug's effectiveness while the other believed in its potency. The doctors and the patients were unaware which pills were meprobamate and which were placebo. Remarkably enough, meprobamate worked significantly better than the placebo only for the physician who believed in it. The skeptical physician's patients received no benefit from the drug. When this experiment was replicated in three separate clinics the same results occurred in two of the clinics. The drug was effective when administered by a physician who believed in it and not so when administered by a doubting physician[24].

The same result, corroborating the power of physician's belief in the treatment, occurred in three double-blind studies which evaluated the use of vitamin E in treating angina pectoris. A doctor who enthusiastically believed in the power of vitamin E found it to have a significant effect while two studies conducted by a skeptical physician suggested that it had no effect[25]. Studies cited by Dr Alfred Berg[9] show that a physician's expectations of a drug's efficacy can alter the 'outcome of therapy by about 25 to 30% in either direction'.

The placebo effect

A physician's encouragement and belief in a treatment to help empower the elderly patient is a significant part of the largely unexplored healing dynamic known as the activation of the *placebo effect*. Benson and Friedman clearly distinguish the placebo effect, which they refer to as the 'symbolic significance of a treatment in changing a patient's illness', from the medical use of *a placebo*[26]. The placebo effect is 'the aspect of treatment not attributable to specific pharmacological or physiologic properties'. A placebo, on the other hand, is a harmless treatment thought to have no measurable effect on the condition to which it is being applied. Benson and Friedman suggested that three components are required to manifest the placebo effect:

- positive expectation on the part of the patient
- positive beliefs on the part of the physician
- a good relationship between the patient and physician.

They also suggested that the placebo effect should really be renamed 'remembered wellness' because of the incredible capacity for people to become healthy as a result of the non-pharmacologic or physiologic aspects of treatment.

In fact, much of what passes for acceptable medical practice today already makes use of the placebo effect. Hunt refers to a leading pharmacology textbook's estimate that 35–45% of present day prescriptions are unlikely to have specific effects on the diseases for which they are prescribed[27]. For 20 years Herbert Benson has documented the incredible range of disorders that are amenable to the placebo effect[28,29]. This research has demonstrated that medical and surgical treatments for diverse conditions such as heart disease, chronic pain, and psychiatric disorders can be enhanced by the placebo effect.

For example, a recent study by Archer and Leier (1992)[30] investigated the effects of placebo medication in 24 patients suffering with varying degrees of congestive heart failure. The patients were randomized into an experimental group who received a placebo plus the standard treatment and a control group who received simply the standard care. At the conclusion of the study, the patients who were in the experimental group showed a significant 81 second improvement in endurance on the exercise treadmill.

Hope

Another important reason to offer a patient encouragement is to facilitate hope. In elderly people in particular, disease can be a frightening experience and the visit to the physician an emotional challenge. Research has shown that elderly people require a greater degree of psychological support when hospitalized compared with younger people but, in fact, they receive less psychological care than do their younger counterparts[31]. This is despite the finding that increasing mental health services for the elderly generates greater monetary savings than providing such support for younger adults. For example, a study of 452 elderly patients with fractured hips, who also had a psychiatric consultation as part of their work up, revealed that up to 70% of the patients had emotional distress significant enough to warrant intervention[32]. When that intervention was administered, hospital stay was reduced by an average of 2 days and costs were significantly reduced. The psychiatric consultation not only reduced cost and length of hospital stay but also speeded the healing rates of the fractured hips.

Similarly, there is evidence to indicate that patients who are optimistic and confident fare better when undergoing medical procedures and have reduced morbidity and mortality compared to their less hopeful peers[20]. A study to evaluate the effects of two distinct personality traits, optimism and pessimism, in an elderly population demonstrated the effects of personality on immune function. Those with a pessimistic view of life, who exhibited a lack of hope, were shown to have a lower ratio of T-helper cells to T-suppressor cells and had poorer T-lymphocyte response when their immune system was challenged[33]. Martin Seligman confirmed these findings showing that optimists had a healthier, more responsive immune system in a study of 300 elderly people, with an average age of 71. A study from the University of Pennsylvania evaluating the immune response of a healthy elderly population demonstrated that hopeful people had a more robust immune system[34].

Clearly, fostering hope can be an important treatment goal for a physician. A physician's encouragement can help an elderly person remain hopeful and optimistic about both their health and their prognosis when hospitalized. Furthermore, a physician aware of the importance of hope will know which depressed or pessimistic patients to refer for further help and when such a referral would be most appropriate.

Evaluating the studies which deal with hope and healing can provide physicians with new insights into the limitations of their responsibility for the patient's health. In the current medical delivery system the psychosocial components of care are largely absent and the physician's biomedical model encourages them to try and 'cure' the patient of the disease. This responsibility places a significant and stressful burden on the physician. Adopting a biopsychosocial model which encourages a physician to diagnose and treat appropriately, but also to encourage, believe and support the patient, makes it clear that it is ultimately the patient who must mobilize their resources to claim their own health. It is difficult for a patient to mobilize their own resources for recovery when advised by a physician who ignores their emotional life. A mind–body approach creates more of a partnership between doctor and patient, with the physician offering both expertise and support and experiencing less strain.

EVALUATING PERSONAL BELIEFS ABOUT AGING

Another critical aspect physicians should address when dealing with elderly people, is the effect their own experiences with aging and the beliefs they hold about the aging process have on treatment. We live in a youth oriented culture which fears the changes that aging is presumed to bring[35]. Many of the images that we have about old people are filled with the dread of reduced physical capacity and approaching mortality. Clearly, physicians are not immune to the effect that negative stereotypes about aging can have on treatment decisions. Even more important are the unexplored beliefs or theories that physicians hold about the aging process itself. If the physician conceptualizes aging as an inevitable decline in function of all the bodily systems leading to an unfortunate end in death, treatment decisions will follow that unexpressed and unexplored theoretical viewpoint.

An editorial in the *Journal of the American Medical Association* suggests that medical treatment decisions are often made on the basis of advanced age and not on a realistic appraisal of the physical condition of the particular patient[36]. Wetle suggests that this is a form of age discrimination and reflects cultural prejudices about aging. Studies have shown that in some countries admission into the intensive care unit of a hospital[37], or into a renal dialysis unit[38], have been age rationed, even though age by itself gives no indication of how well the patient will tolerate the treatment. Elderly people in good health generally tolerate intensive care as well as younger people. Interestingly, there is some evidence to suggest that elderly patients are more grateful for the life-saving interventions than are younger patients[39].

Early research into the aging process contributed to the generally negative views many people have about what happens as we age. The early research supported the culturally posited axiom that aging is a guaranteed process of mental and physical decline. These studies on aging were to a large degree completed on hospitalized patients[3] which biased the sample and missed the huge numbers of elderly individuals out in the community who were aging in relatively good health. These and other early studies showed a universal decline in both physical and mental function. More recently, longer term, and generally more representative, studies have been conducted. The most influential has been the Baltimore Longitudinal Study on Aging. When data were first collected by this study they showed some steep average declines in function. In particular people were shown to metabolize glucose less efficiently, develop cardiovascular problems and have reduced kidney function. However, when the data were reanalyzed excluding people with clearly delineated disease, a large proportion of elderly population were found to have minimal or no decline in function.

A specific example from the Baltimore Longitudinal Study of Aging looked at creatinine clearance as a measure of renal function[40]. Reduced glomerular filtration rate (GFR) was assumed to be concomitant with aging. However, when people with established renal disease were excluded, one-third of older subjects had no decrease in GFR and creatinine clearance. Thus, a large number of the elderly population did not follow the expected course of declining function. This suggested that physicians need to re-evaluate their assumptions about inevitable declines in ability associated with the aging process. Similar results were found in studies examining cardiovascular function. For example, there was no age-related decline in stroke volume and cardiac output if an elderly individual was free of coronary artery disease and the observed age-related increase in blood pressure, body weight and cholesterol levels did not occur in many non-industrial societies[41].

Age-related changes in all aspects of the cardiovascular system do occur, but age-mediated decline in functional capacity is not inevitable. With increasing age the mitral valve tends to close more slowly, the left ventricle thickens and the arteries become stiffer. However, current thinking is that these changes allow successful adaptations to other physiological changes and are not the result of or an indication of a disease process[3].

Current theories of aging

In a seminal article by Rowe and Kahn, the authors discuss two kinds of aging. They distinguish between successful and usual aging[42]. They define usual aging as the 'dominant pattern of aging in a particular society.' Usual aging would include the elderly who, because of a disease process, have vastly diminished functional capacity. Rowe and Kahn, while not ignoring usual aging, focus their attention on the evidence that a process of successful aging exists for a significant number of adults. They offer that successful aging is the ability of older people to retain physical and mental capacity and function without having to experience the dramatic changes brought about by disease. They therefore separate out, from the normal aging process, the steep functional decline in elderly people suffering from specific disease conditions. Furthermore, they suggest that through the judicious use of lifestyle modifications such as nutrition, exercise, stress management and social support, aging does not have to involve significant functional decline at all and in some cases may involve regeneration of capacity.

Aging as a result of disuse

Bortz suggests that it is disuse and not age that causes many of the changes in function thought to be a consequence of aging[39]. He goes so far as to suggest that in the inactive and overfed lifestyle of industrialized western society what is considered a normal lifestyle may actually, when measured, be contributing to the development of disease. His claim is that our inactivity is a change in the way people have lived throughout history and that we violate our genetics because we are designed, as a species, for considerable activity and exercise. He posits that the consequences of such gross inactivity lead to many of the diseases we label a consequence of aging. For an example, he shows that while a normal cholesterol count for the USA is 200 mg%, for the Kalahari Bushman it is 77 mg%. Normal blood pressure in the USA is considered at 120/80 mm Hg while for aboriginal people it is 105/70 mm Hg. These differences, Bortz suggests, are indicative of the consequences of disuse and not suggestive of either age-related deterioration or disease.

It has also been assumed that aging is associated with significant cognitive deterioration. However, the evidence suggests that intellectual deterioration is not as inevitable as previously thought. Schaie and Willis compared an elderly population with an age-related decrease in fluid intelligence to elderly individuals with stable intelligence[43]. Both groups then received five training sessions and were able to sustain substantial improvements in memory. This would suggest that part of the deterioration seen in intelligence is the result of disuse and not simply a decline in functioning capacity.

In contrast, earlier work suggested that the declines in intellectual performance could be explained by differences in education[44]. Subsequent research re-analyzed cross-sectional data which had shown dramatic age-related deterioration in intelligence[45]. When re-evaluating the data using longitudinal methods there was a clear-cut cohort effect. Thus the changes previously thought to be age-related were actually due to changes in the relative ability of each successive age group and not due to aging per se.

Social context of aging

Beyond the concepts of aging as being either successful or usual a third model exists which takes as its starting point the theory of psychosocial stages as developed by Erikson[35]. In Erikson's theory people pass successively through eight stages of development[46]. Each stage combines the compelling need for personal growth with the social implications of that growth, its social context and its expression. Erikson hypothesized that each of the eight stages involved the resolution of a challenge inherent in that stage of development. The challenges inherent in the last two stages of life can provide some useful insights in understanding the psychosocial changes that the elderly have to cope with. Erikson's stages of life afford a different perspective on aging which puts less emphasis on the maintenance of physical function and more on the exploration of the emotional, social and spiritual experience in aging.

Erikson's seventh stage is referred to as generativity vs. stagnation. Successful achievement during this stage requires the aging adult to continue to be useful by providing encouragement, help and support to the succeeding generations. The challenges of this stage include mentoring, leadership and other forms of care. The leadership provided in the seventh stage by the elderly is no longer for personal gain, but to help develop a sense of continuity in the ever-moving cycle of generations. An unsuccessful experience at this stage leads to a sense of purposelessness as an individual's role in the world diminishes as retirement looms. This unsuccessful resolution can lead to desperate grasping for achievement and money driven by the fear that the opportunity and time for personal gain is becoming sorely limited.

Erikson's eighth stage is called ego integrity vs. despair. In this, the last stage of life, the elderly are challenged to achieve a sense of completeness and self-acceptance that offsets the continuing physical changes. Erikson claims that success in this stage requires an individual to understand the importance of each individual life and how it has contributed to the larger whole. A person comes to see that their life is unique and important because of its contribution to life in general. Each life is seen to have a meaning that is not measured merely by past accomplishments. A failure at this task leads to despair, an exaggerated fear of death and a chilling sense that time is running out.

The meaning of life

Both of Erikson's last two stages require that the aging adult plays a meaningful role in their social environment. This is not simply a matter of carving out an individual niche but requires an acceptance of the changing role required with advancing age. Successful completion of both of Erikson's last two stages hinges on the powerful need for elderly people to establish a coherent sense of meaning and purpose in their lives. This is not a sense of meaning created simply from previous accomplishments but one that is related to the timeless meaning of life itself. To Erikson, a sense of purpose evolves from meaning gained from personal accomplishment in addition to meaning gained from embracing some of life's timeless verities. When an elderly person's life can be viewed as successful, even in the face of physical decline, a significant and important change has occurred.

When the need for meaning becomes more than simply acknowledging accomplishments and acquisitions and planning new ones, then the spiritual aspects of life emerge. Jung agreed with Erikson, in claiming that the second half of life is best used for people to grapple with their mortality and to create new ways of finding meaning in their lives[47]. If this is true then spiritual issues may have to be addressed when working with the elderly. Not all elderly people are grappling with spiritual questions but many are and, unfortunately, most physicians are not prepared to address the spiritual concerns of their patients.

While a survey of family practices revealed that most patients and physicians believed in God (91% for the patients and 64% for the physicians) almost no time was spent during the doctor–patient consultation on spiritual matters[48]. Only when life-threatening illness needed to be dealt with did some physicians (69% by their account, 19% by the patient's account) discuss spiritual matters. This survey found that 40% of patients felt that their doctor should discuss pertinent religious issues with them.

Matthews and Larson (1995)[49] commenting on the study say:

> This useful study confirms the findings of other studies that patients, and the general public, are considerably more religious than health care professionals and that a marked separation between religious practice and medical practice exist for both parties. This separation creates confusion for both groups. Patients are often quite interested in addressing spiritual matters, but physicians rarely do so, except in cases of major, or terminal, illnesses. Many physicians are apparently concerned that addressing spiritual matters may offend patients, but this fear appears unfounded, although its impact upon patient satisfaction has rarely been assessed.

Religion and spirituality

Interestingly, a developed sense of spirituality, which is often measured by the surrogate markers of church attendance or religious practice, is associated with improved outcomes in a variety of medical situations. Both mortality and morbidity are affected positively[50]. Church attendance and other forms of measurable religious practice are not the same as spirituality but both have been shown to have salutary health benefits. In a study of 300 hospitalized patients, those individuals with the greatest sense of spirituality were the most emotionally healthy[51]. In this study of the terminally ill, those who possessed a greater spiritual understanding had far less fear of death, decreased loneliness, and less discomfort. Reed also suggested that a spiritual perspective emerges in many terminally ill people and facilitates acceptance of their imminent physical demise.

A similar study of more than 100 elderly patients demonstrated that individual religious commitment correlated with greater health on a variety of measures[52]. People with little religious activity had higher rates of cancer, anxiety, depression and cigarette and alcohol use. In a larger study involving 2800 elderly people, researchers found that religious activity was inversely related to subsequent disability over a 3-year period even when levels of disability were controlled for at the beginning of the study. The elderly who did become disabled experienced less depression if they had more religious activity[53]. A study by Zuckerman found that elderly people who were forced to relocate from their homes had less distress if they had a strong religious connection[54].

Finally, prayer, one of the commonest manifestations of spiritual or religious practice, has been demonstrated to be an important and valuable activity for elderly patients[55]. In the famous prospective randomized double-blind study by Byrd, 192 hospitalized cardiac patients who were prayed for had significantly reduced need for antibiotics, diuretics and ventilation than did the control group who were not prayed for[56]. In this study, conducted over a 10-month period, between three and seven people prayed for each patient throughout the duration of their hospital stay. What was remarkable about the study was that the people doing the praying only knew the name and the severity of the condition of the people they were praying for. Somehow the prayers were effective, producing a small but significant improvement in clinical outcome.

Life and death

Schachter-Shalomi and Miller (1995)[35] take the idea of spiritual health and follow it to its logical conclusion. They suggest that the physical changes and decline in function associated with aging may be necessary to ensure an optimally lived life. They make the case that aging is the natural culmination of life and the physical decline is not a mistake. They note, as does Hayflick (1994)[57], that change and dissolution are inherent to the process of life. To them the physical changes can be seen as necessary preparation for increased emotional and spiritual growth.

Inherent in their view is the idea that it is only when individuals fully embrace their mortality that the true potential of the human being emerges. Instead of running from the changes that aging brings they suggest accepting the opportunity that emerges. They suggest that 'eldering' may be a good term for someone who embraces the end of life with the same courage and passion as the beginning. An elder then is someone who is successfully negotiating the psychosocial stages that Erikson has postulated.

The authors reinterpret Freud's theory where he posits there are two primordial drives which energize human experience. Freud named them thanatos, the death urge, and libido, the life urge. In Freud's conception life is a ceaseless struggle between these two forces. Libido is the force that causes people to search for pleasure and delight in new experience. It is what makes youth such a passionate experience. Thanatos is the force which resists change and yearns for cessation of all activity. In Freud's view thanatos ultimately wins out over libido as everyone is destined to die.

Thanatos and libido

Schachter-Shalomi and Miller suggest that we live in a culture obsessed with the power of libido and terrified by the power of thanatos. During youth libido is in its ascendancy. People crave movement and excitement and have a need to leave their mark on the world. However, as life progresses the force of thanatos begins to assert itself. At first its stirrings are muted. People experience more of a desire for quiet, they want less stimulation and their energy levels often become diminished. In a culture not terrified of death or thanatos, these changes could be seen as life's call to engage in greater contemplation and maybe less action. It might also be seen as the call to replace quantity of experience with quality of experience. Finally, it could be seen as a inner prompting to begin the formal practice of meditation. Meditative practices are designed to help people achieve focused attention whose goal is greater appreciation and acceptance of their moment to moment experience[58].

If an elder were to heed the call of thanatos and deeply contemplate the inevitable changes aging causes, it might free their remaining libido power to be used in the service of generativity and mentoring as Erikson has suggested. When an elder actually accepts their diminishing physical power and inevitable death, what is more appropriate than doing a small part to help something outside of themselves which may survive their demise? If mortality were embraced, and accepted as normal what would be more important than making peace with the way life is? If the striving for everlasting personal physical existence, in a physical world which does not grant immortality, were seen as a form of insanity, then the later stages of physical life might take on a whole new meaning. Insanity in this context means, to paraphrase Albert Einstein, the folly of doing the same thing over and over and expecting the result to be different.

The argument that aging might have a spiritual purpose in no way diminishes the important work involved in successful aging. Lifestyle decisions are critical and affect both mortality and morbidity. Since a good percentage of elderly people suffer minimal functional decline it is imperative that physicians become aware of the lifestyle factors that give the elderly the greatest chance of maximizing their lives. After all, it is easier to contemplate life's mysteries when one is in good health than in pain or disabled. There are many mind–body approaches to pain control and physical disability and that in fact is one of the benefits of mind–body medicine[58]. What is clear is that a physician will treat elderly patients differently depending on how each views the purpose and possibilities inherent in aging.

The sick role and the dying role

In the first place, as Eisner and Osmond (1996)[59] suggest, in our death denying culture we need to understand the difference between the sick role and the dying role. Parsons (1951)[60] has elucidated the four components which make up the role of a sick person that appear to be consistent in many cultures: (1) the sick person is allowed to skip some or all normal responsibilities; (2) the illness is not the fault of the sick person; (3) the sick person wants to get well as soon as possible; (4) the sick person will seek aid and cooperate with the helper. In the sick role all possible means are taken to achieve health and the patient's personal, family and cultural resources are coordinated to help restore health. The dying role is more difficult to define exactly because different people have different expectations. From the author's point of view, when handled appropriately the dying role is characterized by an acceptance of the end of physical life and concomitant concentration on quality of life, care and pain management.

Parsons states that there are usually three methods by which a patient can leave the domain of the sick role: (1) by becoming well; (2) by becoming disabled; (3) by entering into the role of a dying person. Eisner and Osmond state that the transition from sick person to dying person is currently a difficult one. Sometimes, because of the need to protect themselves from malpractice claims, physicians continue to aggressively treat and assess people who are clearly ready for the dying role. More commonly, the boundaries between the sick and dying role are unclear and often remain so until the end of life.

The authors acknowledge the 'medical-legal warfare that assigns primary importance to life and staying alive'[59]. This emphasis on remaining alive at all costs can make the transition from sick person to dying person difficult if not impossible. Clearly the two are different stages of life and require different approaches to management. If the stage of dying is handled as simply a continuation of being sick then appropriate care may not be given. Clearly, one of the ways that physicians could assist in this transition from sick person to dying person is to use a variation of the models presented above of successful aging and eldering.

When an elderly patient is sick and has a reasonable hope for recovery then the goal of treatment is to provide optimal care so that whatever libido power remains may be harnessed. An optimal intervention prepares the elderly person to remain as physically successful as possible. When the possibility of resurrection of physical power is minimal or nil then the appropriate care honors the power of thanatos and helps the patient to surrender their libido. Making peace with one's family, coming to terms with past failures, and impending death, and the management of pain could then become the medical standard of care. This is not a radical idea and is practiced in hospices. However, the distinction between a sick patient and a dying patient is one that is useful to accentuate. It is one that is useful to share with the family of the patient as well. When incorporated with acceptance that the innate process which leads to death is a normal one, spiritual health may emerge and lessen the burden on all involved.

PATIENTS MENTOR THE DOCTOR

One further way that a physician may assist the elderly patient is to allow the elder to mentor the physician. If handled properly this can help heal both doctor and patient. Fostering mentoring by the physician acknowledges that both patient and doctor are on different points on the same road called life and that each has something to offer the other. While it is eminently clear what the physician has to give to the patient it may be less clear what a sick and elderly person may offer a physically healthy doctor.

If the elderly are understood to have navigated more of life's journey than their younger counterparts, and that their experience often leads to greater learning of life's lessons, then a physician always has something to hear about where the journey leads. And if the summative experiences of life are to integrate contemplative and mentoring experiences with personal accomplishment, then what better opportunity to begin than by the physician who deals daily with life, death and illness. Besides offering an incredible kindness to the elderly patient, which must not be minimized, listening and offering to be taught may allow the physician to personally gain from the interaction. It is possible that allowing the elder to help the physician in this way could minimize some of the strain inherent in medical practice and minimize some of the reasons for burnout.

As Dr Remen says[61]:

> One of the reasons that many physicians feel drained by their work is that they do not know how

to make an opening to receive anything from their patients. The way we were trained, receiving is considered unprofessional. The way most of us were raised, receiving is considered a weakness.

The irony is that for each one of us it is simply a matter of time before we confront the inevitable diminishment of our physical abilities and mortality. The question is not if this will happen but when. While a significant number of elderly people will not suffer disability, everyone at some point has diminished function or dies. The effect of this aging process on the mind and body of each person is both similar and unique. Regardless how it occurs, it will happen to us all. Since physicians see the myriad of physical changes as a regular part of their jobs what better gift can they give both themselves and their elderly patients but their attention, understanding and compassion. In effect they are offering these qualities to themselves because we are all just time away from becoming elderly.

MIND–BODY MEDICINE

The final trait the physician interested in mind–body care is asked to entertain is an openness to the research which suggests that specific mind–body techniques such as meditation and martial arts have disease-fighting effects. Mind–body techniques have been defined as 'an approach that sees the mind, our thoughts and emotions, as having a central impact on the body's health'[62]. This leads by implication to the tenet that for a physician it is advisable to treat the whole person and not just the physical body. Another tenet is that people should be supported in becoming active participants in their own health care and may be able to shorten the course of disease or prevent it outright by the management of their psychological states.

Inherent in the practice of mind–body medicine is the idea of prevention which forms a crucial component of the patient assuming a role in his or her own health. Physicians can aid in this process of prevention by encouraging and supporting alternative forms of treatment such as imagery, meditation and martial arts. Today many physicians recommend dietary and exercise regimens to patients as both prevention and treatment modalities. This is certainly a step in the right direction but still misses the psychosocial aspects of activities a patient can do for him/herself. And for elderly people they have their own specific contraindications for certain treatment recommendations.

First, recommending exercise to elderly patients can be problematic. Some patients may have some form of heart disease which restricts them from rigorous forms of exercise. Walking, which may benefit some people, may be threatening to elderly people who don't live in neighborhoods which are conducive to walking. Some patients may be resistant to changes in diet or have no-one to prepare their meals. Or, patients may make changes in diet and exercise and still continue to come to the doctor complaining of symptoms which may be better treated by focusing on the mind and body. The need still exists for treatment which specifically addresses the direct emotional and psychological experience of the elderly patient.

Scientific studies and reviews of such mind–body techniques as relaxation, social support, imagery, visualization, meditation, yoga and qigong, to name a few, are currently taking place in the USA at major research universities under the direction of the Office of Alternative Medicine at the National Institute of Health. This chapter arises in part from a review whose charter is to examine the effectiveness of mind–body therapies on aging.

Qigong

One mind–body approach, used widely in China for its 'anti-aging' effect, is a practice from traditional Chinese medicine called qigong. Qigong is an exercise practice which combines meditation, body movement and breathing exercises with the goal of unblocking, or making more fluid, one's internal *chi*, or vital energy force. This force has no direct physiological correlate, but is a prime tenet of most forms of Eastern medicine. The body is viewed as a series of energy conduits and when a person is ill the energy balance is considered to be altered. The practice of qigong is designed to be both preventative and restorative[63].

Some of the anti-aging effects claimed by qigong practitioners are reduced hypertension, reduced incidence of stroke and mortality, better heart functioning, increased bone density, sex hormone level changes, and increased blood flow to the brain. A multitude of studies on hypertension by Wang (1993)[64] at the Shanghai Institute have demonstrated these results by instructing patients to practice qigong for 30 minutes twice a day. Qigong may be an ideal adjunct or even alternative approach for hypertension in elderly patients as there are no side effects reported[65].

Yoga, relaxation and meditation

Another study evaluated a yoga-based regimen for treatment of osteoarthritis (OA) of the hands. (Garfinkel et al, 1994)[66] randomly assigned groups of OA sufferers to a yoga group and a control group receiving no therapy. The yoga program was effective in providing significantly more relief with less pain and tenderness, and increased strength, motion, and hand function. Although this program was not compared with another type of therapy, the significant results still present an alternative for traditional medical treatment of arthritis which can be costly and inconvenient. The other advantage to yoga therapy is the self-efficacy which develops from managing one's health through one's own means.

One of the psychosocial hazards of aging, loneliness, has been examined in conjunction with stress in one Ohio State University study discussed in *The Alternative Health Medicine Encyclopedia*[67]. Thirty residents from a retirement home were divided into three groups. One received relaxation training three times per week, one received individual 'social contact' three times per week, and one had no contact with researchers. Those who received relaxation training and social contact had increases in white blood cell levels while those with no contact had decreased levels and showed the least resistance to herpes virus infections.

Another interesting study showed that nursing home residents, average age 81, who learned transcendental meditation (TM) performed better on many measures of learning and mental health than did subjects in two different kinds of control groups. The experimental group had as controls a group receiving relaxation training and another receiving no treatment. Interestingly, after 3 years all of the meditators were still alive, while only 63% of the control group was still alive[68].

Meditation training can be helpful in more ways than just boosting the immune system or improving mental functioning. Meditation techniques have been shown to decrease blood pressure, lower heart rate, and reduce O_2 consumption. Other effects are an increase in alpha waves on the EEG and an increased synchronization of different cortical areas. Also meditation has been shown to positively effect changes in anxiety, depression and many other symptoms common among the elderly[69].

A study on TM practice and its relationship to aging conducted by Wallace et al. (1982)[70] compared groups of TM practitioners. By measuring biological age (which includes measurements of hearing, vision and blood pressure) in comparison with chronological age, TM practitioners were found to have significantly lower biological age, up to 12 years, as compared with chronological age. This effect was dose specific and was directly related to how long a person had been a practitioner of TM. This study suggests biological functioning, presumably related to aging, can be affected by the practice of TM. TM is a simple technique that can be utilized with minimal cost or risk.

Mind–body techniques may forestall some of the deterioration of function associated with age. As we have referenced, studies on mind–body interventions are beginning to demonstrate effective ways to prevent and treat such common conditions as arthritis and hypertension. These two conditions are statistically the two most common found in elderly patients.

They are also the greatest causes of disability in the elderly. Therefore, recommending a martial arts or yoga or meditation practice to elderly patients can allow the patient to benefit in both body and mind. Another benefit is the increase in self-efficacy that occurs when patients can manage their own diseases[71]. Finally, many of these practices help patients connect to the spiritual dimensions of existence which we have shown are often of critical importance to the elderly.

SUMMARY

Some fundamental qualities inherent in a physician practicing mind–body medicine have been explored in this chapter. Evidence from the literature has been presented which affirms the value of this type of treatment approach with elderly patients. Evidence has also been presented showing the efficacy of specific mind–body interventions in the facilitation of healing in elderly populations. Research clearly demonstrates the effect of psychosocial variables on the course of disease.

Not covered directly, and difficult to measure, may be the subjective response of individual elderly patients who are in need of care while they are sitting in the offices or on the phone with their physician. The basic question in medicine remains: How can I help my patient? Surveys have shown that patients are often dissatisfied with their care, particularly in hospitals[1]. Listening, introduced at the beginning of this chapter, may not only be a quality necessary in the promotion of the healing process, but an integral part in the understanding of what constitutes effective care.

The mind–body practices and principles discussed in this chapter are by no means the only practices which have been shown to be efficacious with elderly populations. There are many mind–body techniques discussed in the literature which we have not touched upon. There also exist many techniques which have been evaluated as effective by subjective means but have not been scientifically studied with randomized, controlled trials. With our ever-growing elderly population and their unique and often more compelling need for health care, physicians are advised to arm themselves with information that will enable them to serve this population which may make up the majority of the patient pool in the next 20–30 years.

The qualities discussed in this chapter are important and valuable components of a mind–body approach to elderly care. However, true human connection and healing is much more complex than what we have covered and does not end with what has been discussed. This chapter suggests to physicians some starting points, a necessary packet of tools with which to work more effectively within the healing process. We hope physicians interested in the mind–body interaction will continue to evolve in their ability to help heal their patients' minds and bodies by continuing their own personal growth both as a physician/healer and as an individual.

CONCLUSION

Everything that this chapter has to offer can be summarized by the following statement: As a physician working with an elderly patient it is critical to remember that there are two individuals with two separate minds, bodies and spirits which must join forces to create the optimal healing environment.

Acknowledgement

The preparation of this chapter was supported in part from a grant from the Office of Alternative Medicine, National Institute of Health (Grant # AG 43558).

REFERENCES

1 Moyers B 1993 Healing and the mind. Doubleday, New York

2 AARP 1995 A profile of older Americans. AARP Program Resources, Washington DC

3 National Institute on Aging 1994 Hearts and arteries: what scientists are learning about age and the cardiovascular system. US Department of Health and Human Services, Washington DC

4 Beckman HB 1984 The effect of physician behavior on the collection of data. Annals of Internal Medicine Nov:692–6

5 The SUPPORT Principal Investigators 1995 A controlled trial to improve care for seriously ill hospitalized patients. Journal of the American Medical Association 274(20):1591–8

6 Dossey L 1991 Meaning and medicine: a doctor's tales of breakthrough and healing. Bantam, New York

7 Ornstein R, Sobel D 1987 The healing brain. Simon and Schuster, New York

8 Achterberg J, Lawlis GF 1984 Imagery and disease: diagnostic tools? Institute for Personality and Ability Testing, Champaign, Ill

9 Hafen BQ, Karren KJ, Frandsen KJ, Smith NL 1996 Mind-body health: the effect of attitudes, emotions and relationships. Allyn and Bacon, Needham Hights, Mass

10 Amick TL, Ockene JK 1994 The role of social support in the modification of risk factors for cardiovascular disease. In: Shumaker SA, Czajkowski SM (eds) Social support and cardiovascular disease. Plenum, New York

11 Seeman TE, Kaplan GA, Knudsen L, Cohen R, Guralnk J 1987 Social network ties and mortality among the elderly in the Alameda County Study. American Journal of Epidemiology 126(4):714–23

12 Depner CE, Ingersoll-Dayton B 1988 Supportive relationships in later life. Psychology and Aging 3(4):348–57

13 Dreher H 1993 Why did the people of Roseto live so long? Natural Health 23(5):72–9, 130–1

14 Pilisuk M, Parks S 1986 The healing web. The University Press of New England, Hanover, NH

15 Pennebaker JW 1990 Opening up: the healing power of confiding in others. William Morrow, New York

16 Bandura A 1994 Self-efficacy: the exercise of control. International Universities Press, New York

17 Cummings NA, VandenBos GR 1981 The twenty years Kaiser Permanente experience with psychotherapy and medical utilization: implications for national heath policy and national insurance. Health Policy Quarterly 1:59–75

18 Kroenke K, Mangelsdorff D 1989 Common symptoms in ambulatory care: incidence, evaluation, therapy, and outcome. American Journal of Medicine 86:262–6

19 Uchino BN, Cacioppo JT, Kiecolt-Glaser JK 1996 The relationship between social support and physiological processes: a review with emphasis on underlying mechanisms and implications for health. Psychological Bulletin 119(3):488–531

20 Justice B 1988 Who gets sick: thinking and health. JP Tarcher, Los Angeles

21 Arnetz BB, Thorell T, Levi L, Kallner A, Eneroth P 1983 An experimental study of social isolation of elderly people: psychoendocrine and metabolic effects. Psychosomatic Medicine 45:395–406

22 Dossey L 1993 Healing words: the power of prayer and the practice of medicine. Harper Collins, New York

23 Uhlenhuth EH, Cantor A, Neustadt JO, Payson HE 1959 The symptomatic relief of anxiety with meprobamate, Phenobarbital and the placebo. American Journal of Psychiatry 115:905–10

24 Uhlenhuth EH, Rickels K, Fisher S, Park LC, Lipman RS, Mock J 1966 Drug, doctor's verbal attitude and clinical setting in the symptomatic response to pharmacotherapy. Psychopharmacologia 9:392–418

25 Toone WM 1973 Effects of vitamin E: good and bad. New England Journal of Medicine, 289:689–98

26 Benson H, Friedman R 1996 Harnessing the power of the placebo effect and renaming it 'remembered wellness'. Annual Review of Medicine 47:193–99

27 Hunt M 1991 Faith, hope and placebos. Longevity May:68–74

28 Benson H, Epstein M 1975 The placebo effect: a neglected asset in the care of patients. Journal of the American Medical Association 232:1225–7

29 Benson H, Starg M 1996 Timeless healing: the power and biology of belief. Scribner, New York

30 Archer TP, Leier CV 1992 Placebo treatment in congestive heart failure. Cardiology 81:125–33

31 Mumford E, Schlesinger G, Glass V, Patrick C, Cuerdon T 1984 A new look at evidence about reduced cost of medical utilization after mental health treatment. American Journal of Psychiatry 141:1145–58

32 Strain JJ, Lyons JS et al. 1991 Cost offset from a psychiatric consultation liaison intervention with elderly hip fracture patients. American Journal of Psychiatry 148:1044–9

33 Kamen-Siegel L, Rodin J, Seligman MEP, Dwyer J 1991 Explanatory style and cell-mediated immunity in elderly men and women. Health Psychology 10(4):229–35

34 Ranard A 1989 The world through rose colored glasses. Health 8:58

35 Schachter-Shalomi Z, Miller RS 1995 From age-ing to sage-ing: A profound new vision of growing older. Warner Books, New York

36 Wetle T 1987 Age as a risk factor for inadequate treatment. Journal of the American Medical Association 258:516

37 Knaus WA, Legall JR, Wagner DP 1982 A comparison of intensive care in the USA and France. Lancet 2:642

38 Westlie L, Umen A, Nestrud S et al. 1984 Morality, morbidity and life satisfaction in the very old dialysis patient. American Society Artificial Internal Organs 30:21–30

39 Bortz WM 1989 Redefining human aging. Journal of the American Geriatrics Society 37: 1092–6

40 Lindeman R, Tobin J, Shock N 1985 Longitudinal studies in the rate of decline of renal function with age.

Journal of the American Geriatric Society 33:278–85

41 Waldron I et al. 1982 Cross-cultural variation in blood pressure. Social Science Medicine 16:419–30

42 Rowe JW, Kahn RL 1987 Human aging: usual and successful. Science 237:143–9

43 Schaie KW, Willis SL 1986 Can decline in adult intellectual functioning be reversed? Developmental Psychology 22:223–32

44 Green RF 1969 Age-intelligence relationship between ages sixteen and sixty-four: a rising trend. Developmental Psychology 1:618–27

45 Schaie KW, Labouvie-Vief 1974 Generational versus ontogenetic components of change in adult cognitive behavior: a fourteen-year cross-sequential study. Developmental Psychology 10: 305–20

46 Erikson E, Erikson J, Kivnick H 1986 Vital involvement in old age. Norton, New York

47 Jung CG 1965 Memories, dreams, reflections. Vintage Books, New York

48 Maugans TA, Wadland WC 1991 Religion and family medicine: a survey of physicians and patients. Journal of Family Practice 39(4):349–52

49 Matthews DA, Larson DB 1995 The faith factor: an annotated bibliography of clinical research on spiritual subjects. Volume III. National Institute for Healthcare Research, Washington, DC

50 Sagan LA 1987 The health of nations. Basic Books, New York Resources, Washington, DC

51 Reed PG 1987 Spirituality and well-being in terminally ill hospitalized adults. Research in Nursing and Health 10:335–44

52 Koenig HG, Moberg DO, Kvale JN 1988 Religious activity and attitudes of older adults in a geriatric assessment clinic. Journal of the American Geriatric Society 36(4):362–74

53 Idler EL, Kasl SV 1992 Religion, disability, depression and the timing of death. American Journal of Sociology 97(4):1052–79

54 Zuckerman DM, Kasl SV, Ostfeld AM 1984 Psychosocial predictors of mortality among the elderly poor. American Journal of Epidemiology 119:410–23

55 Aldridge D 1993 Is there evidence for spiritual healing? Advances 9(4):4–19

56 Byrd RC 1988 Positive therapeutic effects of intercessory prayer in a coronary care unit population. Southern Medical Journal 81(7):826–9

57 Hayflick L 1994 How and why we age. Ballentine, New York

58 Kabat-Zinn J 1990 Full catastrophe living. Delta, New York

59 Eisner BG, Osmond H 1996 The sick role vs. the dying role. Advances 12(2):67–70

60 Parsons T 1951 The social system. The Free Press, Glencoe, Ill

61 Remen RN 1996 Stories to heal by. New Age 13(4):78–81, 145–51

62 Goleman D, Gurin J 1993 What is mind-body medicine? In: Goleman D, Gurin J (eds) Mind-body medicine: How to use your mind for better health. Consumer Reports, New York

63 Eisenberg D 1985 Encounters with Qi. Norton, New York

64 Wang C et al. 1993 Effects of qiqong training on preventing stroke and alleviating the multiple cerebrocardiovascular risk factors- A follow-up report on 242 hypertensive cases over 30 years. Proceedings, Second World Conference for Academic Exchange on Medical Qiqong, Beijing, China

65 Sancier KM 1996 Anti-aging benefits of qigong. Journal of International Society of Life Information Sciences 14(1):12–21

66 Garfinkel MS, Schumacher HR et al. 1994 Evaluation of a yoga based regimen for treatment of osteoarthritis of the hands. Journal of Rheumatology 21:2341–3

67 Marti JE 1995 The alternative health medicine encyclopedia. Visible Ink Press, Detroit, MI pp 299–314

68 Alexander C et al. 1991 Growth of higher stages of consciousness. In: Alexander C, Langer E (eds) Higher stages of human development. Oxford University Press, New York

69 Walsh R 1993 Meditation research: the state of the art. In: Walsh R, Vaughan F (eds) Paths beyond ego: the transpersonal vision. Putnam, New York

70 Wallace RK, Dillbeck M et al. 1982 The effects of transcendental meditation and TM-Sidhi program on the aging process. International Journal of Neuroscience 16:51–3

71 Lorig K, Morzzonson PD, Holman HR 1993 Evidence suggesting that health education for self-management in patients with chronic arthritis has sustained health benefits while reducing health care costs. Arthritis and Rheumatism 36(4):439–46

CHAPTER CONTENTS

14

Self-care: Stress and the practitioner

David Peters

INTRODUCTION

A new arrival in Heaven, strolling near the pearly gates, spotted a white-coated figure wearing a head-mirror who was clearly rushing off, black case in hand and stethoscope flailing at his neck, on some urgent mission. Curious to know who the important and preoccupied figure might be, he asked a nearby angel who said 'Oh that's just God, sometimes He likes to play doctor.'

If doctors have fantasies of being more than human, it is a triumph of hope over experience that patients believe it too. Despite patients' traditional projections, doctors are not a special case. In fact they are particularly at risk; doctors' mental health is poorer, and their suicide rates, levels of alcoholism, and drug abuse higher than any other profession's. Long before Drs Faust and Jekyll stalked our imagination, 'impaired physicians' were with us, yet they have only been a cause for organized concern in last 20 years. Similarly, the impact of the stresses and strains of medical education and everyday practice has only very recently been recognized. As the century ends, it is clear not only that the conceptual high ground of late modern medicine is in difficulty, but that many of its practitioners are too. If the two problems are related, mind–body medicine may represent an emerging theoretical and practical way forward for a stressed profession and its increasingly strained biomedical model.

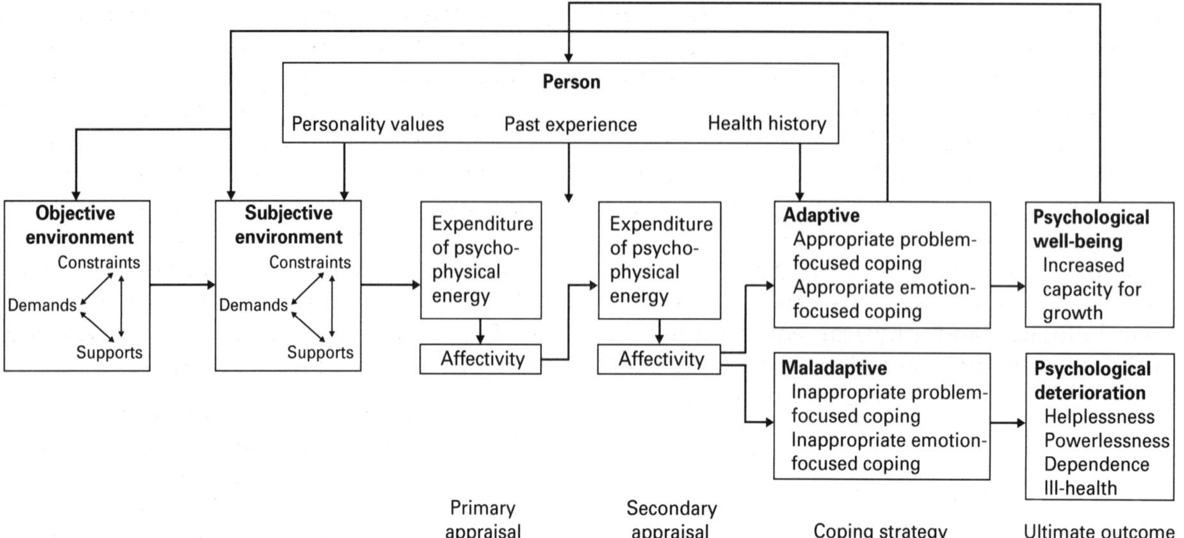

Figure 14.1 A stress-strain coping framework. Reprinted by permission of J Wiley and Sons.

ADAPTATION TO STRESS

The language of 'stress' derives from the world of engineering. Comparing the person to a bar of metal under strain, it depicts outside forces changing and reshaping us; implying that like metal, a person will either bend or break, according to 'what he is made of'. But people are not just malleable inanimate material, and the stress metaphor implies a capacity to adapt. So whether a person facing 'crack-up', breaks-through or breaks-down, depends on what limits and what facilitates adaptation. Payne and Firth-Cozens' excellent summary of the problems health professionals face[1] uses a model that clarifies how the factors involved interact, the Supports Constraints Model (Fig. 14.1).

This basic model of the stress process takes into account that how individuals respond to stressors depends on their susceptibility and resilience, and how well they are supported by buffering factors or constrained by factors that limit adaptation.

The factors constraining or supporting adaptation might be physical, cognitive, emotional or social and organizational; obvious examples are the need for rest or respite, insight, and personal support. If there are excessive constraints or inadequate support for adaptation, then meeting life's demands will be at the expense of any reserve capacity, and coping will become increasingly difficult. Withdrawal from the predicament would be a sensible option then, but circumstance, beliefs, or attitudes often mean a person continues to struggle on despite increasingly poor performance (Fig. 14.2).

In this supply and demand model, the currency is the mental and physical energy needed for adaptation. A stress-free existence is not the aim though, for people have an innate

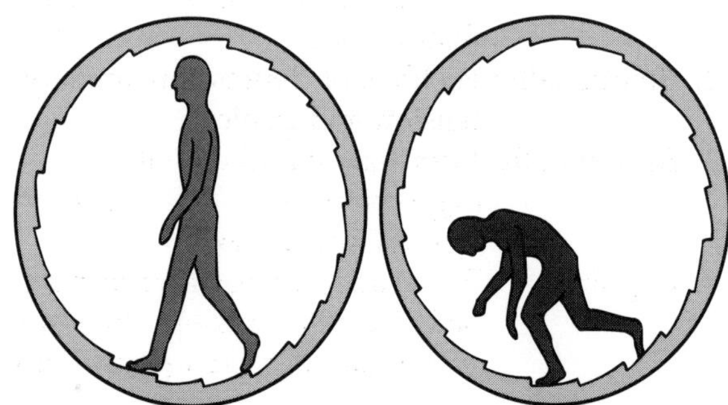

Figure 14.2 The treadwheel is a useful image for considering the factors which determine the ability to cope with heavy effort over long periods of time, and the consequences of success or failure.

need to learn and grow, and humans are challenge-seeking creatures; evolution and psychodynamics have made it so. Human development unfolds as we learn to deal with inevitable and potentially traumatic hurdles in infancy and childhood. Because the human condition is such a rich source of predicaments, living is stressful, and demands will out-strip resources from time to time. The process of adaptation continually disturbs and restores psychological and physical equilibrium. But this capacity for restoration is not unlimited; some tasks or predicaments are impossible. The available inner or outer resources can be inappropriate or inadequate and constraints too powerful. People differ in their reserves of coping capacity and ways of responding to pressure and levels of tolerance. Moreover some survival strategies eventually undermine coping.

THE EFFECTS OF STRESS

The concept of 'stress-related symptoms' relates certain functional disturbances — physical, mental-emotional, behavioral — to the strain of adaptation. Diverse as the warning signals can be, certain patterns are common. Managing stress effectively, means recognizing the warning signs, and dealing with their cause; ideally at an early stage.

The strain of adaptation ('stress') typically affects a person in four ways:

1. Physically: pain, digestive disorders, cardiovascular instability, sleep disturbance.
2. Emotionally: Feelings of depression, anxiety, tension and panic.
3. Behaviorally: Withdrawal and denial, aggression, substance abuse of alcohol and drugs.
4. Cognitively: Poor concentration and memory, bad decision making, poor reasoning and mistaken perceptions.

Burn-out

One description of the how stress affects health professionals and their care of patients involves the idea of 'burn-out'. Defined as 'a loss of concern about the people for whom one is working, in response to job related stress'[2], it has four identifiable stages: the scene is set by idealistic enthusiasm; this is followed by stagnation and disappointment when expectations about one's work are not met; then comes frustration as one's own needs and one's patients' needs are no longer satisfied; finally apathy sets in. The personal consequences of 'burn-out' follow a predictable route:

1. **Personal resources and work demands become imbalanced:** longer working hours, little time with family, hurried meals, frequent minor illnesses, sleep disturbance.
2. **Short-term response to stress:** angry outbursts, tired all the time, irritability, anxiety about physical health.
3. **Terminal burn-out:** balance between demands and personal resources cannot be re-established, deals with people and tasks mechanically, by the book, late for appointments, derogatory about patients, uses superficial stereotypes, communication is authoritarian.

Although the notion of 'burn-out' arose from nursing studies, it obviously applies to doctors as well: their occupational demands and expectations are high, and how they cope will influence their approach to patient care. Yet doctors' self-esteem and job satisfaction also depend on how well they deal with patients. So doctors' ability to cope gracefully with high demand both shapes their approach to patients, and affects how they feel about themselves.

However, medicine encourages doctors — financially and organizationally — to take on a large number of patients and to work quickly. Because the constraint of needing to work quickly tends to undermine patient care, this constraint which is a stressor in itself also tends to undermine support factors — locus of control, job satisfaction and self-esteem — all of which exert a protective effect. This is an example of how demands and responses can interact in ways that further impair the ability to cope.

The 'wounded doctor'

Although certain 'normal' pressures and conflicts are inherent, a medical life can be a good one, despite having to strike a balance between accessibility and time out, responsibility and delegation, uncertainty and medico-legal issues, vulnerability and omnipotence, expectations, needs and resources, job and home. To the outsider it might seem strange if many doctors appeared to be unhappy; the medical life looks like a perfect opportunity to do good for others, to enjoy people's gratitude, to exercise authority and be given high status while doing interesting and demanding work. As Glynn Bennett puts it in the introduction to his excellent book *The Wound and the Doctor*[3]

> Doctors are privileged people; allowances are made for them on the assumption that they live their lives poised in readiness to dash to the bedside of a sick person. They have a high status, high income, carry complete security and a pension at the end, and it is exceptional to find one unwillingly out of work. There is no other group in society which is quite so well placed in terms of opportunities of a satisfying and well-rewarded life.
>
> The private lives of doctors contrast sharply with their professional style. Some difference between the outward image and private life is to be expected, but not in an extreme degree nor in those whose job it is to maintain the health of the population. They should know what makes for a good and healthy life and how the hazards can be avoided, but doctors taken collectively compare badly with their patients when it comes to managing their private lives. So, if in return for privilege, doctors face stressful situations and demanding work, this may be the nature of the job itself. But medical decision-making and patient contact, the possibility of round-the-clock responsibility, the conflict of being doctor and neighbour in one's community, the juggling of work and home life, the one interfering with other, are not new aspects of medical life.

DOCTORS AT RISK

If a medical career can be highly demanding it is also potentially well buffered. Why then is the balance so often lost? Let us consider the question of medical stress and the possibility of enhancing protective factors, starting with the evidence that doctors are a high risk group.

If stress is unrelenting, the long-term pathological consequences associated with that stress, which we can assume to be indicators of excess demand and inappropriate adaptation, are predictable. The medical profession's pattern of stress-related disease and mortality certainly suggests there is a problem which needs attention.

A 1992 report *Stress and the Medical Profession*[4] points out that statistics on doctors' high rates of alcoholism,[5] drug abuse[6] and suicide[7] are a continuing cause for concern. Although as a relatively wealthy and high status profession, doctors have a lower mortality ratio than the population in general, certain causes of death are notably high: cirrhosis and chronic liver disease, suicide and death by drugs and other substances of abuse in particular[8] (although statistics might not be entirely reliable; the stigma of death from substance abuse or suicide may mean doctors are reluctant to certify them as the cause of a colleague's death). Male doctors in the UK are twice as likely and female doctors three times more likely to commit suicide than members of the general public, about 10 times more likely than MPs and senior civil servants, and six times more likely than university teachers and clergymen. They are also twice as prone to alcoholism compared with other members of social class I, and their wives commit suicide more often than the wives of other professional people.

Occupational factors

Various studies suggest that doctors' stress-related sickness is only the tip of an iceberg. Beneath the surface there are unseen strata of

Box 14.1 General sources of occupational stress[4]

1. Factors intrinsic to the job
2. Factors related to the organizational structure and climate
3. Factors related to career development
4. Factors related to role within the organization
5. Relationships at work.

exhaustion, boredom, poor job satisfaction and depression — in fact 'burn-out'. A 1994 survey of GPs in Aberdeen for instance, revealed that 87% felt exhausted at times, that 64% found work stressful, 50% were enduring boredom, 30% lacked work enjoyment and 11% experienced depression[9].

Occupational sources of stress, although they are inevitably intertwined with the personal and social stresses that impact on professional life and coping, are of particular concern (Box 14.1). Medical work is clearly rich in stressors intrinsic to the job: long unsociable hours, shift work, new technology, danger of injury or infection, work overload, repetition, and excessive difficult tasks mean that the practice of medicine is intrinsically fraught with high demand. However, doctors' work also has a quite unique profile of difficult and potentially conflicting tasks (Box 14.2).

Changing times

We cannot be sure whether medical strain and distress have always been such a problem; only lately has it been widely discussed and studied. Was it formerly too uncomfortable to believe that doctors have wounds and human frailties? In our culture's collective imagination, doctors have to be like good and strong parents, therefore doctor distress, like child abuse and middle-class family violence, had to be denied. But the levels of mortality and impairment have provoked public examination; and it appears that these levels are rising. In fact all studies conducted in the past 10 years indicate that the casualty rate is rising, and pressures are worse[4]. An interweaving of factors must be responsible — increased susceptibility, more trigger events and fewer buffering influences — some personal, some specifically occupational, some because of more general and cultural change.

In the late 20th Century there are more and different pressures on doctors: rising expectations, and the problems of managing increasingly technologized investigations and treatments; a substantial demographic shift; rapidly changing organizational aims and imperatives; increased uncertainty over resources and outcomes. All impose new strains, but the scene for eventual health break-down and impairment will be set by susceptibility — internal strains and conflicts, and a lack of coping skills. And it will depend on particular circumstances to set the cascade of burn-out and break-down in motion. Whether working life for instance, actually becomes damaging will be determined by the human and technical resources available, and by how well work is organized, supported and managed.

Rapid and unpredictable change is particularly stressful, and many UK doctors have found the sweeping Health Service re-organization of the early 1990s more than they could cope with. It is significant that the UK spends less of its gross domestic product on health care than in most other developed countries — 6.1% in 1987[11], for under-resourced organizations demand more of their staff and are less able to support them. The British Medical Association (BMA) has this to say about the UK's National Health Service (NHS) as an employer:

Box 14.2 A consensus on stressful aspects of doctoring[10]

- Face to face contact with patients, colleagues and superiors
- Dealing with death and dying
- Dealing with physical suffering and long-term disability
- Long hours and shift work
- Necessary but traumatic, invasive, intimate medical procedures
- Advances in medical technology leading to increasing moral and ethical dilemmas
- Responsibility for people rather than objects
- Self-doubts about responsibility for medical failure
- Enormous consequences of wrong decisions, threat of litigation
- Exposure to occupationally acquired illness (esp HIV, HBV), toxic chemicals and hazardous processes
- Risk of physical violence, especially in psychiatry, mental handicap and accident and emergency
- Public expectation and demand
- Renumeration differences between team members causing tension
- Interference by government and management
- Inflexible unpredictable career path, uncertainty of reaching consultant status
- Conflict between professional role and personal values/conscience
- Conflicts in loyalty to employers, colleagues and patients.

Almost three quarters of NHS expenditure is on staff, and yet the NHS has been called a terrible employer. Many staff are on low rates of pay, training may be poor and drop out rates among, for instance, nurses are high. The salary structure of most staff does not allow better pay for better performance. Some groups work absurdly long hours in often poor conditions. Career development is chaotic for some, sickness and accident rates are high and occupational health services are often non-existent[12].

Their report concludes that for many doctors in the UK, the work-culture and environment are a prodigious source of stresses which the organization does too little to alleviate. All grades are affected. On the bottom of the career ladder at the front line of health care delivery, the UK's junior hospital doctors experience severe strain. One study showed that 25–35% of pre-registration doctors (interns) were clinically depressed[13]. Junior hospital doctors work legendary hours in the UK; typically over 100 hours a week for residents. Sleep deprivation and exhaustion lead to depression and confusion, yet the amount of time junior hospital doctors spend in patient contact has, until very recently, increased year on year.

In the UK there are new NHS imperatives: health-screening and prevention in general practice; increased pressure for rapid patient turnaround in hospital practice; business practices and evidence based medicine are the new by-words; an internal market in the provision and purchasing of health technology has brought an element of competition to health care; the need to evaluate all health care activity has imposed new uncertainties.

It seems these new policies and bureaucratic working methods have caused a sharp decrease in job satisfaction. Doctors say these changes have increased their sense of being driven by forces beyond their control even at the top of the profession. One survey of consultants revealed that although 91% of respondents did not regret having taken up a career in medicine, two-thirds felt that the NHS changes would erode their job satisfaction[14]. Levels of distress rose in family practice too. GPs questioned in 1990 said all occupational stress factors were more difficult to deal with than 3 years before, and this study by Cooper and Sutherland also found rising levels of mental illness among doctors[10]. In a 1990 survey of GPs in Sheffield UK, more than half were thinking seriously about alternative employment, and most found life more stressful than before the NHS re-organization[15]. A 1996 survey conducted for the British Medical Association's *News Review* confirms this depressing picture (Box 14.3)[16].

Box 14.3 Stress in UK General Practice 1996: key findings

- 88% of GPs say doctors have more stressful lives than 5 years ago
- 68% believe a stress counseling service for doctors would be welcomed
- 69% have suffered from stress-related problems

Of those reporting stress-related problems:

- 91% say their stress was caused by work pressures
- 70% believe that stress adversely affected their work
- 35% say stress caused them to increase their alcohol consumption
- 4% say stress led to drug misuse
- 21% say stress caused them to contemplate suicide.

Staff wastage

As the medical task becomes more challenging, and resources more limited, then we can predict the consequences: more stress-related illness, practitioner impairment and staff wastage. The signs are clear enough; one disturbing figure reveals that 40% of female doctors and 10% of male doctors leave the profession within the first 5 years of qualification[5]. Training a medical student in the UK costs the state around £80 000, so the wastage of some 25% of qualified personnel from the system is an enormous loss. Many women doctors leave to start families, but many do not return; the medical career structure and culture were not evolved by men and women who wanted to spend more time with their family rather than in practice. Even in family medicine being a part-timer is far from an easy option.

Though more rigorously managed medical

services and an efficient 'evidence based' market in health technology might in the long term improve health care, in the short term the injection of a business ethic and the commodification of medicine has adversely affected morale. It remains to be seen whether 'managed care' will have a negative impact on this and other important facets of human resource management. However, if doctors continue to feel the health care agenda is moving out of their hands it is predictable that job-related stress and staff wastage will become even more prevalent.

Are there solutions to the impending crisis?

The huge loss of qualified personnel alone calls for urgent preventive measures, but the deteriorating health of doctors has more far-reaching effects. The Nuffield Provincial Hospitals Trust published a succinct summary of the problem of sick doctors in 1995[17]. Their report — much referred to in this chapter — is a far reaching critique of the underlying problems. It promotes the case for better occupational health services for doctors and it outlines the organizational and educational reforms needed, to prevent damage.

> The work of the doctor means that the person who practices medicine is specially placed. She/he is a high cost resource whose practice by its nature is bound by an ethic to do no harm. When the health of a doctor is impaired, it must not be allowed to impede that practice. She/he must be recognized as not only subject to the same rights of employment as any other health care worker but also as entitled to them. To ensure that patients continue to receive safe and effective medical care and that doctors receive proper health care for themselves, it is essential that steps are taken to improve the supports available to them[17].

Organizational change is another important prescription, as a recent leader in the *British Medical Journal* reiterated:

> The current crisis in recruitment and retention in medicine adds to the urgent humanitarian need to provide help for sick doctors. Equally important are the unquantified effects of doctors' stress on care of patients ... But the real question remains. If the job is making doctors sick, why not fix the job rather than the doctors?[18]

Prevention is better than cure. Relaxation techniques, holidays and training in stress management, though necessary first aid for relief from personal stress, could only partially protect doctors from truly unrealistic work demands. The authors of one key text point out that adequate resources and good management protect well-being in a more general way than individual psychodynamics and coping skills[1]. No such political and organizational revolution is in the offing though; in fact it may be that health care delivery will run into even more difficulties; for the way it is conceptualized, the national policies affecting its financial base and how organizations manage it will all continue to change rapidly. Throughout the Northern world, resources are likely to remain constrained, and concepts such as 'managed care' will present doctors with difficult and unfamiliar choices.

STRESS MANAGEMENT

For the forseeable future, individual psychological factors and individual coping skills training are likely to exert a more positive influence than any longed for improvement in health care resources. Nonetheless, damage limitation will also depend on available staff support programs and improved occupational health services.

In the face of doctors' stress-related casualty figures, implementing individual or group approaches to stress management could seem like rearranging the deck chairs on a sinking Titanic. But there are successful examples of stress management programs in both undergraduate and postgraduate training[13], and they could be incorporated more widely. These programs usually comprise a short series of brief, focused small group sessions aimed at sensitizing participants to behavioral and cognitive signals of stress; to their own susceptibility profiles; the relevance of lifestyle buffers (e.g. diet and exercise); training in the practice of simple coping strategies and techniques for relaxation. These simple mind–body interventions deserve to find a place at every level, from pre-clinical training to advanced postgraduate practice. Their rationale is outlined in a later section, but before exploring approaches to individual self-care we will consider some organizational responses to the problem of doctors and stress.

ORGANIZATIONAL SOLUTIONS

The challenge of difficult work is partly what attracts people into medicine. No doubt doctors put a lot of pressure on themselves. So if we accept the general thesis that some uncertainty, intensity, and ambiguity is inevitable, then how should medical education change so as to prepare medics more appropriately? Are there models of good practice we can look towards? One interpretation of medical 'busy-ness' sees it as an individual and organizational defense against the difficult humanistic issues implicit in doctors' day to day contact with patients. This may be the seed of an omnipotence which pervades the biotechnical medical philosophy. Will a post-biomedical theory be required to re-humanize medical practice? Some hidden agendas are explored at the end of the chapter.

Reforming undergraduate education

Everyone has an Achilles heel. Whether a doctor is protected from it will depend on circumstances and also on the presence of elements that provide resilience. It is not pre-determined that some doctors are going to become impaired. It has been suggested that candidates who might not handle stress ought not to go into medicine. However it is the more empathic students, and those bringing high expectations who are more vulnerable to the pressures and constraints of practice[19]. Should they be deselected? Empathy is important in medical practice and patients value it highly; high standards drive the profession forward. How then might medical education help empathic students harness their sensitivity? Bennett argues that doctors who feel more comfortable with their own vulnerability are better able to help patients, and captures this paradox in his notion of the 'wounded healer'. He reminds doctors that they are surrounded by vulnerability, limitation and dependency, and if they deny these elements of the human condition in their own make-up, they will find it difficult to accept them in their patients. Medical education in its present form, along with the rigors of practice, probably selects out more empathic doctors or forces them to adjust by losing their sensitivity or by lowering their standards.

Recall too that the quality of idealistic enthusiasm coupled with unrealistic expectations sets the scene for 'burn-out'. Despite this, realistic limits to therapeutic ambition and the importance of acknowledging limits to medicine are topics seldom tackled in the undergraduate (or postgraduate) curriculum. Furthermore, medical training makes it difficult for students to show weakness. Students are aware of doctors' high public esteem when they begin medical training, and of the very high expectations that go with it. They see their seniors enjoying their status and they emulate them, by working long hours without asking for help or support from their seniors, by denying feelings, and by learning to to be less than curious about their own and their patients' predicaments.

New medical students have humanitarian ideals; initially curious about their patients' inner lives, they communicate better with patients in their first than in their last clinical year[20]. Medical students are aware of the strain their training imposes[5] and of their needs for help in managing them. One exemplary undergraduate program developed with this in mind is a peer-led scheme established at the University Medical School in Louisville[21]. Staffed by final year students who have themselves been through the program, it uses small group teaching and mentoring to help students grapple with ethical issues and values, communication skills, and stress management techniques. Although voluntary, it now attracts over 75% of the student intake.

The Nuffield Hospitals Trust's Report[17] suggests that medical schools should move away from emphasizing scientific knowledge and learning by rote. Problem solving, communication and interpersonal skills are more relevant, especially when first moving out into practice — which can be a time of profound disillusion and strain. Pointing out that many medical students and doctors deny themselves even elementary personal health care and often have no personal physician of their own, the report insists that medical training should develop students' self-awareness and their understanding of stress management. The observation that airing ethical issues, teaching communication skills, management training, and support groups all lead to improved standards of care, points to one way forward for medical education. But endemic influences shape an organizational culture of denial and competitiveness in medicine, and the report points out that only established practitioners can take responsibility for bringing about the necessary corporate change in this culture.

Improved occupational health services for doctors

Medical schools and hospitals have a curiously 'macho' culture, one that the media reflects in an increasingly unglamorous way. The Nuffield Report comments on this unyielding, hierarchical, elitist ethos and some of its consequences:

> These attitudes have prevailed over many decades and prevent doctors in training from learning humility. They need to be taught to accept that they can be ill and that they are allowed to be patients by understanding their own frailties ... they must address the fact that they have high personal expectations which cause the stress and that they cannot be expected to be always right or superhuman; that stress does not mean failure and to dispel the myth that careers end due to illness[17].

The care of doctors has always been erratic, and this has stifled their own notions of self-care. Generally they hide their own experiences of stress and its impact; one reason why the understanding of stress amongst doctors is so incomplete. They are reluctant and troublesome patients; slow to seek help, they often short-circuit the usual routes, and typically prescribe for themselves. A study published in 1991 revealed that the average delay in seeking treatment was almost 7 years amongst 144 doctors with drug or alcohol dependency[22]. The cynical observation that an alcoholic is a man who drinks more than his doctor, reminds us once again that doctors often ignore the kind of instructions they offer their patients: anodynes about diet, exercise, striking a balance between work and family life, and moderation with alcohol. Stereotypically workaholic, doctors tend to soldier on, even when ill.

Eight-hundred GPs were surveyed in 1996, and 70% said they had suffered stress-related problems. Most of these doctors believed their work had been adversely affected, but only 15% sought professional help, and only 17% had time off work. Thirty-five per cent said they had increased their alcohol consumption[16].

According to Professor Sidney Brandon, the Chairman of the National Sick Doctors Counselling Service in the UK[23]:

> This failure to seek proper care and advice applies to all illnesses, but when the problems are psychiatric or emotional it becomes even more marked. Insight is often lacking and even if present, the stigma is such that the doctor will go to inordinate lengths to conceal his or her difficulties. When drink or drugs are involved the fear of their removal from the Register is so great that concealment is almost inevitable.

For many years the British Medical Association has recommended an overhaul of doctors' occupational health services. Confidentiality is a central issue here, and hospital doctors are particularly reluctant to use occupational health services based in the work setting, feeling that these services are confidential in theory only. Their worries about confidentiality may actually reflect the way doctors treat confidentiality amongst themselves. Though it breaches medical confidentiality when a doctor discusses the health of one colleague with another, the boundaries do become blurred. Traditionally doctors handle this conflict by seeking help outside their area, especially where psychiatric problems or

Box 14.4 Constraining factors when doctors seek help[17]

- Uncertainty about confidentiality
- Anxiety over professional consequences
- Professional loyalty and collusion
- Medical training, failure to legitimize vulnerability
- Stigma of illness
- Underdevelopment of occupational health services
- Customary self-treatment and casual consultations
- Poor insight.

sexually transmitted diseases are involved (Box 14.4).

The Nuffield report concludes that the way medical services are provided for doctors will have to change; that a broad approach is needed, and that it should include prevention (Box 14.5). This prevention has to be more than individually focused, and organizational change is essential, so that support systems can be put in place. Ways have to be found to identify and appraise doctors in need, but without stigmatizing them. Confidentiality is crucial, and a profound change of ethos will be required if doctors are to feel safe enough to admit illness and allow themselves to get help. Changing the way doctors conceptualize health, the aims and limits of medicine, and their own role will be a part of this process. It will demand a broad ranging overhaul of medical education and organizational culture to bring this about.

Box 14.5 Nuffield Provincial Hospitals Trust's Report: summary of recommendations[17]

- Better access to medical services for all doctors with more certainty of confidentiality.
- Support for hospital residents and an inspection system to see that posts and workloads are appropriate.
- Greater emphasis in medical education on humanistic aspects; communication and interpersonal skills.
- Training should help students deal with the emotional impact of medical practice.
- The identification of personal stress — elements widely ignored and consequently marginalized in medical culture — which harm doctors and patients.
- A change in attitude that allows a pastoral structure to develop at all levels of medical education, post-graduate as well as undergraduate.
- Problems should be routinely reviewed and appraised by a formal mechanism.
- Senior hospital doctors should be trained in management skills to ensure this happens.

INDIVIDUAL SOLUTIONS

Doctors' stresses and their sources are obviously wide ranging, and dealing with them demands organizational and cultural change to underpin individual efforts at improving coping and resilience. But what might doctors themselves actually do?

Stress management skills

Stress management models interpret disturbed thoughts, feelings and function as signs of impaired adaptation to *current* stressors. Tension accumulates around powerful unexpressed emotions that have to do with the 'here and now' — for instance work problems, daily life hassles and relationship issues. But *current* feelings of anger, worry or sadness may overlie psychic substrata that contain rage, fear and despair. So *current* distress about the present is only partly distinct from *archaic* distress linked to earlier experience. Consequently current emotion-filled situations can resonate with more disturbing psychological bedrock. Such reverberations make coping unaccountably more difficult — perhaps because apparently inappropriate feelings surface, or because it becomes harder to think or act rationally. In psychodynamic terms these are the layers of the unconscious where psychological and psychosomatic disorders originate. The sources of these feelings may be unclear; but whether acted out, repressed or denied, they can still precipitate bodily and psychological problems — potentially, professional problems too. For any doctor suffering frank depression, panic or personality disorder, it is vitally important to recognize what is happening and to seek professional help. Simple stress management techniques are not appropriate when formal psychiatric help is needed. In these circumstances, professionally problematic though it

Table 14.1 A systems approach to stress management

Personal	Organizational	Cultural
Recognize own 'stress symptoms' or illness	Improve occupational health care	Validate possibility of doctors as being vulnerable
Review support needs, consider supervision?	Facilitate support structures	Develop pastoral ethos
Appraise coping skills: time management? relaxation response? exercise/fitness? communication?	Introduce skills training	New educational forms
Appraise own practice model, incorporate new approaches?	Innovation, team care	Humanize medical models
Appraise management skills, learn relevant methods	Ensure competent management	Incorporate modern management theories
Nutrition, sleep, leisure?	Recognize staff support needs, ensure adequate breaks, provide adequate recreation	Appropriate expectations, attainable goals and limits to medicine

might seem to seek help, the consequences of avoiding it would be worse.

Feelings of pessimism, cynicism, burn-out and isolation are not as some medics believe, 'part of the territory'. They do not 'come with job'. In fact they may mean a doctor is clinically depressed — the evidence shows that many are. Psychotherapy is an important option to consider here. 'Humanistic' approaches emphasize creativity, wholeness, growth, spirituality and self-realization; analytic models explore the shaping effect of early experiences and trauma; cognitive-behavioral approaches consider irrational and limiting beliefs that perpetuate distress, and teach ways of breaking free from them.

Box 14.6 Personal stress management

- self-awareness: recognizing the symptoms
- begin to define the underlying problem
- consider what help is needed to deal with the problem
- consider time management skills: clear sense of goals and resources
- rest, respite, recreation: learning to initiate a relaxation response
- bodily resilience: exercise and fitness
- emotional resilience: catharsis, psychotherapy
- interpersonal resilience: assertiveness, communication
- personal needs including: support, intimacy, love and care
- transpersonal needs including spiritual concerns, creativity, existential questions

Having made these provisos, there are still ways of increasing one's resilience (Table 14.1).

Personal stress management has four core steps (Box 14.6). The essential first step is *self-awareness*, the ability to recognize that one is not coping adequately. The signs could be psychological, physical or interpersonal; but something will have to change for coping to improve, and initiating change will require time and effort.

Rest and recreation may be needed to prime the pump and provide room for the second skill which is *time management*. This means setting realistic goals, and organizing feasible ways of achieving them.

Thirdly, the ability to make and sustain effort depends on cycles of rest. Although the *relaxation response* is physiologically as basic as flight, fight and freeze reactions, the ability to relax deeply without using recreational or prescribed chemicals becomes, once lost, a skill that has to be re-acquired. Techniques can help here: progressive muscular relaxation, work with breathing, or more structured methods — autogenic training, biofeedback and self-hypnosis, systems of meditation and exercise such as yoga or tai chi. If bodily tension seems hard to release, then aerobic exercise might help express it or massage may calm it down. In some programs cathartic release of feelings is encouraged too.

Finally, *communication skills* are transferable: active listening and assertiveness skills let one respond more effectively to others, and convey one's own needs more clearly. Once learned, they are relevant to professional practice, and in personal relationships that are probably under strain too; for the impact of burn-out never limits itself to life at work.

Stress counseling programs

Until very recently there were no formally organized projects delivering support services to doctors in the UK, but several are now under way. One pilot scheme for GPs was set up in 1994 in the Midlands county of Staffordshire under the Royal College of General Practioners' auspices[24]. The scheme is open to any GP who is 'under stress, in distress, depressed, over-anxious, not coping, drinking too much, or worried about themselves in any other way'. Seven psychologists, a marital counselor and 14 GPs are available to offer advice and counseling, and if necessary a psychologist will visit practices as stress consultant[30]. This project began after a 1994 survey of 620 GPs in the area showed that 26% of GPs had symptoms of depression, and 41% of anxiety.

Dr Graham Curtis-Jenkins Director of the Counselling in Primary Care Trust (CPCT) believes as many as 15% of GPs have suicidal thoughts at some time and that perhaps 25% are more depressed than their patients. In October 1995 CPCT helped launch GP Care, a support network in South-East England providing stress counseling to 2200 family doctors[25]. The project provides a 24 hour helpline staffed by professional counselors, and face to face counseling is available through a free service supported by charitable funds, with contributions from the NHS and the BMA. Recognizing the need for some organizational space between its clients and doctors' employers (an important consideration given doctors' concern about confidentiality) GP Care contracted an organization specializing in occupational programs, whose counselors have no links with the NHS[25]. With levels of distress rising, calls for the development of a nation-wide service for GPs, were eventually answered in April 1996 when the British Medical Association set up its own national pilot 24 hour counseling service for doctors.

Support groups

Shocking critical incidents, and unrelenting strain can be part and parcel of medical life, so dealing with their impact makes obvious sense. Supervision has a bearing on this, because it provides an opportunity for professionals to appreciate some of the uncomfortable feelings that are inescapable when working with patients and in organizations. Despite the need for supervision, far less is made of it in medicine than in social work or nursing training.

Perhaps the most widely known model of doctor supervision and support is the Balint Group. Conceived in the 1950s under the influence of Michael Balint, they have shaped one important strand in UK postgraduate GP training. Balint groups explore a psychoanalytic understanding of everyday practice, offering ways forward for practitioners struggling to manage difficult patients and intractable problems of chronic disease, psychosomatic, stress-related and functional disorders. Balint challenged doctors' attitudes and their therapeutic ambitions and encouraged them to face transferential issues — to be more aware of how current relationships and situations resonate with significant but unconscious earlier experiences.

General practitioners influenced by Balint's interpretation of the GP role, see the therapeutic relationship — Balint named it 'the doctor as drug' — as their main strength[26].

These case discussion groups aim to analyze the doctor–patient relationship, but they also allow doctors to talk more openly with one another, so a parallel element of peer-support is entwined with the intellectual task. Critics of Balint groups say they limit their attention to some mythical 'professional' self, as if it could be separated from personal concerns. Some post-Balint models have developed, notably through the British Post Graduate Medical Federation in the early 1980s, under the influence of John Heron and Patrick Pietroni[27], at a time when Heron was developing his concept of 'emotional education' for doctors. The notion of doctors' personal and professional growth has been taken up internationally; for instance one dynamic support and supervision group for GPs was described in the *Journal of the American Board of Family Practitioners*[28]. A member describes the process:

> Members wanted help in facing the psychological, political and economic challenges of daily medical practice, in order to avoid the disillusion that seemed to be prevalent among older physicians. Over the years the focus of the group has evolved from the discussions of patient care to explorations of personal values and feelings. It became apparent that our problems with patients, had their roots in our personalities and experiences which extend beyond the immediate practice setting. Feelings have gradually replaced intellectualization as we find the issues critical to our professional performance to be related more to our own marital discords, fears of death, failure to live up to our own goals as parents and persons and feelings of incompetence or uncertainty or self esteem.
>
> It seems that to work well we find we must deal with our own unfinished business. Personal insights and support have become instrumental in moving us towards our original goals and strengthening our work, improving our ability to deal with difficult patients and turning the stress of practice from a burden into a stimulus for personal growth.

This broad, non-specific, humanistic approach affirms — if anyone still doubted it — that doctors are ordinary people with ordinary needs. Could it be that relatively happy doctors are relatively good doctors? Though there is no scientific basis to confirm this, there may be an essential truth in the idea; one study of 255 male doctors assessed for hostility and cynicism in medical school and then followed up for 25 years showed that those with hostility scores over the median suffered 6.4 times the death rate of those scoring at or below the median[29].

Recovering impaired doctors

The Nuffield Provincial Hospitals Trust's report draws attention to the predicament of women in medicine. Their levels of distress and rates of suicide are disturbingly high; a fact that has largely been ignored. For male and female doctors alike, there are few established options should they need to get help with professional recovery. Collusion, denial, and ostracism are common responses to the doctor who is breaking down, who abuses substances or patients or who is psychiatrically ill. Could the absence of targeted, non-stigmatizing programs be a message about how impairment still remains unacceptable to the profession?

The Physician Prescribed Education Program at the University of Syracuse in New York State is a notable exception. This rigorous program takes impaired physicians (some self-referred, but the majority referred by the Office of Medical Conduct) into the program for 'a complete professional rebuild', beginning with a week's psychosocial and skills assessment, after which doctors are effectively retrained under supervision[30]. Dr Bill Grant, the psychologist who initiated the program, agrees that though expensive, the New York Medical Licensing Authorities and medical defense organizations believe the program is cost-effective; for it is impaired doctors against whom medico-legal claims are most commonly made. The program is still being evaluated, but it seems the cost of preventing error and law suits will be money well spent, for this new program has so far rehabilitated 75% of the impaired physicians enrolled.

PREVENTION OF DOCTOR DISTRESS

The buffer of hardiness

Susan Kobasa, an occupational psychologist in the USA, describes a group of factors which together constitute what she names 'hardiness'[31]. These attributes predicted the executives whose health did not break down when they were faced with rapid unrelenting organizational change. Kobasa named the qualities challenge, choice, commitment, stress management skills and social support in the work setting (Box 14.7). Executives with these attributes thrived under pressure; those who did not, had much higher levels of physical and mental ill health.

Kobasa studied business executives. Her findings may not fully apply to doctors, but they provide a framework for exploring 'salutogenic' (the opposite of pathogenic) attitudes and why some organizational cultures apparently buffer staff against health breakdown. Commitment for instance has always been a strong protective factor in medicine: the commitment to one's medical school or hospital, and especially a commitment to the ideals of medicine. Altruism may be a buffer too[20], but it is one that could be undermined by the rise of internal markets, and imperatives for competition and cost-benefit.

There is no similar research into the value of doctors' traditional protection — the respect, trust and deference which their patients and society as a whole award them. Patients have in the past seen the medical role as 'extra-ordinary'. Even in the more litigious and adversarial medical milieu of the USA, a sense of the special social contract between the medical profession and society persists. But this is no longer something the profession can take for granted. Our increasingly violent society has not left health care professionals untouched, and according to some well placed observers, the contract is breaking down in the face of managed care and doctors having to act as unwilling agents of government. If medicine loses its customary altruism and vocation the professional role will become more 'ordinary'. Might this fading of their 'magic cloak' be contributing to the rising level of assaults on doctors? Whether it is or not, such a potent cause of lost belief — over and above doctors' shrinking locus of control — adds to a growing vulnerability that could further undermine their ability to cope[32].

If the element of commitment is under attack then so too are Kobasa's components of choice, and challenge — and probably of support too. A lack of adequate resources will erode them all. Stress management skills are not encouraged either in medical training or by the macho values and workaholism endemic in the organizational culture. Where personal coping skills training has been offered to hospital doctors the uptake has been poor[40], so too has the uptake of the newly established stress counseling services for GPs in the UK. There have been few attempts to research the impact of personal coping skills among doctors although their general value in increasing resilience has been widely studied elsewhere. For instance one study comparing the coping ability of three groups — using exercise, relaxation and time-management skills — showed that all three were significantly more effective than control[41]. The case for a wide variety of preventive 'mind–body medicine' approaches — including biofeedback, exercise, autogenic training, and relaxation techniques — is substantial. The research literature on the benefits of meditation (both TM and Vipasana) is now extensive too. So there is no shortage of data for doctors requiring evidence-based stress management,

Box 14.7 The buffer of hardiness?

- Choice: Locus of control. Having a sense that options are available for dealing with situations that arise.
- Challenge: Seeing problems as creative opportunities for growth and development.
- Commitment: A sense that work is meaningful and coherent.
- Stress management: An awareness of when one is feeling or performing badly, and of personal options for dealing with the situation.
- Support at work: Having peers who empathize, encourage and commiserate.

and the problem is rather one of how to implement appropriate strategies.

'Emotional education'

John Heron was assistant director of the British Postgraduate Medical Federation in the early 1980s. His approach to postgraduate education and the program he initiated (which included courses in stress management for doctors) was humanistic[34]. According to Heron a stultifying traditional approach to education makes doctors see the human condition in the light of a catastrophically out-dated medical model. Bennett touches on similar themes in his book *The Wound and the Doctor*[3]. For Heron the educationalist and for Bennett the psychiatrist and doctor-observer, medicine's cultural perspective is problematic, and its expression in practice potentially destructive. Along with other writers (e.g. De Vries[35], Leder[36]) they argue that the mind–body split, scientific reductionism and rationalism, though they provide a solid foundation for scientific advance, have also undermined the role of the intangible; the mind, feelings, values and spirituality. Heron also discussed medical education as harming doctors because:

> It is exclusively concerned with the development of intellectual competence. In the traditional educational model the incidental function of the intellect is to control feelings, this can lead to perfectly healthy control but also to repression and denial of grief, fear and anger and denied distress which significantly distorts behavior[34].

Heron pointed out that the working world of the doctor is full of strong emotions — their own as well as their patients'. And since anger, anguish, sadness, pain and distress are inevitable, doctors will either find ways of living with these feelings or they will repress them. Such denial, said Heron, shapes a medical culture of professional objectivity which in turn determines the stereotypical medical persona; so repression of feelings is carried into the professional role. Here it can be acted out through technical interventions legitimized by a view of the body as mind-less; and thus medicine becomes applied biotechnology. Heron and Bennett also argue that the overvaluing of objectivity has led to a devaluing of subjectivity, and that thereby the lived experience of both doctor and patient is invalidated. This sustains the doctor's position of omnipotence and invulnerability (though leaving the patient weak and mute), but if practitioners rely on this strategy then their approach to medicine will deny the very emotions their work inevitably involves. This neglect of 'emotional education' makes doctors less competent, not only when dealing with the reality of the medical milieu and its demands, but also in coping with their own lives. Heron called on emotionally shut-down doctors to resensitize themselves to their own feelings and the capacity to relate. His favored intervention was small group-work, drawing on techniques paralleled in Fritz Perls' Gestalt approach and Assagoli's Psychosynthesis[34].

THEORY AND PRACTICE: THE NEED FOR A NEW MEDICAL MODEL

Conventional medicine may have reached the peak of its biotechnological trajectory. Many commentators believe conventional medicine's sense of inexorable progress is no longer justifiable. Effective though the approach has been — in infectious and deficiency diseases, in anesthesia and surgical technique — it has not had the hoped for impact on the epidemic diseases of the West. The problems doctors now encounter are stress-, environment- and lifestyle-mediated diseases, as well as addiction and psychological disorders. Modern biotechnical medicine has failed to cure them; nor does it deal easily with 'undifferentiated disease', ordinary unwellness, and the complex impact that learning, behavior and lifestyle have on health. Although such problems are rarely seen in the teaching hospitals, where students' ideas about illness are shaped, they are, more than end-stage pathology, what primary health care is confronted with. Furthermore, patients are dissatisfied with approaches that marginalize their experiences and beliefs; that disempower or patronize. They share with many health professionals a deepening uncertainty about causes and cures, and a justifiable concern about pharmaceutical side-effects. This unease has encouraged a lively complexity of new notions and a growing interest in non-conventional therapies. Many doctors feel left behind by these developments; even threatened or rejected by apparently consumer-led attempts to turn away from conventional practice. It is important then, for doctors to realize that new discourses are emerging from *within* medicine and nursing. They include mind–body medicine, and holistic health care. The growing professional interest in complementary therapies, bodywork and new approaches to psychotherapy all reflect attempts — perhaps naive or misguided at times — to put these important theories into practice.

Holistic health care

George Engel, Professor of Psychiatry at Rochester NY developed his critique of biomedicine in the 1970s[37]. Setting out the reasons for its undeniable success, he went on to explore its de-humanizing influence and its theoretical limitations where complex psychological factors are at work — which is arguably in most health care situations. The sociological ramifications of this theme — which he refers to as the 'the biologization of medicine' — are explored in Foucault's extraordinary book *The Birth of the Clinic*[38]. Engel's work is a call for more holistic approaches, and he does not discuss the impact of the biomedical approach on the inner life of doctors. Bennet's critique of medical theory, culture, the attitudes and the practice it shapes, is more explicit though. Heron, Balint and Bennet, along with Engel and Foucault provide us with a wider cultural and philosophical perspective on doctors' distress. They articulate how poorly doctors are prepared for their role, having learned to relate to patients in ways that are often technically and psychologically inappropriate. Moreover they relate the medical problem to a deeper crisis in our cultural notions of the mind and body as being separate. Other philosophers, notably those in the European streams of anthropological medicine and phenomenology warn against an exclusive emphasis on a rational-technical approach. Late-modern medicine they insist, has enshrined at its core a theory of the person which does not comprehend the intertwining of mind and body, and so marginalizes emotion and ignores lived experience. Some authors, such as Illyich[47] also assert that it ignores significant local and global eco-political threats to well-being.

One response to late-modern medicine's fragmention of patients and their health care, is holism. Holism can be interpreted as an applied biopsychosocial approach whose three dimensions are concerned with reintegrating into health care what biotechnical medicine has historically divided. The three sundered dimensions are mind from body (the psychosomatic), predicament from disease (the behavioral), and the person who is healed from the person who is healing (the humanistic).

The *psychosomatic* dimension explores mind–body interaction, acknowledging individuals who are related to and shaped by, a social order. Psychological and physical factors are seen as interdependent, mutually influencing self-regulation. It sees that psychosocial pressures are met by physiological and potentially pathophysiological responses. One of its theoretical underpinnings is psychoneuroimmunology (itself a triumph of hi-tech reductionism), whose project may eventually map the biochemical pathways that take happiness or sickness into cells[40].

Behavioral medicine tries to take account of a person's own power over their health, and the possibility of using a broad range of interventions to enhance well-being. It harnesses a capacity consciously to influence homeostasic processes, and extends its interest into ways that social factors — for instance housing, isolation, and education — influence health. Examples of behavioral medicine's more general interventions would be attempts at improving lifestyle and nutrition — by educational rather than political strategies (though these are of great relevance to public health) — or by encouraging exercise and relaxation skills; the interventions of mind–body medicine — meditation, visualization, autogenics and biofeedback, for instance are related specific methods, whose psychophysiology is only partly understood.

The dimension of *humanistic medicine* provides holism with a necessary theory of what the person is. It is explicitly concerned with the influence of inner life, of lived experience and inter-personal factors. The practitioner/client dynamic is centrally important; attitudes, power and empowerment issues are crucial too. It considers the well-being of practitioners as significant, and holds that values and spirituality have a legitimate impact on well-being and relationships.

A less alienating medical model could help the medical profession heal itself. A more patient centered theory would for instance subvert the illusion of medical objectivity, the inter-personal equivalent of Newton's motionless observer, surely inappropriate at a time when the wider culture is struggling to embrace relativity and complexity. Given the current levels of distress and impairment, the challenge for medicine to develop new approaches will have to be taken seriously. It will mean constructing a person-centered perspective and incorporating a mind–body approach to understanding and practicing health care, but without eroding the immense benefits of late-modern medicine's technological triumphs.

CONCLUSION

The project of helping doctors manage stress has barely begun. Medicine stands at a threshold; the morbidity figures, the crisis reflected in theoretical, educational and organizational upheaval and the failure of current practice to meet rapidly changing expectations, make further developments inevitable. Although they represent an opportunity for eventual transformation, the turbulence and uncertainty eddying out from upheaval at the macro-level have already become unbearable for many doctors. Self-care and support groups, though only micro-solutions, are a way of surviving such 'interesting times'. The profession, in seeking ways forward, should bear in mind an early prescription — perhaps one that expresses the stress management advice of its era. It was written over the entrance to the healing temple of Aesclepios at Delphi: 'Know Thyself'.

REFERENCES

1 Payne R, Firth-Cozens J 1987 Stress in health professionals. Wiley, Chichester
2 Maslach C 1982 Coping strategies, causes and costs. In: McConnell EA (ed) Burnout in the nursing profession. CV Mosby, St. Louis
3 Bennett G 1987 The wound and the doctor. Secker and Warburgh, London
4 British Medical Association 1992 Stress and the medical profession. British Medical Association, London
5 Alibone A, Oakes D, Shannon HS 1981 The health and health care of doctors. Journal of the Royal College of Practitioners 361:328–331
6 Valient G, Brighton J, Macarthur C 1970 Physicians use of mood altering drugs. New England Journal of Medicine 282:365–370
7 Office of Population Center and Surveys 1986 Occupational mortality 1970–1980, 1982–1983: Decennial supplement. HMSO, London
8 Harrington JM 1990 The health of health care workers. Journal of the Royal College of Physicians 243:189–195
9 Morrice JKW 1984 Job stress and burnout. Bulletin of the Royal College of Psychiatry 8:45–46
10 Cooper V, Sutherland C 1992 Job stress, satisfaction and mental health among general practitioners before and after the introduction of the new contract. British Medical Journal 304:1545–1548
11 Organisation for Economic Cooperation and Development 1987 Proportion of Gross Domestic Products spent on health. Operation for Economic Cooperation and Development, Paris
12 British Medical Association 1991 Leading for health: a BMA agenda for health. British Medical Association, London
13 Firth Cozens J 1989 Stress in medical undergraduates and house officers. British Journal of Hospital Medicine 41:161–164
14 Caplan RP 1994 Stress, anxiety and depression in hospital consultants, general practitioners and senior health services managers. British Medical Journal 309:1261–1263
15 British Medical Association 1991 Reforms and doctor's morale. BMA News Review, June = Sheffield survey?
16 British Medical Association 1996 Doctors under stress. British Medical Association News Review, April 10

17 Silvester S et al 1994 The provision of medical services for sick doctors. Nuffield Provincial Hospitals Trust, London
18 Chambers R, Maxwell R 1996 Helping sick doctors. British Medical Journal 312:722–723
19 Allen I 1988 Any room at the top? A study of doctors and their careers. Policy Studies Institute, London
20 Johnson WDK 1991 Predisposition to emotional distress and psychiatric illness amongst doctors: the role of the unconscious and experiential factors. British Journal of Medical Psychology 64:317–329
21 Benor DJ 1995 The Louisville programme for medical student health awareness. Complementary Therapies in Medicine. 3(2):93–99
22 Brooke D, Edwards G, Taylor C 1991 Addiction as an occupational hazard: 144 doctors with drug and alcohol problems. British Journal of Addiction 86:1011–1016
23 Brandon S 1991 Doctors who need help. Medical Monitor, 16 August, p 13
24 Chambers R 1995 Paper at Royal College of General Practitioners' Conference on stress and GPs. May
25 General Practitioners Counselling and advisory trust. 3a Majestic House, High Street, Staines, Middlesex. TW18 4DG. UK
26 Balint E, Courtenay M, Elder A, Hull S, Julian P 1993 The doctor, the patient and the group: Balint revisited. Routledge, London
27 Pietroni P 1984 Training or treatment? A new approach. British Journal of Holistic Medicine 2:109–112
28 Eubank DF, Zeckhausen W, Sobelson GA 1991 Converting the stress of medical practice to personal and professional growth: five years of experience with a psychodynamic support and supervision group. Journal of the American Board of Family Practitioners 4(3):151–158
29 Williams, Barefoot, Shekelle 1985 The health consequences of hostility. In: Chesney MA, Rosenman RH (eds) Anger and hostility in cardiovascular and behavioral disorders. McGraw-Hill, New York
30 Grant W 1995 An individualised educational model for the remediation of physicians. Archives of Family Medicine 4:767–773
31 Kobasa S 1990 Stress resistant personality. In: The healing brain: a scientific reader. Guilford, New York, pp 219–239
32 Curtis-Jenkins G, personal communication
33 Bruning FS, Frew DRF 1987 Effects of exercise, relaxation and time management skills training on physiological stress indicators: a field experiment. Journal of Applied Psychology 4:515–21
34 Heron J 1984 Holistic aspects to medical training. British Journal of Holistic Medicine 1:80–85
35 DeVries M 1985 The redemption of the intangible in medicine. Psychosynthesis Trust
36 Leder D 1992 The cartesian corpse and the lived body. In: Leder D (ed) The body in medical thought and practice. Kluher Academic, Dordrecht
37 Engel G 1977 The need for a new medical model: the challenge for biomedicine. Science 196:129–136
38 Foucault M 1976 The birth of the clinic: an archeology of medical perception. Tavistock, London
39 Illyich I 1976 Limits to medicine. Medical nemesis: the expropriation of health. Pelikan, London
40 Ornstein R, Swencionis C 1990 The healing brain: a scientific reader. Guildford, New York

CHAPTER CONTENTS

15

Putting mind–body care into practice

Alan Watkins
George Lewith

INTRODUCTION

There is now a substantial amount of sound scientific evidence demonstrating that an individual's thoughts, feelings and spirit can have a profound effect upon their endocrine, autonomic, cardiorespiratory, gastrointestinal and immune systems. This book has attempted to draw together much of this research and has argued that physicians need to adopt a mind–body approach to patients. They need to shift from a biomechanical viewpoint, which only addresses the biological factors of disease, to a biopsychosocial approach, which can incorporate information about the patient's resilience, spirit, emotional intelligence, hardiness and their social support.

There is no doubt that the reductionist approach of biological medicine has provided some truly remarkable technological advances and treatments. However, there is also little doubt that the biological approach has certain limitations and its technological power must be balanced with the human qualities of care, compassion and empathy. Such humanistic qualities are not mere niceties, they can have significant physiological effects[1]. A physician's attitude and approach can profoundly influence a patient's mental, emotional and physical well-being; either stimulating or handicapping recovery.

Adopting a mind–body approach means recognizing that illness is not merely a biological malfunction of one organ or one bodily system, but a breakdown in a wide variety of defenses be they immunological, physiological, emotional or spiritual.

Therefore, if physicians are to deliver high quality care on all levels, not merely technological and pharmaceutical, into the 21st Century it is necessary for them to broaden their understanding of how the different systems within the body interact and fully embrace the evidence demonstrating that taking care of the mental, emotional and spiritual aspects of a patient's life is just as important as correcting physiological derangements, for all these aspects are inseparable. Such notions are not fanciful, they are based on very sound scientific evidence, as laid out in the chapters of this book.

Furthermore, adopting a broader, more holistic mind–body approach to patients is not unrealistic. It has been argued that physicians have insufficient time to do anything other than patch up the physiology. Such arguments are fallacious. Embracing a mind–body approach shifts emphasis away from time-consuming and relentless technical investigations in the pursuit of physiological derangements and places emphasis on a more judicious and prudent use of investigative resources, thereby freeing more time to care.

The adoption of a mind–body and biopsychosocial approach changes the way a physician takes a history, examines a patient and ultimately manages their problem. It also allows for more creativity and scope to respond to the human dilemma of illness and minimizes the tendency to see individuals as biological subjects to be fitted into treatment protocols. Scope for creativity is rarely encouraged in the management of illness in traditional medical circles. The overriding philosophy is for 'one size fits all' treatments, but clearly no two illnesses are the same, and no two patients possess the same social support and powers of recovery. Creative solutions to individual dilemmas need to be considered, and these may not necessarily come from traditional sources. Complementary and alternative approaches may have much to offer, particularly in the absence of effective conventional approaches.

Need for change

However, in order to embrace a mind–body approach physicians must first recognize the need for change; the need for a new model of illness that can more effectively address all the needs of the patients, not just the physical manifestations of ill health. If the need for a more holistic, biopsychosocial approach encompassing mind–body interventions is recognized, then physicians will need the energy, motivation and education to embrace such an approach. It is all too easy, in the face of excessive work commitments, to return to habitual ways of practicing, to methods and models that are known to be inadequate but which have a comfortable familiarity.

Motivation and energy for change

The motivation and energy to embrace the mind–body approaches advocated in this book can come from a strong desire to improve the personal quality of medical practice, in addition to a desire to increase the breadth of care patients receive. They can also come from a clear vision of the benefits that both patients and physicians themselves might accrue as a result of adopting a mind–body approach. Holding on to such a vision is difficult, and the pressure not to change is great.

The motivation to embrace mind–body approaches can also come through experience. If a physician has experienced the benefits of such approaches, rather than just visioned them, then they are more likely to be able to sustain the effort required to adopt them. A single experience of the benefits of a mind–body approach is usually insufficient to sustain motivation; repeated experience of mind–body approaches, either personally or through the experience of respected colleagues, is required to overcome inertia and resistance, in addition to the hurdles of complacency and time mismanagement.

In order to embrace mind–body approaches and a biopsychosocial model, it is crucial to be able to change current practice without exhausting vital personal reserves. Burn-out can occur just as easily through an overzealous, misplaced desire to change all aspects of medical practice as it can through stress and overwork. Adopting a broader perspective means integrating mind–body approaches with conventional training and practice. If this is the situation, what changes need to be made in practice and on what level?

INTEGRATING MIND–BODY MEDICINE

The integration of mind–body medicine within conventional medical practice and the adoption of a biopsychosocial approach can occur on a number of levels: personally; within medical teams; within an organizational structure; and ultimately in the cultural environment in which medicine is practiced.

Integrating mind–body medicine personally

Integrating mind–body medicine into conventional practice requires that physicians change their own individual view and adopt a biopsychosocial perspective. This necessitates a fundamental change in their perception of illness and how patients are perceived and managed. In the biopsychosocial model, the mental and emotional characteristics of the patient and their social circumstances are assessed in greater detail, and the potential contribution of these factors to the development and progression of the illness is determined.

Current and previous psychosocial problems are elicited and their contribution to the present situation is established with a view to addressing what factors in the social and psychological makeup enable recovery to take place. Priorities for intervention are determined, and appropriate biomedical and psychosocial investigations are arranged once the physical examination has identified any specific physical issues that need urgent attention.

A physician skilled in eliciting a psychosocial history is able to glean the important mental, emotional and physical features of the illness rapidly and efficiently, without any additional requirement in time. This is facilitated by the physician quickly establishing an empathic bond with the patient who recognizes that their doctor is sincerely interested in them and not just their symptoms.

Addressing all the needs of the patient is not only greatly appreciated by the patient, but is also far more rewarding to the practitioner. The crucial skills required when adopting a biopsychosocial model are the development of a genuine sense of compassion and the avoidance of an overburdening sense of omnipotence. Physicians should not attempt to take responsibility for all the patient's problems and attempt to 'solve' them. Rather, physicians should help patients to understand their illness, provide guidance and advice, and recommend intervention where appropriate. It is important to identify what resources are available to the patient for recovery, and what treatments, traditional or mind–body, can facilitate the recovery and restoration of function.

Integrating mind–body medicine into medical teams

To integrate mind–body approaches into orthodox medical practice effectively requires all members of the health care team to embrace such approaches individually. A single individual within a health care team operating from a mind–body perspective when all other practitioners are operating from a traditional biomedical standpoint is likely to set up tensions within the group that are potentially destructive for the group and confusing for the patients. In contrast, when all members of a health care team are operating from the same theoretical, practical and therapeutic standpoint the environment in which the patient is cared for is likely to be more harmonious and the quality of care is likely to be of a much higher standard.

The importance of cohesion within a health care team is rarely addressed in undergraduate or postgraduate medical education. Indeed team cohesion is often dismissed as managerial jargon and of little relevance to medical practice. In fact, a complete lack of team cohesion is commonplace, particularly in teams containing different health care professions. Amongst physicians the importance of supporting and caring for each other is poorly understood. If anything, the reverse is often found. Medical undergraduates are frequently subjected to psychological abuse, intellectual intimidation and an emotional battering during their training[2]. Such attacks on cohesion and the natural kindred bond trainee doctors might feel towards their profession are not isolated phenomena. In one study up to 80% of undergraduates reported some form of abuse, with 16% saying that they were permanently scarred by such experiences[2]. In another study 'verbal abuse' was so pervasive that 75% said they had become more cynical about their chosen profession, and 65% felt they were worse off than friends in other professions[3]. More than 30% of undergraduates said they had considered dropping out of medical school and 25% said they would have chosen a different profession had they known the extent of the mistreatment they would have to endure[3].

It is a sad paradox that the 'caring profession' is so uncaring towards its fledglings. The ritualistic mistreatment inherent in many undergraduate programs, and the lack of emphasis placed on developing a caring culture may help to explain why record numbers of doctors are leaving the profession and why so many doctors become victims of stress themselves.

Integrating mind–body medicine into organizational structures

A large proportion of general practitioners have received training in mind–body therapies[4–6] and up to 25% of general practices in the UK are already providing some form of mind–body therapy, be it acupuncture, homeopathy or another alternative intervention[7]. If the definition of a mind–body therapy is widened to include formal counseling and psychotherapeutic interventions then a much larger percentage of practices would have to be included.

There are a number of ways of incorporating a mind–body approach into a conventional primary or secondary care setting. Perhaps the most common model presently employed is for physicians to refer patients directly to non-medically qualified practitioners or alternatively to provide one or two clinics a week themselves. Very few general practices are formally restructured to make the provision of such approaches central to the running of the practice.

One general practice where the organization has been completely restructured to integrate a mind–body approach is the well-patronized Marylebone Health Centre in London, UK, founded by Dr Patrick Pietroni. Dr Pietroni's aim when establishing the Marylebone Health Centre, was to bring conventional and alternative medicine closer together in a more holistic, mind–body integration of the best practices from biomedical and biopsychosocial medicine[8]. The Marylebone experiment is described below.

Cultural change: adopting a mind–body approach

It is often assumed that science and medicine are independent from the culture in which they exist; that there is some scientific reality that transcends cultural influence. However, the culture in which medicine is practiced has a profound effect on the way physicians perceive illness, the types of therapeutic interventions employed and the scientific studies that are performed to investigate both disease and its treatment.

For example, the diagnostic and therapeutic criteria used in traditional Chinese medicine are conceptually quite different from those used in conventional western medicine. Thus, a traditional Chinese physician may explain an individual's persistent exhaustion as a kidney xu disease or the invasion of various pathogens into the pi-spleen. Such definitions immediately indicate, to a traditional Chinese physician, that specific therapeutic techniques should be adopted. While such diagnostic and therapeutic language may be completely alien to conventional physicians, they provide an important framework for managing the patient to those with a clear understanding of the concepts of traditional Chinese medicine. They represent a different medical language through which symptoms are interpreted and problems diagnosed; this results in a treatment regime which, even though it may primarily be eliciting non-specific effects, has been used with a great deal of empirical success for the last 2000 years.

Thus, an individual's beliefs, be they a physician, scientist or health care worker, are culturally determined. It must be remembered that the culture which molds these beliefs is itself constantly evolving. Therefore, changing the overriding culture in which medicine is practiced is not such an enormous undertaking as it might at first seem, for it is already in a constant state of flux. The speed of change and the direction of change can be influenced but usually by different forces.

Speed of change

The speed or momentum for change depends on a critical mass of individuals, who desire the change, working to bring it about. This is true in society and medicine, since one reflects the other. While the number of physicians embracing a mind–body approach has not yet reached a critical mass, conventional clinical medicine is increasingly moving towards a biopsychosocial approach to illness. This shift is being driven by an increasing awareness that the communication between different bodily systems, e.g. mind and body, is crucial to understanding health and disease. For example, the development of neurocardiology, neuroendocrinology, neuroimmunology, neuropsychology, psychophysiology, immunopsychiatry and psychoneuroimmunology indicates that there is an increasing number of individuals who recognize that the interactions between the different systems is the key to understanding how the human organism operates as a complete living system. As the critical mass of individuals working in these areas increases and the number of individuals who embrace an integrated mind–body approach increases, then the speed of change will accelerate.

Rapid change in the practice of science and medicine is not only brought about by a critical number of individuals working towards a new vision; it can also be brought about by disease itself. For example, the explosion in HIV disease brought about a very rapid change in the way research was funded around the world. Similarly, technical breakthroughs can accelerate our understanding of disease.

Direction of change

Perhaps the most crucial factors in determining the direction in which medical practice evolves are the results of medical research. Certain research findings act as watersheds in our understanding and critically change the direction of much of the research that follows, by providing whole new insights into the pathogenesis and progression of disease. The medical literature is littered with such examples. For instance, the discovery, in 1975, that the immune system could be classically conditioned helped to spawn the whole field of psychoneuroimmunology[9].

MIND–BODY CARE IN PRACTICE: THE MARYLEBONE EXPERIENCE

With the appropriate individual, group and organizational reorganization, it is possible to integrate mind–body medicine into a community or hospital-based practice. The approach adopted in primary care by the Marylebone Health Centre was to provide patients with access to a wide variety of highly skilled mind–body therapists. Fully qualified general practitioners worked alongside these therapists and acted as gatekeepers in the system.

Physician as gatekeeper

Experience suggests that patients are reassured by the fact that the doctor advising them about treatment options, conventional and mind–

body, is medically qualified. For example, the discussion of an individualized management plan for breast or bowel cancer may be severely limited by a non-medical practitioner's knowledge and understanding of the conventional treatment options available. Anti-cancer drugs might be seen as a uniformly poor option for the patient, when in fact they may have much to offer in a number of malignant illnesses.

Similarly, few patients have sufficient knowledge of mind–body therapies to determine which approach may be most appropriate for their needs. They may find the process of choosing a treatment confusing and unsettling, particularly when the language used by a therapist may be quite alien.

In some circumstances, such as 'undifferentiated' illness, it may prove impossible to make a clear conventional diagnosis[10]. In such situations an understanding of alternative conceptual models and treatment options such as acupuncture or psychotherapy may prove to be of great help in unraveling a patient's problem and even arriving at a diagnosis and subsequent treatment plan. The treatment plan may be based on a familiarity with the evidence base for mind–body therapies, previous clinical experience with mind–body therapies and a theoretical understanding of such approaches[11].

Assessing a mind–body approach

All medical teams and organizations, whether based in a primary, secondary or tertiary care setting should audit their practice. This is perhaps more important for holistic practices working from a biopsychosocial model and embracing mind–body therapies to do since such centers are advocates for a change in the status quo. However, the supply of a single mind–body therapy on an ad hoc basis by an interested physician is unlikely to generate sufficiently robust data that could be used to make a strong argument for either expanding such a service or demonstrating efficacy. Similarly a center offering a wide variety of mind–body therapies to a wide range of patients in an informal way runs the risk of being inappropriately assessed[12].

The scientific evaluation of either a single mind–body therapy or a practice providing mind–body therapies requires specialist knowledge and collaboration with a center of excellence which can provide the appropriate expertise for the evaluation. The Marylebone experiment was not formally assessed, but the experience of the individuals working there provided very valuable insights and helped to identify many of the difficulties inherent in restructuring an organization to embrace a mind–body approach. Some of these difficulties were generic and some were due to the specific approach adopted by Marylebone (see below).

Larger primary or secondary care practices able to provide sufficient patient numbers with specific conditions such a fatigue, cancer or allergies would be more valuable sites to investigate mind–body approaches.

Problems of organizational restructuring

The organizational restructuring of the Marylebone Health Centre generated practical difficulties on a number of levels which had to be addressed:

- **The patients:** Could a primary care facility designed to provide a wide variety of mind–body therapies meet the various and often very disparate needs of a general practice population?
- **Efficacy:** Would the problems presented by the patients be more effectively managed by the range of approaches provided by a multidisciplinary health care team compared with the management of the same problems by physicians alone in a standard general practice? And could such disparate interventions be evaluated and the treatment outcomes be appropriately assessed?
- **Health care practitioners:** How well would practitioners working with different illness models and therapeutic approaches work together in the management of individual patients?

- **Financial viability:** Could such a multidisciplinary practice be financially viable and cost effective, and act as a model for other practices to follow?
- **The media:** How would the Marylebone model of mind–body medical practice be reported by the media and received by other physicians and the general public?

Much has been written about the strengths and weaknesses of the Marylebone Health Centre, both in the medical and the lay press[8]. While the caring environment developed and the approach espoused by Pietroni and his colleagues have been well received by many of the patients, whether it is the optimum model for delivering mind–body medicine in a primary care setting remains unclear.

Furthermore, because of its innovative approach, the Marylebone Centre attracted a group of highly experienced mind–body practitioners whose breadth of skills and research ability were too great for the patient population attending. As a consequence the wide-reaching facilities available to the Marylebone Centre became less applicable to general practice than might have initially been intended. Nevertheless, it certainly raised awareness, within the medical and lay community in the UK, of a variety of alternative approaches to ill health, and showed how a more holistic mind–body approach could be integrated into a traditional general practice setting.

Common language

One of the key issues, and most fruitful areas for research, raised by the Marylebone experiment has been the identification of communication problems between members of a multidisciplinary health care team[13]. The diverse models employed by different professionals within the team can generate conflict. An evaluation of the communication difficulties revealed that the doctors and complementary practitioners were both very 'territorial animals', and often had great difficulty understanding each other's concepts and values in the diagnosis and management of illness. Furthermore, many of the non-medically qualified practitioners appeared to have difficulty communicating with each other, each viewing their therapy as the best approach to a particular problem while having few skills and little knowledge with which to consider the advantages and disadvantages of other conventional or complementary medical approaches.

Thus, it is clear that reorganizing a primary care practice and adopting a mind–body approach does not itself ensure the cohesive functioning of that practice. Organizational change which has not embraced individual and group change is likely to fail. In order for organizational change to work all individuals within that organization have to understand the changes and share the same vision of the new order.

Financial viability

It is clear that the financial viability of a primary care center in the UK offering the services of a wide variety of mind–body therapists in addition to highly qualified doctors, as exemplified by the Marylebone Health Centre, is dependent on charitable money, and is not sustainable within the financial structure of the NHS. While the holistic approach produced some savings in drug expenditure and high-tech investigations, these were largely outweighed by the increased costs involved in providing a whole range of therapeutic interventions free of charge.

Recently, a degree of flexibility has been introduced in the funding structures in the UK and the USA to enable the cost of mind–body therapies to be covered either by private health insurance or the NHS. This is in line with the recommendations of the 1994 European Parliament[14]. However, such financial reimbursement is still limited and as yet cannot match the demand for such approaches by the general public. Such restrictions may limit the implementation of mind–body medicine in primary and secondary care settings.

There are organizational implications for covering the cost of mind–body approaches.

For example, back pain could be managed by chiropractors and osteopaths in a primary care setting as opposed to rheumatologists and orthopedic surgeons in hospital. This raises the question of who will provide the service. Will it be non-medically qualified practitioners or multi-skilled GPs? If it is to be non-medically qualified individuals, then issues of competence and medical responsibility will need to be addressed far more coherently than they are at present. While it is beyond the scope of this chapter to address the issue of 'competence to practice', this debate is of primary importance to health care provision, particularly within a state-funded system such as the NHS. If GPs are increasingly going to provide mind–body interventions such as acupuncture, homeopathy or psychotherapy in addition to their normal practice commitments, without any formal structural reorganization, then clearly some aspect of care will suffer. Furthermore, how will the competence of the general practitioner's skills in mind–body medicine be assessed? There is likely to be a huge diversity of skill and experience amongst GPs trained in mind–body therapies. Some may be less competent than non-medically qualified practitioners. Furthermore, some physicians and alternative practitioners may consider themselves therapists after a weekend course in massage. Hopefully the recent legitimization of a number of professional organizations through statutory regulations will help clarify these issues.

CENTERS OF INTEGRATION

A number of centers have contributed to the momentum to integrate a more biopsychosocial, mind–body approach into primary care in the UK. The Blackthorn Trust began 10 years ago offering an anthroposophical approach to the management of chronic illness and its holistic concepts have facilitated the rehabilitation of both young and old alike. Those practicing within the Blackthorn Trust have been able to provide a truly holistic approach to general practice[15].

A different approach has been utilized by both Liverpool and Lewisham. Liverpool has developed a community-based facility for the provision of complementary medicine which has been described by both its development officer[16] and from the perspective of the therapists working within the center[17]. Many issues were raised by the Liverpool experience, including the medicalization of the therapists and the limited facilities available to fulfill the apparent demand from general practitioners.

The Sheffield survey confirms the increasing demand from general practitioners for the provision of mind–body therapies within the NHS. However, Liverpool's experience suggests that such environments can very rapidly become overloaded with chronically sick patients pursuing a maintenance therapy that temporarily alleviates their symptoms[14].

The establishment of a clinic at Lewisham clearly demonstrated that demand from general practitioners far exceeded the clinic's capacity to provide a service and fairly stringent guidelines were rapidly developed for both referral and treatment in order to avoid the service becoming overwhelmed[18].

A similar study in West Yorkshire evaluated a Health Service-based project which looked at the provision of acupuncture, massage, homeopathy, aromatherapy, osteopathy and yoga in general practice[19]. This study again demonstrated that many primary care physicians, responsible for purchasing and providing care within the NHS, believe that mind–body interventions have value despite a sparse evidence base for their effectiveness. Whether this reflects a simple response to patient demand or a more deeply held belief on the part of physicians in their actual value, is unclear.

In line with the Marylebone experiment, the Yorkshire study reported a number of communication difficulties amongst the various complementary practitioners and between the complementary practitioners and general practitioners. These difficulties necessitated the rapid development of a team approach to the patient with both doctors and complementary practitioners having to re-evaluate their opinions of each other and develop better mechanisms through which they could communicate.

Outreach clinics and secondary referral centers

There is an increasing trend towards specialist physicians running outreach clinics within primary care. This model lends itself particularly well to the provision of mind–body therapies within general practice. Not only does it provide a facility for the management of acute problems, but it would provide large enough patient resources to address issues of efficacy in the management of chronic illness with mind–body therapies. Such a service would need to be designed and coordinated by a physician with a broad based but specialist interest in mind–body medicine. The specialist mind–body physician would need not only to act as a provider but also to supervise and direct the employment of other mind–body therapists and to evaluate the needs of particularly complex and difficult patients. An alternative to running specialist mind–body outreach clinics is to provide a centrally-located secondary mind–body referral center where administrative and clinical support could be condensed. Such a center could also act as a central focus for clinical audit, outcome evaluation and other clinical research.

While a single mind–body practitioner in primary care could provide front line management, a more coordinated and systematic approach involving outreach clinics or secondary referral centers may help to provide the appropriate level of mind–body medical services required by primary and secondary care physicians.

Centers of excellence

At present there are six major secondary referral centers operating in the UK: the Glasgow Homoeopathic Hospital, the Bristol Homoeopathic Hospital, the Royal London Homoeopathic Hospital, the Tunbridge Wells Homoeopathic Hospital and the Centres for the Study of Complementary Medicine in Southampton and Manchester. These centers provide a clinical service and act as a focal point for research into mind–body therapies. These centers mirror the centers of excellence set up by the Office of Alternative Medicine (OAM) at the NIH in the USA and are likely, in line with the increased funding of the US centers, to receive increased governmental support in the coming years.

Centers staffed by non-medically qualified practitioners

In addition to the six centers of excellence in the UK, staffed by qualified doctors, there are numerous 'centers' offering a wide selection of mind–body therapies in almost every major city in the UK. These 'centers' have usually been based around one individual purchasing a building, initially to house their own practice, and then renting out rooms to other therapists. Occasionally, doctors practicing complementary medicine have joined such groups but, in the majority of cases, these groups involve non-medically qualified practitioners such as acupuncturists, counselors, chiropractors, reflexologists and aromatherapists. Because each individual practitioner is keen to promote and develop their own private practice, there is very little advantage in developing a coherent management plan for an individual patient within the practice. Instead, the choice of intervention is patient-driven and these choices may be encouraged by the therapist, for either clinical or economic reasons. For example, two or three consultations aimed at appropriate nutritional and dietary advice might resolve an individual's migraine, while it might take 10 or 12 sessions with an acupuncturist. If the patient chooses acupuncture as their preferred approach for migraine, then while an acupuncturist may competently treat the migraine, it may be more cost effective to utilize other approaches.

At present there is no mechanism for incorporating independent complementary practitioners, working outside the NHS and within their own isolated and individual private practices, into mainstream medical practice to meet the increased demand for complementary medicine. Moreover, it is unlikely that such private practices will ever become part of the NHS, even on a contractual basis, unless there is much greater economic and clinical control over their work. Improved communication between the various non-medically qualified complementary practitioners is vital if coherent management plans for individual patients are to be designed.

It is probable that the future development of mind–body medicine within the NHS will increasingly occur in the context of primary care and through the employment of properly trained, non-medically qualified individuals at a primary care level. However, mind–body medicine will not be put into practice until there is a better evidence base.

EVIDENCE BASE

A recent survey by the National Association of Health Authorities and Trusts in the UK suggested that the lack of information on the effectiveness of mind–body therapies was the single most important factor affecting NHS funding of these therapies[20]. However, the scanty evidence base or the lack of a valid mechanistic explanation for many mind–body therapies does not seem to have retarded its rise in popularity and certainly does not invalidate its efficacy. In the absence of a sophisticated conventional or biopsychosocial explanation for a symptom complex, as occurs in food intolerance for example, an empirical mind–body approach that may alleviate symptoms should not be perceived as any less valid than an empirical allopathic treatment. Dismissing any mind–body therapy because of its lack of an adequate evidence base closes down potential therapeutic options which could be explored in a responsible manner.

While the arguments about the evidence base for many mind–body techniques will persist until a more systematic scientific investigation in centers of excellence has taken place, the fundamental philosophies and concepts that underpin mind–body medicine can provide interesting philosophical and therapeutic insights. A mastery of mind–body medicine can be an excellent way of understanding the idioms and implicit social assumptions that exist within conventional medicine.

Ridsdale's text on evidence-based general practice provides us with great insight into the day-to-day problems that confront the professional family physician; perhaps one of the most telling aspects of Ridsdale's text is that it only runs to 130 pages, suggesting that the evidence base for much of what is done in a primary care setting is limited[21].

All too often, clinical decision making is based on flawed arguments, limited information and often inadequate and inappropriate interpretation of the evidence that does exist. The setting up of Cochrane collaborations targeting key areas of medicine is an attempt to put the whole of medicine on a more evidence-based footing. However, Cochrane defines evidence only in terms of randomized controlled trials and other forms of evidence are not included.

While there is a large evidence base for complementary medicine much of the research is poorly designed, inadequately controlled and of insufficient sample size to generate meaningful results. However, there are some areas, such as the use of acupuncture in nausea, where the evidence is much stronger[22]. In other areas, such as the use of homeopathy in the treatment of allergies[23] preliminary data look promising but require large-scale independent replication. Apart from a few particular therapies for specific conditions such as eczema and traditional Chinese medicine[24,25] most reviews of the evidence base for complementary therapies have concluded that more research is required before conclusions can be drawn, and complementary medicine can be integrated into conventional medical practice. Until this research has been performed it is likely that resources will not be committed to the widespread and wholesale support of complementary medicine in general practice or elsewhere in spite of increasing public pressure to provide such a service.

Randomized controlled trials (RCT)

Conventional medicine tends to regard only objective, quantifiable evidence as valid. It views subjective evidence as suspicious and often uses the term 'subjective' in a pejorative sense in the same way as it uses the concept of a placebo response to discredit a therapeutic intervention. It disregards personal experience as anecdotage and has developed an obsession with the randomized double-blind placebo-controlled trial. However, the quantification of clinical trial results in conventional medicine is a fairly recent discipline. Bradford-Hill's first studies on tuberculosis after the Second World War represent western medicine's first attempts to subject treatments to proper scientific scrutiny. Until that time, reports of therapeutic intervention were based on an individual physician's or surgeon's enthusiasm, often associated with a series of uncontrolled case reports.

Despite a tradition that puts much greater emphasis on experience than objective measurement, it would be wrong to think that complementary practitioners base their interventions solely on theory and philosophy and make no attempt at objective measurement. Ever since the first Royal Commission into Boyd's Emanator in the early part of this century, complementary medical practitioners have continually tried to measure and evaluate the changes in subtle energies which they believe underpin many of their interventions. For example, the acupuncture measurement instrument (AMI) is designed to measure changes in skin impedance over acupuncture points. Other diagnostic machines exist (Figs 15.1 & 15.2) that attempt to measure electrical disturbances, both before and after specific electrical stimulation. More recently, sophisticated machines have been developed that can measure electro-

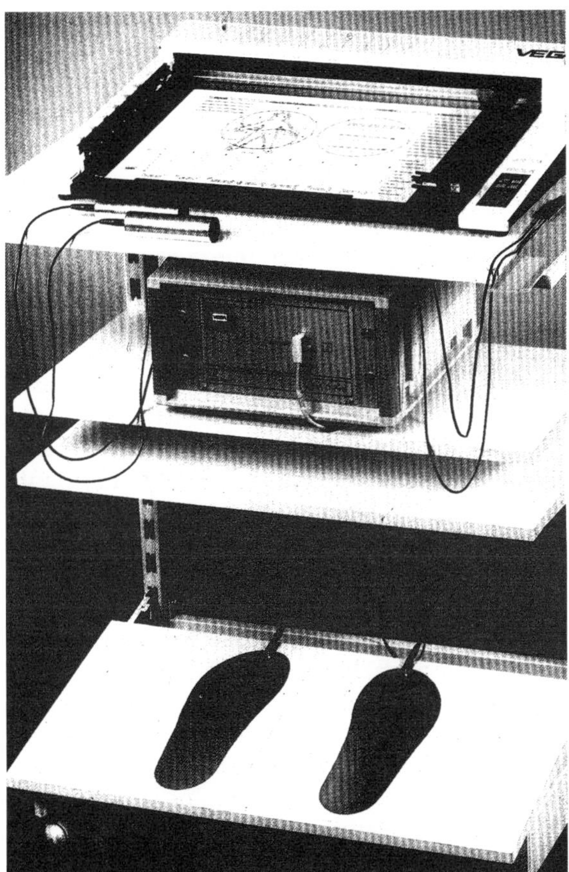

Figure 15.1 The DFM purports to give a fast survey of energetic disturbances within the patient together with regulatory capabilities.

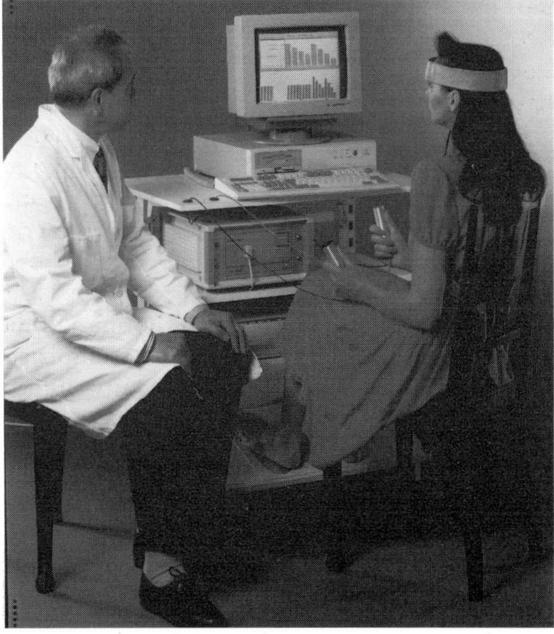

Figure 15.2 The Segmentelectrogram (SEG) purports to measure the body's segmental energetic balance and also acts as a diagnostic aid.

magnetic energy away from the body surface in addition to electrical energy close to the body surface[26,27].

Complex treatment packages may be very difficult to dissect in the context of randomized controlled clinical trials. Furthermore, the whole process of randomization denies, by its very assumption, the concept that patient preference may have a significant impact on outcome. These problems can be addressed in a rational manner, but it would take time, vast resources and very clearly focused hypotheses alongside carefully designed investigative protocols if clear-cut answers are to be obtained. Many mistakes have been made in the development of clinical trial methodology to assess mind–body therapies[28] and these will need to be addressed coherently if better trial design is to be developed which can provide clearer results.

Furthermore, the more vitalistic mind–body therapies do not easily lend themselves to randomized clinical trials, because of the nature of their very subtle and subjective effects. Similarly, the individualization of treatment which is central to many mind–body interventions makes it difficult to subject such approaches to randomized controlled trials. For example, Atherton's studies on a standardized herbal mixture for eczema[24], while effective, suffered from a number of problems as far as traditional Chinese medicine is concerned. The herbalist working with Atherton selected the most common form of eczema occurring in the UK and then designed an appropriate herbal mixture; if the eczema appeared to fit a slightly different traditional diagnosis then the mixture needed to be changed. While this was possible in clinical practice, it was not possible within the constructs of the placebo-controlled trial carried out by Atherton. To some extent many of these problems may be overcome by better trial design[29]. In other areas the assessment of best practice involving treatment packages and simple outcome data may also provide valuable information. While it is possible to construct appropriate clinical trials within many areas of mind–body medicine, it requires considerable expertise and knowledge of the problems inherent in such research.

Multiple therapies

The assessment of the evidence base within complementary medicine is not the only problem. Many complementary therapists will employ a constellation of activities during a therapeutic consultation, and may seek to enhance a placebo or non-specific response as well as utilizing a specific therapy. It is the difficulty of separating the placebo response, the therapeutic relationship and the specific therapy and controlling for these variables that makes research in this area so fraught with problems. However, these difficulties must be overcome in order to answer questions of efficacy.

Asking the right question

Many of the difficulties in conducting research into mind–body therapies are generated from the trial hypothesis. Too frequently the question asked of complementary therapy is 'does it work?' More specific and appropriate questions need to be posed, such as 'does homeopathic immunotherapy using house dust mite allergen reduce the symptomatology in house-dust allergic asthmatics?' Such specific questions can be subjected to RCTs, but cannot then be used to address more generic questions about whether therapies 'work'. Rigorous clinical trials, while completed to a high standard of scientific accuracy, are always far less generalizable in terms of clinical practice than more pragmatic studies; unfortunately pragmatic studies are often less scientifically rigorous. Thus, despite the difficulties posed by the RCT for mind–body therapies, they remain the best method of assessing efficacy and will be required if mind–body therapies are to be integrated into conventional medical practice.

Interim evidence

The construction and running of large-scale RCTs to assess efficacy is time-consuming, expensive and requires considerable expertise, not only in the therapy under scrutiny, but also in trial methodology. There are very few centers that have the necessary expertise to perform this work. Until these centers receive sufficient funding to conduct robust scientific studies, decisions as to whether there should be increased service provision within this field will have to be based on forms of evidence other than randomized controlled trials. Smaller scale studies designed to assess quality of life, patient preference and subsequent patient satisfaction, as well as other simple outcome data can contribute important evidence in the short term on which decision-making can be based. Thus, if large numbers of patients report significant improvement in symptoms or quality of life following the use of complementary medicine, associated with high degrees of satisfaction, then this is a strong argument for re-examining our assumptions about the distribution of medical resources.

Although there is an abundance of basic scientific evidence demonstrating that higher perceptual centers and limbic emotional centers regulate immunity and all the major physiological defense systems, research into the clinical efficacy of mind–body interventions, which seek to harness the natural healing forces, is in its infancy. Few resources and little expertise have been invested in mind–body medicine. Therefore, if it is to be integrated into conventional medicine and mind–body therapies are to be provided as a service within health care services, then it is incumbent upon those responsible for coordinating the service to develop an appropriate research agenda. This must clearly run in parallel with appropriate national research agendas such as those established in the UK by various Health of the Nation documents and priorities set for NHS research. Since the expertise required to conduct this work is in short supply, there is a strong argument for taking a proactive approach, as has occurred in the USA, and establishing specific centers of excellence. Without these, funding will likely fall into the hands of physicians with experience of clinical trials, but without experience of the specific problems of mind–body research, or alternatively physicians with an interest in mind–body therapies, but little experience in clinical trial research.

IN CLINICAL PRACTICE

The approach utilized by one of the authors (GTL) in practice in Southampton is therefore to make the best possible diagnosis using both a conventional medicine and a mind–body approach. The aim is not only to utilize conventional biomechanical descriptions and investigations, but also to develop and evaluate a variety of different mind–body measurement techniques which may ultimately lead to a better understanding of an individual's illness process.

Having made the diagnosis employing a variety of different conceptual models, it is then necessary to explore an appropriate management plan with the patient. They may, for instance, have come seeking acupuncture for their problem and while this may be both a relevant and appropriate approach to their condition, our clinical experience might lead us to suggest that other approaches might be more effective. A process of negotiation begins in which the patient is encouraged to develop realistic expectations of what to expect from a mind–body approach; one consultation is unlikely to solve a problem that has been present for years. Such discussions enable appropriate and individualized treatment plans to be developed. As always, management plans require modification as the treatment progresses, so if three or four sessions of a particular acupuncture technique have failed to produce benefit in the management of an individual's back pain, then the problem will need to be re-evaluated and either the acupuncture technique will be changed or a different therapeutic approach will be adopted. Most patients receive a treatment package based on their clinical response to a variety of different interventions. While an approach based on acupuncture or manipulation may be all that is required to treat a simple spinal problem, chronic fatigue syndrome may require a treatment package that involves several mind–body therapies.

The interested conventional physician

The approach adopted in Southampton is based on nearly 20 years' clinical experience. But where should an interested conventional physician begin in adopting a mind–body approach to the patient? What can be done in his or her own hospital or general practice?

The first step is undoubtedly a conceptual and philosophical one. There has to be a willingness to take on board the idea that there may be other approaches to illness than those which have been taught at medical school.

Step two is to acquire some first hand knowledge of different mind–body therapies. Being on the receiving end of an individual treatment is a useful starting point. Most conventional physicians will have only very limited experience of mind–body interventions. Their view of osteopathy may be changed significantly by receiving treatment for a bad back or bad neck.

Step three is to expand the knowledge base from a simple curiosity to a more extensive education into the history and philosophy of specific therapies. This will undoubtedly involve some background reading as well as a few more visits to a skilled mind–body therapist.

If there is still a desire for more understanding, then the physician has a series of decisions to make. Is their interest purely in learning about a single therapy, or do they wish to develop therapeutic skills themselves? Employing a complementary medical practitioner within their own medical practice, or adopting a policy of regular referrals for certain specific problems may be the next logical step. This should involve learning to work with a specific individual who will help manage the patients in close consultation with the conventional physician. Through this process an understanding of the advantages and disadvantages associated with a particular mind–body approach will become apparent by discussing and evaluating individual patient needs and response to treatment.

CONCLUSION

As we approach the millennium we have an ideal opportunity to evaluate our medical practice. Why did we enter a caring profession? What was our vision then and what is it now? Are we providing the best care we can, which addresses all our patients' needs and embraces all the therapeutic options available?

This chapter has argued that we need to embrace the biopsychosocial model and adopt a mind–body approach to our patients. This suggests that all the aspects of an individual are important, not just the physical, and they all need care and attention. It is no longer sufficient to be a competent manager of physical ailments and a dispenser of pharmaceutical remedies. We need to embrace whatever interventions help to maintain the health of those who seek our help, and work sincerely to create a positive environment of support to promote recovery. A working environment of care, compassion and empathy should be part of our vision for our practice. Such emotions can themselves have a profound physiological impact on our patients as well as ourselves and those we work with. This is not only good common sense but good scientific sense.

REFERENCES

1 McCraty R, Atkinson M, Tiller WA, Rein G, Watkins AD 1995 The effects of emotions on the short term power spectral analysis of heart rate variability. Am J Cardiol 76(14):1089–93

2 Silver HK, Glicken AD 1990 Medical student abuse: incidence, severity, and significance. JAMA 263:527–32

3 Sheehan HD, Sheehan DV, White K, Leibowitz A, Baldwin DC Jnr 1990 A pilot study of medical student 'abuse'. JAMA 263:533–7

4 Wharton R, Lewith G T 1986 Complementary medicine and the general practitioner. British Medical Journal 292i:1498–1500

5 Anderson E, Anderson P 1987 General practitioners and alternative medicine. Journal of the Royal College of General Practitioners 37:52–55
6 Thomas K B General practice consultations: is there any point in being positive? British Medical Journal 294:1200–1202
7 Thomas K, Fall M, Parry G, Nicholl J 1995 National survey of access to complementary health care via general practice. University of Sheffield, Sheffield
8 Pietroni P 1990 The greening of medicine. Gollancz
9 Ader R, Cohen N 1975 Behaviourally conditioned immunosuppression. Psychomatic Medicine 37:333–40
10 Lewith GT 1988 Undifferentiated illness: some suggestions for approaching the polysymptomatic patient. Journal of the Royal Society of Medicine 81:563–5
11 Brown M, Gibney M, Husband PR, Radcliffe M 1981 Food allergy in polysymptomatic patients. Practitioner 225:1651–4
12 Chilvers C, McElwain T 1990 Survival of patients with breast cancer attending the Bristol Cancer Help Centre. Lancet 2:606–10
13 Reason P 1991 Power and conflict in multidisciplinary collaboration. Complementary Medical Research 5:3
14 Lannoye P 1994 The state of complementary medicine. European Parliament Committee on the Environment, Public Health and Consumer Protection Draft Report
15 Logan J 1994 The Blackthorn Trust: expanding a national health practice. Complementary Therapies in Medicine 2:154–7
16 Whelan J 1995 Complementary therapies and the changing NHS: a development officer's view. Complementary Therapies in Medicine 3:79–83
17 Donnelly D 1995 Integrating complementary medicine within the NHS: a therapist's view of the Liverpool Centre for Health. Complementary Therapies in Medicine 3:84–7
18 Richardson J 1995 Complementary therapies on the NHS: the experience of a new service. Complementary Therapies in Medicine 3:153–7
19 Hooper J, Ruddlesden J, Heyes A 1995 Introducing independent complementary therapists into GP practices in Huddersfield and Dewsbury. West Yorkshire Health Authority
20 National Association of Health Authorities and Trusts 1993 Research Paper 10: Complementary Therapies in the NHS. NAHAT Publications, Birmingham
21 Ridsdale L 1995 Evidence-based general practice. A critical reader. WB Saunders, London
22 Vickers A 1994 P6 acupuncture point stimulation as an anti-emetic therapy, a report commissioned by North East Thames Regional Health Authority
23 Reilly D, Taylor MA, Beattie NGM et al. 1994 Is evidence for homeopathy reproducible? Lancet 344:1601–6
24 Sheehan MP, Atherton DJ 1992 A controlled trial of traditional Chinese medicinal plants in widespread non-exudative atopic eczema. British Journal of Dermatology 126:179–84
25 Sheehan MP, Rustin MHA, Atherton DJ et al. 1992 Efficacy of traditional Chinese herbal therapy in adult atopic dermatitis. Lancet 340:13–17
26 Stroink G 1989 Principles of cardiomagnetism. In: Williamson SJ, Hoke M, Stroink G, et al. Advances in biomagnetism. Plenum Press, New York, pp 47–57
27 Jessel-Kenyon J, Cheng N, Blott N, Hopwood V 1992 Studies with acupuncture using a SQUID biomagnometer: a preliminary report. Complementary Medical Research 6(3):142–52
28 Lewith G, Vincent C 1995 Evaluation of the clinical effects of acupuncture. A problem reassessed and a framework for future research. Pain Forum 4(1):29–39
29 Lewith GT, Aldridge D 1993 Clinical research methodology for complementary therapies. Hodder and Stoughton, London

Index

Page numbers in bold type refer to illustrations and tables.

A

D

E

F

G

H

I

J

K

L

M

N

O

P

Q

R

S

T

U

V

W

Y

Z